Promoting Health Care Transitions for Adolescents with Special Health Care Needs and Disabilities

University of Colorado at Colorado Springs
Kraemer Family Library

**KRAEMER FAMILY LIBRARY
ENDOWMENT**

El Pomar Center

Promoting Health Care Transitions for Adolescents with Special Health Care Needs and Disabilities

edited by

Cecily L. Betz, Ph.D., RN, FAAN

University of Southern California

University Center of Excellence in Developmental Disabilities

Children's Hospital Los Angeles

and

Wendy M. Nehring, Ph.D., RN, FAAN, FAAIDD

Rutgers, The State University of New Jersey

College of Nursing

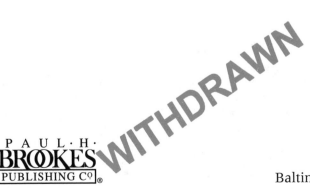
·P A U L·H·
BROOKES
PUBLISHING C.O. ®

Baltimore • London • Sydney

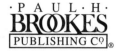

Paul H. Brookes Publishing Co.
Post Office Box 10624
Baltimore, Maryland 21285-0624
www.brookespublishing.com

"Paul H. Brookes Publishing Co." is a registered trademark of
Paul H. Brookes Publishing Co., Inc.

Typeset by Graphic World Inc., Maryland Heights, Missouri.
Manufactured in the United States of America by
George H. Buchanan Printing, Bridgeport, New Jersey.

The individuals described in this book are composites or real people whose situations have been masked and are based on the authors' experiences. Names and identifying details have been changed to protect confidentiality.

Library of Congress Cataloging-in-Publication Data

Promoting health care transitions for adolescents with special health care needs and disabilities / edited by Cecily L. Betz and Wendy M. Nehring.
  p.   cm.
  Includes index.
  ISBN-13: 978-1-55766-860-8
  ISBN-10: 1-55766-860-4
  1. Teenagers with disabilities—Medical care—United States.
  I. Betz, Cecily Lynn. II. Nehring, Wendy M., 1957–
  [DNLM: 1. Adolescent Health Services—United States. 2. Adolescent—United States.
  3. Continuity of Patient Care—United States. 4. Disabled Children—United States.
  5. Health Services Needs and Demand—United States. WA 330 P965 2007]
  RA564.5.P738 2007
  616.00835—dc22
                                      2006035714

British Library Cataloguing in Publication data are available from the British Library.

Contents

About the Editors

Cecily L. Betz, Ph.D., RN, FAAN, Director of Nursing Training and Director of Research, University of Southern California, University Center of Excellence in Developmental Disabilities, Children's Hospital Los Angeles, 4650 West Sunset Boulevard #83, Los Angeles, CA 90027

Cecily L. Betz serves as Director of Nursing Training and Director of Research at the University of Southern California's University Center of Excellence in Developmental Disabilities, located at Children's Hospital Los Angeles. She has worked with ill children, adolescents, and families for more than 30 years in a variety of roles as a clinician, educator, administrator, and researcher. For the past 20 years she has served as Editor-in-Chief of the *Journal of Pediatric Nursing,* the official journal for both the Society of Pediatric Nurses and the Pediatric Endocrinology Nursing Society. She has published extensively on health care transition planning for adolescents with special health care needs and on issues related to pediatric nursing. Her textbook, *Pediatric Nursing Reference,* is in its sixth edition. This textbook, along with others she has authored, has been translated into three languages. She has been the principal investigator of a number of extramurally funded federal and state grants. She is the principal investigator of South Los Angeles Youth and Young Adult Self-Determination Project, a youth information and referral center for youth and young adults with developmental disabilities funded by the Administration on Developmental Disabilities. In addition, she is testing a health care transition planning intervention funded by the National Institutes of Health. She has served on a number of regional, state, and national professional committees representing the interests of pediatric nurses and children and adolescents with special health care needs and disabilities. She is a fellow of the American Academy of Nursing of the American Nurses Association and was formerly Chair of the Child and Family Expert Panel.

Wendy M. Nehring, Ph.D., RN, FAAN, FAAIDD, Associate Dean for Academic Affairs, Director of the Graduate Programs, Associate Professor, Rutgers, The State University of New Jersey, College of Nursing, 180 University Avenue, Ackerson Hall Room 102A, Newark, NJ 07102

Wendy M. Nehring is Associate Dean for Academic Affairs, Director of the Graduate Programs, and Associate Professor at the College of Nursing at Rutgers, The State University of New Jersey. She joined the faculty at Rutgers in July of 2003. Previously, she held administrative and faculty positions at Southern Illinois University at Edwardsville and the University of Illinois at Chicago, as well as a faculty position at Illinois Wesleyan University. Dr. Nehring received a doctorate in nursing science from the University of Illinois at Chicago, a master's degree in pediatric nursing from the University of Wisconsin–Madison, and a bachelor of science in nursing from Illinois Wesleyan University. Dr. Nehring is nationally and internationally known in the field of intellectual and developmental disabilities. In addition, she wrote the only nursing history book in the field of intellectual and developmental disabilities. Dr. Nehring and her colleagues revised the scope and standards of this specialty practice in 2004, and these were published by American Nurses Publishing and the American Association on Mental Retardation. Dr. Nehring is also the editor of a core curriculum for nurses and health professionals specializing in the field of intellectual and developmental disabilities, as well as an evidence-based practice book on specific health promotion topics. She has written, presented, and consulted widely on this nursing specialty. She is a fellow of the American Academy of Nursing and the American Association on Intellectual and Developmental Disabilities.

Contributors

Lioness Ayres, Ph.D., RN
Assistant Professor
University of Iowa
College of Nursing
50 Newton Road
Iowa City, IA 52242

Kathleen B. Blomquist, Ph.D.,
M.P.H., M.S.N., B.S.N., RN
Consultant
Healthy & Ready to Work National
  Resource Center
Kentucky Commission for Children
  with Special Health Care Needs
333 Waller Avenue, Suite 300
Lexington, KY 40504

Eric B. Christeson, J.D.
Captain, U.S. Army
OIC Area IV Clients Services, USFK
Area IV Legal Center
19th ESC, Unit 15015
APO AP 96218

Nicole Garro, M.P.H.
Research Associate
University of California at Los Angeles
Center for Healthier Children,
  Families & Communities
1100 Glendon Avenue, Suite 850
Los Angeles, CA 90024

Robert W. Gibson, Ph.D., M.S.,
  OTR/L
Associate Professor
Medical College of Georgia
1120 15th Street
School of Allied Health Sciences
Department of Occupational Therapy
EC 2320
Augusta, GA 30912

Linda M. Graham, B.S., LBSW
Social Worker
Alabama Department of Rehabilitation
  Services
Children's Rehabilitation Service
2127 East South Boulevard
Montgomery, AL 36116

Stanley D. Handmaker, M.D.,
  D.Phil., FAAMR
Professor of Pediatrics and Psychiatry
Department of Pediatrics
University of New Mexico Health
  Sciences Center
ACC-3012
Albuquerque, NM 87131

Theodore A. Kastner, M.D., M.S.
President
Developmental Disabilities Health
  Alliance, Inc.
1285 Broad Street
Bloomfield, NJ 07003

Susan W. Ledlie, Ph.D., CPNP
Assistant Professor of Clinical Nursing
Columbia University
630 West 168th Street
New York, NY 10032

Debra S. Lotstein, M.D., M.P.H.
Visiting Assistant Professor of
  Pediatrics
University of California at Los Angeles
Department of Pediatrics
Center for Healthier Children,
  Families & Communities
1100 Glendon Avenue, Suite 850
Los Angeles, CA 90024

Judy Reichle, M.A.
Formerly Program Coordinator
California School to Work Interagency
Transition Partnership
Sacramento, CA 95814

John G. Reiss, Ph.D.
Associate Professor
University of Florida
1329 Southwest 16th Street,
  Room 5133
Gainesville, FL 32610

Roberta Ross, M.A., CRC, NCCC
Rehabilitation Consultant
South California Transition Coalition
33922 Marta Court
Dana Point, CA 92629

Teresa A. Savage, Ph.D., RN
Assistant Professor of Research
Maternal–Child Nursing
University of Illinois at Chicago
College of Nursing
845 South Damen Avenue, Room 841
Chicago, IL 60612
and
Associate Director
Donnelley Family Disability Ethics
  Program
Rehabilitation Institute of Chicago
345 East Superior Street #1375
Chicago, IL 60611

Kathryn Smith, M.N., RN
Visiting Assistant Professor of Clinical
  Pediatrics
Keck School of Medicine
Department of Pediatrics
University of Southern California
and
Associate Nursing Director
University Center for Excellence in
  Developmental Disabilities
Children's Hospital Los Angeles
4650 Sunset Boulevard, Mailstop #53
Los Angeles, CA 90027

**Joseph Telfair, Dr.P.H., M.S.W.,
M.P.H.**
Professor, Public Health Research
  and Practice
University of North Carolina at
  Greensboro
1408 Walker Avenue
437 HHP Building
Greensboro, NC 27402

Jennifer Thomas, B.S.
State Youth Consultant
Children's Rehabilitation Service
Alabama Department of Rehabilitation
  Services
2129 East South Boulevard
Montgomery, AL 36116

Kevin K. Walsh, M.A., Ph.D.
Director of Quality Management
  and Research
Developmental Disabilities Health
  Alliance, Inc.
1527 Forest Grove Road
Vineland, NJ 08360

Preface

The purpose of this book is to provide the reader with comprehensive information about the health care–related aspects of transition planning—an area of transition planning practice that is often overlooked. It is intended to provide educators and health care and non–health care professionals with extensive information about addressing the health care needs of youth with special health care needs and disabilities as part of the transition planning process, whether the youth are students in special or general education. We anticipate that this book will be used by a number of different primary audiences besides educators. These audiences include physicians, nurses, occupational and physical therapists, nutritionists, social workers, psychologists, speech and language specialists, rehabilitation specialists, dentists, youth themselves, and parents.

This book focuses on the health-related aspects of transition planning for adolescents with special health care needs and disabilities. This is an area of emerging practice that has reached a critical mass, as evidenced by the increase in the numbers of articles published on the topic in the last few years. A book on the topic would be a most timely addition to the literature.

Not much is well understood of what is meant about health and health-related aspects of transition planning by professionals no matter their disciplines. This lack of understanding is based on the scant amount of evidence available and the lack of clinical and educational resources that exist to assist professionals in addressing the health and health-related transition needs of youth with special health care needs and disabilities. This book provides the reader with the content, resources, and tools to better understand the meaning and scope of transition health care planning as well as increase their knowledge and skills in addressing these unique needs to better prepare youth for adulthood.

This book is divided into three sections: Health Care Transition Planning Best Practices, Health Care Transition Plans, and Interagency Services. The themes of self-determination and person-centered care are integrated within each chapter, along with clinical examples and vignettes as appropriate. Relevant tools, guides, or other clinical materials are included in the appendices to the book.

The first section, Health Care Transition Planning Best Practices, includes the first six chapters. An introduction to health care transition is the focus of Chapter 1. Betz and Telfair provide an overview of the components of health care transition planning, including the importance of integrating health care recommendations into interagency approaches and services. In Chapter 2, Kastner, Walsh, Savage, and Christeson discuss service, legal, and ethical issues related to the health care transition process. Smith and Garro discuss health insurance options along with the issues associated with insurance coverage for adolescents and adults with special health care needs and disabilities in Chapter 3. In Chapter 4, Betz and Ayres examine the education of health care self-care, long-term disability management skills, and health advocacy of adolescents and adults with special health care needs and disabilities. Next, in Chapter 5, Lotstein describes strategies for finding adult and specialty physicians, as well as obtaining and evaluating the quality of medical referrals from Independent Living Centers, disability organizations, and Internet chat rooms. In Chapter 6, Nehring presents information on the types of health-related accommodations that are used in school and work settings.

The second section covers health care transition plans. In Chapter 7, Ledlie describes the process of assessment in determining the adolescent's needs that should be identified for intervention in transition plans in health care settings. Specific assessment methods for the purpose of developing an individualized transition plan, 504 plan, and/or an individualized plan for employment are discussed. Reiss and Gibson follow with Chapter 8, which covers strategies for implementing a transition plan. In Chapter 9, Blomquist, Graham, and Thomas focus on the identification of transition health outcomes that could be used as benchmarks to determine the effectiveness of the strategies selected to implement the transition plan.

The third section, Interagency Services, covers specific topics related to working with a variety of service agencies that include school and/or work. In Chapter 10, Betz and Nehring discuss individualized education programs and 504 plans. In Chapter 11, Handmaker discusses the role of the health care professional in school and health care settings that work with 504 teams to integrate health-related needs into such plans. In Chapter 12, Ross and Nehring provide information for health care professionals in ways to work with job developers and employers in identifying health-related accommodations in work settings. The role of the Department of Rehabilitation and mentors is emphasized. In Chapter 13, Ross and Reichle provide pragmatic information about forming interagency partnerships with non–health agencies that health care professionals do not typically partner with, such as Workforce Investment Act (WIA) One-Stops, WIA Youth Programs, and Independent Learning Centers. In the final chapter, Smith describes care coordination strategies for working with adolescents with special health care needs and disabilities. The focus of these strategies is on health-related components of transition planning and how such planning is integrated into a comprehensive transition plan that addresses the adolescent's postsecondary goals for education, employment, and community living.

Our experience with health care transition planning has taught and sensitized us to the needs of those involved in providing transition services to youth with special health care needs and disabilities. We have learned over the years that our colleagues in non–health service systems did not really understand what is meant by having a special health care need or disability. Living with a chronic illness or disability changes everything for the youth who has the chronic condition. Learning to live with a chronic condition means that beginning in childhood, the youth needs to become skilled at managing it so that its uncomfortable and pervasive effects on daily activities can be minimized if not contained. Living with a chronic condition means dealing with a myriad of uncomfortable physical sensations such as dull, throbbing pain, sensations of lightheadedness, excruciating pain not always relieved by medications, malaise not relieved with additional sleep, and fewer active daily activities while still engaging in the usual daily activities associated with school, work, and recreation.

We wanted to enhance the awareness of colleagues of what life is like learning to live with special health care needs and disabilities. Living with special health care needs and disabilities means learning to do things differently than what other typically developing youth do. Youth with special health care needs and disabilities may need to learn to use mobility aides such as motorized wheelchairs to navigate their college campus or town. Youth with special health care needs and disabilities who have to use external devices such as uterostomy bags for collecting urine or colostomy/ileostomy bags for fecal materials may be on rigid bowel and bladder schedules, enabling them to socialize with friends after school or in the evening without the fear or embarrassment of having an "accident."

In addition, living with a chronic condition means learning the treatment regimen necessary for daily management. The extent to which learning how to manage new tasks is needed on a daily basis will vary for each youth who has a chronic condition. These tasks may be as simple as taking medications on a daily basis to managing complex technological equipment such as ventilators. Sadly, some youth may not have access to the needed services and supports that will enable them to prevent complications or the occurrence of secondary conditions resulting in more frequent exacerbations of their condition, work or school absences, social isolation, and emotional ill health and distress.

Our challenge and purpose in writing this book was to provide our colleagues with the range of topical content on health care transition planning written by recognized experts to improve the quality of transition services provided to youth with special health care needs and disabilities. We believe by doing so, we move a little closer to realizing that goal. There is much to be accomplished in terms of supporting youth with special health care needs and disabilities to achieve their own goals and dreams for the future such as establishing service models based on the best practices.

To Craig L. Betz,
whose courage in facing adversity has been a great inspiration

To the youth and families
who have taught me so very much about health care transition planning

—Cecily L. Betz

To Debbie Reiling,
you are the best!

And to all of the youth with special health care needs and/or disabilities
who are preparing for transition to the adult years,
may your transition go as smoothly as can be
so that you may experience your optimal adulthood.

—Wendy M. Nehring

Health Care Transition Planning Best Practices

CHAPTER 1

Health Care Transitions

An Introduction

CECILY L. BETZ AND JOSEPH TELFAIR

S cientific advances in the health sciences and improvements in medical technology have contributed to remarkable changes in the survival rates of children diagnosed with special health care needs and disabilities (Health Resources and Services Administration [HRSA], 2001; Sawyer, Blair, & Bowes, 1997). Ninety percent of children diagnosed with special health care needs survive into adulthood (Blum, 1995). Although actual survival rate estimates of specific diagnostic populations are difficult to obtain due to numerous factors (e.g., inaccessible populations, late diagnosis, lack of systematic and organized data collection efforts), available survivor estimates suggest that the population of adults with special health care needs is increasing at a rate that is creating social difficulties, quality of life issues, and service system pressures that can no longer be ignored. For example, according to recent studies

- There are approximately 270,000 adult survivors of childhood-acquired cancer in the United States (National Cancer Policy Board & National Institute of Medicine, 2003)

- The mean survival rate of individuals with cystic fibrosis is 36.5 years (Cystic Fibrosis Foundation, 2006)

- Adult survivors of congenital heart disease are calculated to be at least 787,000 (Warnes et al., 2001)

- Approximately 75% of children with spina bifida are predicted to survive into early adulthood (Bowman, McLone, Grant, Tomita, & Ito, 2001)

- About 60% of individuals with sickle cell anemia survive into their fourth and fifth decades (National Institutes of Health, National Heart, Lung, and Blood Institute [NHLBI], 2002).

Moreover, in addressing transition services for all adolescents with special health care needs and disabilities,

> The severity of the illness or disability, the level of maturity, acceptance and understanding of the patient, additional environmental and family stresses, the need for control by parents or health care provider, a distorted perception (by parents or health care provider) of potential patient outcomes, and lack of patient or family support systems all may contribute to transition stress. (American Academy of Pediatrics [AAP], 1996)

Problems transitioning into adulthood are magnified with chronic health problems (Conway, 1998). Furthermore, adolescents with severe developmental or cognitive disabilities require special consideration pertaining to their lack of medical independence and enhanced reliance on parents or other caregivers. Yet, for many of these young adults, there has been little or no focus on acquiring the needed personal, interpersonal, and social life skills of interaction, independent living, self-advocacy, medical self-management and system negotiation, as well as educational and vocational readiness (Rinehart & Oberg, 1993). As a result, many adolescents with chronic conditions, their primary caregivers, and their health care providers have a difficult time both understanding and successfully navigating the process of competent transition into adult care and life (Blum, 1995; Rosen, Blum, Britto, Sawyer, & Siegel, 2003). While adolescents with chronic conditions vary by disease etiology and manifestation and ethnicity, the health care system for these youth is distinct in its commonality across conditions.

One of the *Healthy People 2010* performance outcomes for children and youth with special health care needs is articulated in Objective 16.23, which states "Increase the proportion of states and territories that have service systems for children with special health care needs" (U.S. Department of Health and Human Services [DHHS], 2000). To meet this objective, the Division of Services for Children with Special Health Needs (DSCSHN) in the Maternal Child Health Bureau (MCHB) developed six core measures to reduce and eliminate barriers to achieving appropriate community-based services systems for children and adolescents with special health care needs, one of which is especially pertinent to this book: "All youth with special health care needs will receive the services necessary to make appropriate transitions to all aspects of adult life, including adult health care, work and independence" (DHHS, 2000). Presently, the health care system is not adequately equipped to respond to the pressing demands for services that this growing population has. At present, there are no formalized service pathways that are designed to facilitate the exit from the pediatric and child health system and entry into the adult health service system. This is unlike the formalized system for special education students. This lack of formalized system linkages between pediatric and adult health care systems results in a patchwork approach developed in local communities. For example, a survey by the National Center for Youth with Disabilities (NCYD) identified the following four models of service that delivery providers are using to support the transition of adolescents with special health care needs from pediatric to adult care:

1. *Disease-focused* model, wherein adolescents are provided transition services from their specialty medical providers

2. *Adolescent-focused* model, wherein service goals are based upon those identified by the adolescent so that the adolescent may be an active planning participant

3. *Primary care* model, wherein the provision of transition services is based on the adolescent's primary care services

4. *Transition coordination* model, wherein a health care professional is designated as the case manager and is responsible for coordinating services and referrals (NCYD, 1995; Scal, Evans, Blozis, Okinow, & Blum, 1999)

In addition, some programs combine models, such as the adolescent-focused and transition coordination model called *Creating Healthy Futures,* which was a pilot transition clinic serving the transition needs of adolescents with special health care needs (Betz & Redcay, 2002, 2003). This lack of uniformity in the provision and structure of services for adolescents with special health care needs has led to large differences in both the quality and receipt of services (AAP, 1996; Conway, 1998; Telfair, Alleman, Dickens, & Loosier, 2005). For example, lack of reimbursement for transition services has been identified as a barrier to implementing transition services, although a national survey of transition programs found that 83% were reimbursed on a fee-for-service basis (Geenen, Powers, & Sells, 2003; Scal, 2002; Scal et al., 1999).

It is unlikely that significant reforms to rectify this service gap will be forthcoming in the near future. Widespread reform would require massive retooling of service systems on a scale similar to the early intervention model. Ideally, an integrated transition service system would embody the components of the early intervention model, such as a formalized planning process leading to the implementation of an interagency adolescent-centered plan, service mandates, and benchmarks to measure progress in the attainment of plan objectives. In the meantime, professionals, youth, families, advocates, and policy makers are struggling to effect modest, albeit necessary, changes in the way transition services are provided. These efforts include the preliminary testing of service models (Bent et al., 2002; Eiser et al., 1993; Kipps et al., 2002) and the development of tools to measure transition needs and readiness (Betz, Redcay, & Tan, 2003; Buran, McDaniel, & Brei, 2002; Cappelli, MacDonald, & McGrath, 1989).

Many health care professionals have collaborated with colleagues from other service systems to replicate their models of transition planning, to collaborate on developing and implementing transition service plans, and to acquire knowledge and skills from experts who have been providing transition services to adolescents (Betz, 1999; Betz & Redcay, 2003; DePoy, Gilmer, & Martzial, 2000; Scal et al., 1999). Interagency colleagues from education, social service, workforce preparation, rehabilitation, and disability service systems have more formalized systems of services for transition-age youth. The advantages these service systems have in the development of transition programs are based on the target populations served, allocation of funding, and legal mandates enacted by federal legislation. For example, transition services for special education students are specified in detail in the Individuals with Disabilities Education Act (IDEA) of 1990 and its amendments (IDEA, 1997, 2004). Similarly, job development programs for youth, including those with disabilities, have been expanded from summer employment programs to more comprehensive year-round programs through the enactment of the Workforce Investment Act (WIA) of 1998.

During the past decade, the DSCSHN has provided national leadership through its federal initiative titled Healthy and Ready to Work (HRTW) to focus attention on the need for health care transition services and programs. Through their efforts, a number of demonstration projects have been funded to plan and implement health care transition programs in local communities, to create the Healthy and Ready to Work National Center to serve as a clearinghouse to disseminate resources, and to convene experts to develop policies related to health care transition planning.

DEFINING HEALTH CARE TRANSITIONS

What is meant by health care transitions? This question can be answered by examining the professional literature and policy statements formulated by several professional associations and governmental agencies. The transition, including health care transition to adulthood, occurs over an extended period time and cannot be considered a discrete event (White, 1997). As will be discussed throughout this book, transition planning is a lifelong process as each successive developmental achievement enables an individual to evolve through the stages of childhood and adolescence and into adulthood. For the purposes of this chapter, health care transition is conceived as a dynamic process (NCYD, 1995) with a beginning, a middle, and an end. The *beginning* phase includes the decision to begin or prepare for the transition. The *middle* phase, transition readiness, includes logistical and other efforts of preparation for and implementation of the transition. *Transition readiness* is defined as the specific decisions made and actions taken in building the capacity of the adolescent and those in his or her primary medical system of support (parental caregivers/family and providers) to prepare for, begin, continue, and finish the process of transition (Telfair, Alexander, Loosier, Alleman-Velez, & Simmons, 2004). The *final* or *end stage* occurs when the adolescent or young adult not only transfers to an adult care setting but also is actively participating in adult care activities, such managing as independently as possible the daily requirements of his or her treatment regimen, working with providers to plan his or her own medical care, deciding if a provider to whom he or she is referred is someone with whom he or she can work, and, if necessary, finding and choosing a different provider.

Given this reality, transition experts have defined the term *transition* from a number of different perspectives depending on their disciplinary focus, research or clinical experience, and time period (see Table 1.1 for a sampling of transition-related definitions). There are several commonalities in these definitions. All definitions agree that transitioning is a process involving the services and support of one or more health care professionals who have specialized expertise in transition planning. Another area of agreement is that the primary goal of health care transitions is the successful transfer of the adolescent from pediatric care providers to adult care providers. Although not explicitly stated, the definitions also imply that the transfer of care entails the establishment of an acceptable, workable relationship between the provider(s) and the new patient. As research has demonstrated, an important measurement of transfer success is continued patient contact with the health care provider—whether it be an adult specialty or primary care physician or nurse practitioner—after the initial office visit.

Beyond these areas of consensus, differences emerge. Some experts view health care transition planning as focused on medical needs (Anderson, Flume, Hardy, & Gray, 2002; Nasr, Campbell, & Howatt, 1992; Pacaud, McConnell, Huot, Aebi, & Yale, 1996) whereas others have more expansive perspectives, suggesting that transition be viewed not just from a sole provider's perspective of transfer of care from the pediatrician to the internist and adult medical specialists, but as a comprehensive approach to learning new developmental competencies and the new systems of care for health, education, employment, and community living (Rettig & Athreya, 1991; Sawyer et al., 1998; Scal, et al., 1999). Those with a more encompassing concept of transition planning embody more fully the

Table 1.1. Transition definitions

Authors	Definitions
Pacaud, McConnell, Huot, Aebi, & Yale, 1996	Transition: Period between the last visit in pediatric care services and the establishment of regular follow-up in adult care services.
Anderson, Flume, Hardy, & Gray, 2002	Transition: Purposeful, planned preparation of patients, families, and caregivers for transfer of a cystic fibrosis patient from pediatric to adult care program.
Flume, Anderson, Hardy, & Gray, 2001	Transfer: The actual responsibility of care of the patient being moved from a pediatric setting to an adult care setting.
Nasr, Campbell, & Howatt, 1992	Transition program: Goal was to ensure patient follow-through and to reduce the incidence of patients dropping out of the health care system.
McDonagh & Kelly, 2003	Uses Blum (1995) definition of transition: "a multifaceted, active process that attends to the medical, psychosocial and educational vocational needs of adolescents as they move from child-oriented to adult-oriented lifestyle and systems" (p. 597). This involvement includes the transition from school to work, from pediatric to adult health care and from family home to independent living in the community.
Rettig & Athreya, 1991	Goals of transition program: 1) Promote continuity of care by way of the systematic transfer of care to an internist rheumatologist; 2) promote independence in the young adult and encourage him or her to take increasing responsibility in the management of the disease; 3) assess impact of disease on the young adult's ability to reach optimal vocational and educational achievement and intervene through appropriate counseling, referral, and follow-up; 4) promote optimal adolescent development by addressing normal adolescent issues regarding sexuality, psychosocial, and future planning concerns; and 5) provide emotional support to the members of the family during the transition period.
Sawyer, Collins, Bryan, Brown, Hope, & Bowes, 1998	"Transfer is an event in the transition process; transition is a process involving the young person and family which takes place over a number of years . . . such a process ideally has the ability to link the young person into a range of services that can address the vocational, psychosocial, general and sexual health, as well as recreational needs of young people." (p. 416)
Scal, Evans, Blozis, Okinow, & Blum, 1999	"The range of services in transition health program should not merely manage physical functioning, but should provide anticipatory guidance for social functioning as well . . . transition health services framework envisions uninterrupted, comprehensive, coordinated, integrated, and developmentally appropriate programs." (p. 260)

(continued)

Table 1.1. *(continued)*

Authors	Definitions
American Academy of Pediatrics, American Academy of Family Practice, & American College of Physicians-American Society of Internal Medicine, 2002	"Transitions are part of normal, healthy development and occur across the life span. Transition in health care for young adults with special health care needs is a dynamic, lifelong process that seeks to meet their individual needs as they move from childhood to adulthood. The goal is to maximize lifelong functioning and potential through the provision of high-quality, developmentally appropriate care services that continue uninterrupted as the individual moves from adolescence to adulthood. It is patient centered, and its cornerstones are flexibility, responsiveness, continuity, comprehensiveness, and coordination." (p. 1304)

emerging consensus of transition experts described in the following section. It is apparent that the question of what constitutes effective transition planning is only beginning to be answered from an empirical perspective. However, the growing interest and attention in the health care system to the issue of transition planning is creating a collective effort to describe the principles of best practices. That is, it is becoming clear that transitioning is more than a transfer process from one provider to another, and the explanatory emphasis of health care transition planning should be placed on the growing evidence of what constitutes best practices.

Several professional associations have taken a leadership role in describing a framework of best practices related to health care transition planning. The AAP, American Academy of Family Physicians (AAFP), and American College of Physicians-American Society of Internal Medicine (ACP-ASIM) issued *A Consensus Statement on Health Care Transitions for Young Adults with Special Health Care Needs* (AAP, AAFP, & ACP-ASIM, 2002). The major provisions of this joint statement include having care coordinator, a transfer health summary, a transition health care plan, provision of adequate primary and preventive care, and health insurance coverage. The details of this joint statement by the AAP, AAFP, and the ACP-ASIM (2002) are displayed below.

1. Have a care manager who coordinates health care planning between pediatric and adult health care providers.

2. Provide transition training to enhance the knowledge and skills of primary care adult physicians.

3. Formulate a medical summary for transfer to adult primary and specialty physicians.

4. Develop a health care transition plan beginning at age 14.

5. Ensure primary and preventive care based on accepted medical guidelines are provided.

6. Ensure continuous health insurance coverage once pediatric eligibility terminates.

Statements of transition practice issued by the AAP (AAP, Committee on Children with Disabilities, 2000, 2001; AAP, Committee on Children with Disabilities and Committee on Adolescence, 1996), the National Association of Pediatric Nurse Practitioners (NAPNAP; 2001), the Society of Adolescent Medicine (Rosen et al., 2003) and the DCSHCN share a number of similar recommendations. These recommendations advocate the following:

- The responsibility for transition service coordination and referral is assigned to one member of the youth's specialized health care team who has expertise in case management (e.g., social worker, nurse).

- Adolescents are active participants and are fully engaged in transition planning, which includes shared decision making, direct input during the planning process, and evolving primary responsibility for managing their condition on a long-term basis.

- Families of transition-age adolescents are provided supports and services to assist them in dealing with their feelings of "letting go" and learning to better support their children's developing self-reliance during the transition process.

- Services are based on the developmental needs of the adolescents, emphasizing strengths rather than deficits.

- Transition planning is a lifelong process with formalized transition services provided beginning at age 14. Transition planning begins at the time of diagnosis based on the belief that goals for adulthood are necessary and achievable based on the skills and capabilities of the adolescent.

- Service coordination includes determination of eligibility and referral to transition and adult services, including Supplemental Security Insurance (SSI) and Medicaid. Referrals to transition and adult services are not relegated to health care needs only but to the comprehensive array of services and programs that will assist the adolescent in achieving his or her goals for the future, such as living independently, being employed, and having a social network of friends and family. The service coordinator assists the youth to identify and obtain needed accommodations based on health/disability-related needs in education, work, and community settings.

- Transition planning ensures a smooth and coordinated transfer from pediatric to adult health care providers and services. This coordination process will involve the active engagement of both pediatric and adult health care providers to achieve success with the transfer to adult care providers and services.

Clinical experts and researchers have contributed to the expanding body of knowledge and have offered a number of suggestions for developing and implementing transition service models. It is widely accepted that health care transition planning needs to be implemented according to a preplanned and structured process incorporating benchmarks of achievement. A best practices approach for transition planning incorporates timelines, identification of goal achievements, and processes for skills and knowledge achievement that can guide the practice of pediatric health professionals. As part of the structure and function of the medical care program, there be must good working relationships and communication between pediatric and adult providers (e.g., primary care providers, specialists, adjunct providers). Such relationships must be tempered with realism for a given setting since such relationships are more easily described than created or maintained (Betz & Redcay, 2002; Clare, 1998). Education of the adolescent, his or her family, other providers from multiple disciplines, and community members needs to emphasize outcomes that demonstrate knowledge and skills obtained. The goals of the program for support in the form of case management need to clearly describe relevant activities (Wojciechowski, Hurtig, & Dorn, 2002). Listening; demonstrating respect for opinions, concerns, and cultural values of the young person, family, and community; providing advice specific to problem solving; and including family and significant others in decision making are all important in providing support to the adolescent in transition.

THREE PRIMARY ELEMENTS OF TRANSITION PLANNING

The primary goal of health care transition planning is to ensure that adolescents continue to receive without interruption the necessary coordinated array of health care services and supports from adult health care providers once they are no longer eligibile for pediatric health care services. In order to realize this health care transition goal, several objectives need to be attained, including 1) accessing adult primary and specialty medical providers, 2) obtaining health insurance coverage, and 3) acquiring the highest level of self-sufficiency possible in managing primary and ongoing chronic health care needs and assessing the potential parameters for the referred system of care.

Accessing Adult Primary and Specialty Medical Providers

Finding adult health care providers who are competent *and* comfortable in providing either primary or specialized services to young adults with chronic conditions is a very real challenge. In addition to research findings, the testimony from adolescents, their families, and pediatric health care professionals convey the difficulties associated with finding and selecting adult physicians and other health care professionals who can continue to provide the assortment of primary and specialized services needed (Geenen et al., 2003; Sawyer et al., 1998; Scal, 2002; Telfair, Myers, & Drezner, 1994). These difficulties range from the scarcity of primary workforce of professionals to care for this population, including physicians and other multidisciplinary providers available to provide specialized care in the community of choice, to the lack of motivation to provide services due to the low reimbursement rates for medical services (Geenen et al., 2003; McDonagh & Kelly, 2003). Other challenges include finding physicians who have the training, experience, and "disability consciousness" to provide the specialized care young adults with chronic conditions require. Logistical specifications include medical environments with disability accommodations, extended office hours to include weekends, and office locations near public transportation lines.

The transfer of care from pediatric to adult medical settings is made all the more difficult because there usually are no formalized service linkages between these two services systems. The health care systems serving children and adults are entirely different with virtually no system or professionally oriented interface between them. Pediatricians and the team of health care professionals who serve pediatric patients have a service philosophical orientation of addressing the needs of their patients from both an individual and family-oriented perspective (Blomquist, Brown, Peersen, & Presler, 1998; Rosen, 1993). Experts refer to this inclusive family service approach as "family-centered care." According to the Institute for Family-Centered Care (2004), "Family-centered care is an approach to the planning, delivery and evaluation of health care that is governed by mutually beneficial partnerships between health care providers, patients, and families." This approach encompasses a comprehensive model of care that is designed to address the diverse needs for these youth.

Pediatricians and other members of the health care team are accustomed to interacting with parents, family members, and the child when providing care. As indicated earlier, the input of family members is critical when making decisions about treatment and long-term management approaches. Information pertaining to diagnostic concerns, test results, and questions about treatment options will likely be shared initially with parents and family members without the child present. Only later, as the child's level of maturity permits and in keeping with family values, will the child be involved in decision making and discussions about medical management.

In addition, means of communicating with children about their illnesses and treatments will be embedded within their world of play and fantasy and their level of cognitive development. The use of play items such as dolls, stuffed animals, and more colorful and simplistic renditions of concepts such as internal organs are used as a means to convey information. Children may even be encouraged to cry, scream, and display other physical acting-out behaviors, such as hitting a doll as a means of expressing pain, fear, and anger in anticipation, during and after painful treatments.

In stark contrast, adult medical care has a different philosophical orientation and approach. Typically, the adult patient is the sole focus of the adult physician's concern, unless the adult has a conservator or is incapable of communicating needs to the physician due to cognitive or sensory limitations. The patient is assumed, if not expected, to be responsible for processing the information communicated to him or her and to adhere to the medical recommendations. The team approach in adult care is less evident, as it is not organized in the same manner. This difference in team approach is, due in part, to the lack of public funding for specialized adult medical teams composed of interdisciplinary health professionals as compared to the Title V Children with Special Health Care Needs Program for children with special health care needs and in part to the differences in the training and orientation of adult and pediatric providers (Telfair et al., 2005). For more information about locating adult primary and specialty care physicians, refer to Chapter 5.

Some experts have asserted that the termination of the relationship with pediatric providers is difficult for adolescents with special health care needs and disabilities and their families. This difficulty with separation has been identified as a rationale for prolonging the physician–patient relationship beyond the usual period for transfer to adult physicians (Hauser & Dorn, 1999; Sawyer et al., 1998). Others suggest that the transfer to adult physicians is less stressful than expected (Eiser et al., 1993; Sharp, McNeil, Wales, Cooper, & Dawson, 1994).

However, experts agree that adequate preparation is needed for transitioning to adult health services (Hauser & Dorn, 1999; McDonagh & Kelly, 2003; Patterson & Lanier, 1999; Sharp et al., 1994).

Obtaining Health Insurance Coverage

Health insurance coverage is one of the most important health-related concerns for adolescents with special health care needs and disabilities and their families (White, 2002). Health insurance coverage for the expenses associated with a special health care need and disability is the driving consideration in making plans for the future as it relates to the life choices of additional education, employment, housing, relationships, and leisure and recreational pursuits. The *fear* of losing health insurance becomes a major impediment to realizing these dreams for the future.

In the past, the default choice for many adolescents with special health care needs and disabilities has been to enroll in SSI with Medicaid health benefits. However, this choice has proven and continues to be an unsatisfactory option for individuals who desire to have the same life options as other typically developing individuals or peers. Although the Social Security Administration (SSA) has instituted programmatic efforts to effect changes in program requirements, such as with the work incentive programs, the challenges of entering the workforce continue. For many entering the workforce for the first time, the health insurance benefits may be limited with only major medical coverage or not offered at all (Newacheck, Inkelas, & Kim, 2004).

Young adults and adolescents with special heath care needs and disabilities will consider their employment prospects much differently than their typically developing peers. Young adults and adolescents with special health care needs and disabilities live with the uncertainty of an unpredictable course of their disease or disability marked by episodes of exacerbations, emergence of secondary conditions and complications, as well as periods of remission. Young adults and adolescents with special health care needs and disabilities are also aware of the "hidden expenses" associated with managing their special needs, such as the additional costs incurred for transportation, supplies, and special dietary needs. Unless a job can offer comprehensive health benefits, young adults with special health care needs and disabilities cannot risk accepting that employment opportunity.

An essential component of transition planning involves exploring with the young adult the range of insurance options available based upon their individual circumstances and needs. Counseling about insurance coverage requires substantial preparation and careful examination of the available benefits, as health insurance plans will vary as to the extent to which specialized ancillary services such as physical and occupational therapy, speech and language, and nutrition are offered. For a more detailed discussion on health insurance coverage, refer to Chapter 3.

Self-Sufficiency with Long-Term Management of Health Care Needs

A transition program has some minimum requirements and should be adequate to address the needs of adolescents with special health care needs and disabilities.

The emphasis on adequacy is based on the reality that nearly every individual with special health care needs and disabilities will have additional, if not extraordinary, daily demands to manage their special needs as compared with their typically developing peers. Additional care will require more time and effort to ensure that they are properly cared for on a daily basis. For some individuals, it will require minimal attention, such as taking additional medications, monitoring their blood pressure, or wearing a leg brace. For others, the treatment regimen is far more rigorous and time intensive. For example, adolescents with Type I diabetes may have to carefully monitor their serum glucose, food intake, and activity levels. Adolescents with cystic fibrosis require daily pulmonary treatments, life-long dietary modifications, and careful monitoring of their activity levels to pre-vent overexertion and excessive fatigue. Adolescents with a colostomy or ileostomy will need to learn to do their own stoma care, learn to use and care for their equipment, perform ostomy irrigation, manage their dietary requirements, and monitor for signs of infection.

An essential component of transition preparation is assessing young adults' health care self-care skills for long-term management of their special health care needs and disabilities. The specification of learning self-care skills can be integrated into the transition plan with benchmarks to measure progress in achieving these new skills. Depending on the type and extent of self-care skills that need to be learned and mastered, arrangements for skills reinforcement and practice can be coordinated with the school nurse and teachers. The individual-ized education program (IEP) and 504 plan are mechanisms support members can use to help young adults with special health care needs achieve skills mastery (Betz, 2001). Coordination with interagency professionals, which is described in more detail in Chapter 14, refers to the process and procedures for implementing skills reinforcement in another setting within which the adolescent functions.

Ideally, learning skills for self-management begins early and is integrated for client-teaching purposes in a developmentally appropriate manner (Betz, 2000). That is, the children assume increasing responsibility for their own special needs self-care as is developmentally and functionally appropriate. For example, a child with epilepsy learns early to describe the symptoms experienced during the aura period immediately before the seizure occurs. By learning to identify the symptoms associated with an aura, the child can respond quickly to ensure that he or she will not sustain an injury during the seizure. Initially the younger child may not be able to adequately describe in words the sensations felt other than to associate them with simplistic, yet age-appropriate terminology such as "feeling funny" and "fuzzy" to name a few. As the child gets older, the aura account will be detailed in more specific terms.

As emphasized previously in this chapter, self-care skill building must be a minimal requirement of a sound transition program. Other self-care skills pertain to assuming more logistic responsibilities, such as refilling prescriptions, setting up medical and dental appointments, and arranging transportation for medical purposes. These skills may not be initially identified and may even be overlooked as they have been performed for prolonged periods of time and in an automatic fashion. However, the ability to independently schedule appointments and procure refill medications and additional supplies should not be taken for granted, particularly if not done previously. For example, one parent remarked that her daughter did not need to learn how to obtain medication refills as "the medications were automatically refilled at the pharmacy." Although initially the adolescent may dismiss the admonition given by the parent, guardian, and/or members of the youth's health care team about the importance of learning the skills needed for self-care management, it is important to be certain that the adolescent can assume responsibilities for them when the occasion arises. For additional information on self-care management, see Chapter 4.

OTHER ELEMENTS OF TRANSITION PLANNING

There are several other elements of health care transition planning. These elements include assisting the adolescent to obtain needed school and workplace accommodations, service referral and coordination with interagency service providers, and access to mentors serving as role models and social supports.

School and Workplace Accommodations

An overlooked area of service need related to an adolescent's special health care needs and/or disability is the identification and arrangement of accommodations for health-related purposes in the school and work settings. The adolescent's ability to function effectively in educational, work, or community settings will be greatly enhanced with the provision of accommodations. The accommodations an adolescent with special health care needs and/or disability requires will be based not only on the individualized needs of the adolescent and his or her willingness to identify those needs but also on the competence of health care professionals who have the level of expertise needed to be thorough, innovative, collaborative with nonhealth colleagues, and sensitive to the needs and preference of the adolescent.

Types of accommodations available address a myriad of needs ranging from those for self-management at the worksite or school, such as rest periods for the fatigue associated with the chronic condition to self-administration of dialysate for peritoneal dialysis. Other accommodations such as time off will be needed for follow-up care requiring outpatient visits during a work day to inpatient hospitalization necessitating several days to weeks off from work. For students, this type of accommodation will necessitate the planning for missed class work, assignments, and tests. Environmental accommodations pertain to the physical modifications needed to ensure the adolescent can perform sufficiently in the classroom or work setting. These accommodations may include software programs enabling enlarged fonts, ergonomic workstations, joysticks for computers, and modified keyboards. Health care professionals have a valuable role in assisting adolescents with special health care needs and disabilities and their families through the transition period and consulting with nonhealth professionals in identifying the need for accommodations and then obtaining them. For more information on accommodations for school and work settings, refer to Chapters 6, 11, 12, and 13.

Parental and Family Support

Transition experts have identified parental support as an important component of transition planning (AAP, Committee on Children with Disabilities, 2000; AAP, Committee on Children with Disabilities and Committee on Adolescence, 1996;

NAPNAP, 2001; Rosen et al., 2003). There is widespread recognition not only of the challenges that adolescents face but also for the difficulties, anxieties, and stress parents undergo as their children become adults (Boyle, Farukhi, & Nosky, 2001; DePoy et al., 2000; Geenen et al., 2003; Hauser & Dorn, 1999; Hauser et al., 1990; Russell, Reinbold, & Maltby, 1996; Sparacino et al., 1997; Westwood, Henley, & Willcox, 1999). Many parents have concerns about their children's ability to make the transition to adulthood. Often they worry about their children's capacity to be self-sufficient and assume the adult responsibilities associated with mature adulthood. More specifically, parents are anxious about their children's ability to obtain and retain a job, manage household and personal finances, and avoid being subjected to some form of exploitation. These legitimate concerns have begun to be studied by researchers to better understand the nature of parents' experiences (Hauser & Dorn, 1999; Patterson & Lanier, 1999; Russell et al., 1996; Stewart, Law, Rosenbaum, & Williams, 2001).

Parents may have concerns about the transfer to adult health care practitioners, especially after having developed long-standing positive relationships with their childrens' pediatrician and pediatric specialists. Parents may have concerns about the professional competence of the adult providers to whom the adolescent has been referred (Hauser & Dorn, 1999). This issue becomes particularly acute in communities wherein the availability of adult specialty and primary care providers who have had previous experience and medical training in providing services to adults with childhood acquired conditions is limited. For example, an adult with sickle cell disease may worry that adult providers may not fully understand or appreciate the need for pain medication (Anie & Telfair, 2005; Telfair et al, 2004). The result is having an adult with sickle cell disease undermedicated during a very painful sickling crisis. In other instances, it may be difficult to find an adult provider who has clinical experience working with adults with autism or a gynecologist who can perform pelvic exams on young women with cognitive limitations or severe spasticity of the lower limbs (Telfair, 2004).

Parents may feel uneasy about the changes in their role as their adolescents' proxies and advocates. During the time the child was seen by pediatricians, the parent served as the historian pertaining to illness episodes, the case manager for handling the child's daily medical and treatment needs, the advocate for ensuring the child received services needed, and the protector in times of stress, discomfort, fear, and pain. With the transfer to adult medical and health care, the parental role is likely to change considerably. The customary pattern of interaction between the parent, child, and pediatrician either no longer exists or is changed. Adolescents become the primary patients assuming the responsibilities and learning the roles once held by their parents. States confer this right and protection to potentially all adolescents who achieve the "age of majority." The age at which this occurs varies according to each state. Generally speaking, age of majority ranges from 18 to 21 years. However, parents can petition the courts for conservatorship for health care decision making, which enables parents to retain authority for their children's health care.

In response to the array of issues parents deal with during the transition process, experts have suggested that parent support programs might be helpful. These programs are designed to support parents with the process of "letting go" of their role as parent to a dependent child to an emerging role of parent to a young adult who has the ambitions and desire to be as independent and autonomous as possible. Other functions of parent groups are to provide information about transition and adult resources and programs as well as enable parents to network with other parents who have gone through or are going through this same experience.

Mentor Programs

Mentor programs enable adolescents to be connected with adults who share a most unique bond of living with a chronic condition or disability. For many youth, meeting an adult through a mentor program who has learned to manage his or her chronic health care needs sufficiently to live productively and independently is the first time they have met an adult with similar needs. Mentor programs are based on the premise that role modeling provided by mentors and peers is an effective approach to educate youth on explicit and implicit behaviors needed for adulthood. Additionally, an adult who knows what life is like to live with a chronic condition or disability has a level of credibility that cannot be matched by other typically developed adults the adolescent knows (Powers, Sowers, & Stevens, 1995; Sinclair, Christenson, & Evelo, 1998; Wortman, 1993).

SUMMARY

This chapter provides an introduction to the concept of health care transition planning for adolescents with special health care needs and disabilities. As described in this chapter, this type of transition planning is focused on addressing three primary health care needs, including finding adult health care providers, obtaining health insurance coverage, and acquiring self-sufficiency in managing long-term disability needs. Other goals of transition planning include obtaining the health accommodations needed for the workplace and in educational settings, providing support for families, and connecting adolescents with special health care needs and disabilities with adult mentors who can serve as role models. Health-related transition planning is an emerging area of practice not only for health care professionals but also for nonhealth professionals who work collaboratively with each other to ensure that adolescents with special health care needs and disabilities achieve their goals for the future.

REFERENCES

American Academy of Pediatrics. (1996). Transition of care provided for adolescents with special health care needs. *Pediatrics, 98*(6), 1203–1206.

American Academy of Pediatrics, American Academy of Family Practice, & American College of Physicians-American Society of Internal Medicine. (2002). A consensus statement on health care transitions for young adults with special health care needs. *Pediatrics, 110*(6 Pt 2), 1304–1306.

American Academy of Pediatrics, Committee on Children with Disabilities. (2000). The role of the pediatrician in transitioning children and adolescents with developmental disabilities and chronic illnesses from school to work or college. *Pediatrics, 106*(4), 854–856.

American Academy of Pediatrics, Committee on Children with Disabilities. (2001). The continued importance of Supplemental Security Income for children and adolescents with disabilities. *Pediatrics, 107*(4), 790–793.

American Academy of Pediatrics, Committee on Children with Disabilities and Committee on Adolescence. (1996). Transition of care provided for adolescents with special health care needs. *Pediatrics, 98*(6), 1203–1206.

Anderson, D.L., Flume, P.A., Hardy, K.K., & Gray, S. (2002). Transition programs in cystic fibrosis centers: Perceptions of patients. *Pediatric Pulmonology, 33,* 327–333.

Anie, K., & Telfair, J. (2005). Multisite study of transition in adolescents with sickle cell disease in the United Kingdom and the United States. *International Journal of Adolescent Medicine and Health, 17*(2), 169–178.

Bent, N., Tennant, A., Swift, T., Posnett, J., Scuffham, P., & Chamberlain, M.A. (2002). Team approach versus ad hoc health services for young people with physical disabilities: A retrospective cohort study. *Lancet (North American Edition), 360*(9342), 1280–1286.

Betz, C.L. (1999). Adolescents with chronic conditions: Linkages to adult service systems. *Pediatric Nursing, 25*(5), 473–476.

Betz, C.L. (2000). California Healthy and Ready to Work Transition health care guide: Developmental guidelines for teaching health care. *Issues in Comprehensive Pediatric Nursing, 23,* 203–244.

Betz, C.L. (2001). Use of 504 plans for children and youth with disabilities: Nursing application. *Pediatric Nursing, 27*(4), 347–352.

Betz, C.L., & Redcay, G. (2002). Lessons learned from providing transition service to adolescents with special health care needs. *Issues in Comprehensive Pediatric Nursing, 25,* 129–149.

Betz, C.L., & Redcay, G. (2003). Creating Healthy Futures: An innovative nurse-managed transition clinic for adolescents and young adults with special health care needs. *Pediatric Nursing, 29*(1), 25–30.

Betz, C.L. (2004). Adolescents in transition of adult care: Why the concern. *The Nursing Clinics of North America, 39,* 681–713.

Betz, C.L., Redcay, G., & Tan, S. (2003). Self-reported health care self-care needs of transition-age youth: A pilot study. *Issues in Comprehensive Pediatric Nursing, 26*(3), 159–181.

Blomquist, K., Brown, G., Peersen, A., Presler, E. (1998). Transitioning to independence: Challenges for young people with disabilities and their caregivers. *Orthopaedic Nursing, May/June,* 27–35.

Blum, R. (1995). Transition to adult health care: Setting the stage. *Journal of Adolescent Health, 17,* 3–5.

Bowman, R.M., McLone, D.G., Grant, J.A., Tomita, T., & Ito, J.A. (2001). Spina bifida outcome: A 25-year prospective. *Pediatric Neurosurgery, 34*(3), 114–120.

Boyle, M.P., Farukhi, Z., & Nosky, M.L. (2001). Strategies for improving transition to adult cystic fibrosis care, based on patient and parent views. *Pediatric Pulmonology, 32*(6), 428–436.

Buran, C.F., McDaniel, A.M., & Brei, T.J. (2002). Needs assessment in a spina bifida program: A comparison of the perceptions by adolescents with spina bifida and their parents. *Clinical Nurse Specialist, 16*(5), 256–262.

Cappelli, M., MacDonald, N.E., & McGrath, P.J. (1989). Assessment of readiness to transfer to adult care for adolescents with cystic fibrosis. *Children's Health Care, 18*(4), 218–224.

Clare, N. (1998). Management of sickle cell disease would improve if doctors listened more to patients. *British Medical Journal, 316*(7135), 935.

Conway, S. (1998). Transition from pediatric to adult-oriented care for adolescents with cystic fibrosis. *Disability and Rehabilitation, 20*(6/7), 209–216.

Cystic Fibrosis Foundation. (2006). *Frequently asked questions.* Retrieved November 14, 2006, from http:www.cff.org/AboutCF/Faqs/#/what_is_the_life_expectancy_for_people_who_have_CF_(in_the_United_States)?

DePoy, E., Gilmer, D., & Martzial, E. (2000). Adolescents with disabilities and chronic illness in transition: A community action needs assessment. *Disability Studies Quarterly, 20*(1), 16–24.

Eiser, C., Flynn, M., Green, E., Havermans, T., Kirby, R., Sandeman, D., et al. (1993). Coming of age with diabetes: Patients' views of a clinic for under-25 year olds. *Diabetic Medicine, 10*(3), 285–289.

Flume, P.A., Anderson, D.L., Hardy, K.K., & Gray, S. (2001). Transition programs in cystic fibrosis centers: Perceptions of pediatric and adult program directors. *Pediatric Pulmonology, 31*(6), 443–450.

Geenen, S.J., Powers, L.E., & Sells, W. (2003). Understanding the role of health care providers during the transition of adolescents with disabilities and special health care needs. *Journal of Adolescent Health, 32*(3), 225–233.

Hauser, E. & Dorn, L. (1999). Transitioning adolescents with sickle cell disease to adult-centered care. *Pediatric Nursing, 25*(5), 479–488, 496–497.

Hauser, S., Jacobson, A., Lavori, P., Wolfsdorf, J., Herskowitz, R., Milley, J., et al. (1990). Adherence among children and adolescents with insulin-dependent diabetes mellitus over a four-year longitudinal follow-up: II. Immediate and long-term linkages with the family milieu. *Journal of Pediatric Psychology, 15*(4), 327–342.

Health Resources and Services Administration. (2001). *Achieving success for all children with special health care needs: A 10-year action plan to accompany Healthy People 2010.* Washington, DC: Department of Health and Human Services.

Individuals with Disabilities Education Act of 1990, PL 101-476, 20 U.S.C. §§ 1400 *et seq.*

Individuals with Disabilities Education Act Amendments of 1997, PL 105-17, 20 U.S.C. §§ 1400 *et seq.*

Individuals with Disabilities Education Improvement Act of 2004, PL 108-446 20 U.S.C. §§ 1400 *et seq.*

Individuals with Disabilities Education Act of 1997 Final Regulations (1998). 34 C.F.R. Part 300, Assistance to States for the Education of Children With Disabilities (Part B of the Individuals with Disabilities Education Act). Retrieved August 7, 2006, from http://www.ideapractices.org/law/regulations/index.php

Institute for Family-Centered Care. (2001). *Frequently asked questions.* Retrieved June 2, 2004, from http://www.familycenteredcare.org/pdf/fcc_qa.pdf

Kipps, S., Bahu, T., Ong, K., Ackland, F.M., Brown, R.S., Fox, C.T., et al. (2002). Current methods of transfer of young people with Type 1 diabetes to adult services. *Diabetic Medicine, 19*(8), 649–654.

McDonagh, J.E., & Kelly, D.A. (2003). Transitioning care of the pediatric recipient to adult caregivers. *Pediatric Clinics of North America, 50*(6), 1561–1583.

Nasr, S., Campbell, C., & Howatt, W. (1992). Transition program from pediatric to adult care for cystic fibrosis patients. *Journal of Adolescent Health, 13,* 682–685.

National Association of Pediatric Nurse Practitioners and Associates. (2001). *Position statement on age parameters for pediatric nurse practitioner practice.* Retrieved October 26, 2002, from http://www.napnap.org/practice/positions/age.html

National Cancer Policy Board & National Institute of Medicine. (2003). *Childhood cancer survivorship: Improving care and quality of life.* Washington, DC: National Academy of Sciences. Retrieved June 14, 2004, from http://www.nap.edu/books/0309088984/html/

National Center for Youth with Disabilities. (1995). *Transition from child to adult health care services: A national survey.* Minneapolis, MN: Author.

National Institutes of Health, National Heart, Lung, and Blood Institute. (2002). *The management of sickle cell disease.* Washington, DC: Author.

Newacheck, P.W., Inkelas M., & Kim, S.E. (2004). Health services use and health care expenditures for children with disabilities. *Pediatrics, 114,* 79–85.

Pacaud, D., McConnell, B., Huot, C., Aebi, C., & Yale, J. (1996). Transition from pediatric care to adult care for insulin-dependent diabetes patients. *Canadian Journal of Diabetes Care, 20*(4), 14–20.

Patterson, D., & Lanier, C. (1999). Adolescent health transitions: Focus group study of teens and young adults with special health care needs. *Family and Community Health, 22*(2), 43–58.

Powers, L., Sowers, J., & Stevens, T. (1995). An exploratory, randomized study of the impact of mentoring on the self-efficacy and community-based knowledge of adolescents with severe physical challenges. *Journal of Rehabilitation, 61*(1), 31–44.

Rettig, P., & Athreya, B. (1991). Adolescents with chronic disease: Transition to adult health care. *Arthritis Care and Research, 4*(4), 174–180.

Rinehart, P.M., & Oberg, C. (1993). Teens can't get by with status quo. *Connections: The Newsletter of the National Center for Youth with Disabilities, 3,* 1.

Rosen, D. (1993). Transition to adult health care for adolescents and young adults with cancer. *Cancer, 71*(Suppl. 10), 3411–3414.

Rosen D.S., Blum, R.W., Britto, M., Sawyer, S.M. & Siegel, D.M. (2003). Transition to adult health care for adolescents and young adults with chronic conditions. *Journal of Adolescent Health, 33*(4), 309–311.

Russell, M., Reinbold, J., & Maltby, H. (1996). Transferring to adult health care: Experiences of adolescents with cystic fibrosis. *Journal of Pediatric Nursing, 11*(4), 262–268.

Sawyer, S., Collins, N., Bryan, D., Brown, D., Hope, M., & Bowes, G. (1998). Young people with spina bifida: Transfer from pediatric to adult health care. *Journal of Pediatric and Child Health, 34*, 414–417.

Sawyer, S.M., Blair, S., & Bowes, G. (1997). Chronic illness in adolescents: Transfer or transition to adult services? *Journal of Pediatrics & Child Health, 33*(2), 88–90.

Scal, P. (2002). Transition for youth with chronic conditions: Primary care physicians' approaches. *Pediatrics, 110*(6, Pt. 2), 1315–1321.

Scal, P., Evans, T., Blozis, S., Okinow, N., & Blum, R. (1999). Trends in transition from pediatric to adult health care services for young adults with chronic conditions. *Journal of Adolescent Health, 24*, 259–264.

Sharp, C., McNeil, R., Wales, S., Cooper, P., & Dawson, K. (1994). Young adults with cystic fibrosis: Social well-being and attitudes. *Australian Nursing Journal, 2*(4), 38–40.

Sparacino, P.S.A., Tong, E.M., Messias, D.K.H., Foote, D., Chesla, C.A., & Gilliss, C.L. (1997). The dilemmas of parents of adolescents and young adults with congenital heart disease. *Heart & Lung: Journal of Acute & Critical Care, 26*(3), 187–195.

Stewart, D.A., Law, M.C., Rosenbaum, P., & Williams, D.G. (2001). A qualitative study of the transition to adulthood for youth with physical disabilities. *Physical & Occupational Therapy in Pediatrics, 21*(4), 3–21.

Telfair, J. (2004). Sickle cell disease: Biosocial aspects. In I. Livingston (Ed.), *The Praeger handbook of black American health: Policies and issues behind disparities in health* (2nd ed.) (pp. 129–146). Westport, CT: The Greenwood Publishing Group.

Telfair, J., Alexander, L., Loosier, P., Alleman-Velez, P., & Simmons, J. (2004). Provider's perspectives and beliefs regarding transition to adult care for adolescents with SCD. *Journal of Health Care for the Poor and Underserved, 15*(3), 443–461.

Telfair, J., Alleman, P., Dickens, P., & Loosier, P. (2005). Quality health care for adolescents with special health care needs: A review of the literature. *Journal of Pediatric Nursing, 20*(1), 1–10.

Telfair, J., Ehiri, J., Loosier, P., & Baskin, M. (2004). Transition to adult care for adolescents with sickle cell disease: Results of a national survey. *International Journal of Adolescent Medicine and Health, 16*(1), 47–64.

Telfair, J., Myers, J., & Drezner, S. (1994). Transfer as a component of the transition of adolescents with sickle cell disease to adult care: Adolescent, adult, and parent perspectives. *Journal of Adolescent Health, 15*(7), 558–565.

U.S. Department of Health and Human Services. (2000). *Healthy People 2010: Understanding and improving health* (2nd ed.). Washington, DC: U.S. Government Printing Office.

Warnes, C.A., Liberthson, R., Danielson, G.K., Dore, A., Harris, L., Hoffman, J.I., et al. (2001). Task force 1: The changing profile of congenital heart disease in adult life. *Journal of the American College of Cardiology, 37*(5), 1170–1175.

Westwood, A., Henley, L., & Willcox, P. (1999). Transition from pediatric to adult care for persons with cystic fibrosis: Patient and parent perspectives. *Journal of Pediatrics & Child Health, 35*(5), 442–445.

White, P.H. (1997). Success on the road to adulthood: Issues and hurdles for adolescents with disabilities. *Rheumatological Diseases Clinics of North America, 23*, 697–707.

White, P.H. (2002). Access to health care: Health insurance considerations for young adults with special health care needs/disabilities. *Pediatrics, 110*(6, Pt. 2), 1328–1335.

Wojciechowski, E.A., Hurtig, A., & Dorn, L.A. (2002). Natural history study of adolescents and young adults with sickle cell disease as they transfer to adult care: A need for case management services. *Journal of Pediatric Nursing, 17*(1), 18–27.

Workforce Investment Act of 1998, PL 105-220 § 112 Stat. 936

Wortman, M. (1993). You've got a friend. *Diabetes Forecast*, 50–54.

CHAPTER 2

Service, Legal, and Ethical Issues Pertaining to the Continuum of Needs of Adolescents with Special Health Care Needs and Disabilities

THEODORE A. KASTNER, KEVIN K. WALSH, TERESA A. SAVAGE, AND ERIC B. CHRISTESON

Although adolescence is an exciting period of life, it also includes rocky and turbulent times. For most adolescents, the challenges during this period consist of establishing independence, gaining a broader perspective of the world, and making important life choices—typically, adolescents don't need to also figure out how to get their health care. For adolescents with special health care needs and disabilities, however, this last challenge may actually outweigh many of the others. For more than a decade, nearly half a million adolescents in the United States have made the transition to adulthood each year (Newacheck & Taylor, 1994; Reiss & Gibson, 2002), and proportionally, more of these individuals have severe disabilities since overall improvements in care have resulted in reduced mortality rates for this population.

Although in many ways, children and adolescents with special health care needs and disabilities are the same as their typically developing peers, they differ in the extent of the health care that they require. The Maternal and Child Health Bureau (MCHB), which is part of the Health Resources and Services Administration (HRSA), considers that "children with special health care needs are those children who have or are at risk for chronic physical, developmental, behavioral or emotional conditions and who also require health and related services of a type or amount beyond that required by children generally" (McPherson et al., 1998, p. 138).

A recent study conducted by HRSA found that 12.8% of the nation's children have special health care needs and disabilities, although approximately 40% of these children are not substantially affected in their general functioning (MCHB, 2001; van Dyck, Kogan, McPherson, Weissman, & Newacheck, 2004). At the time of the survey, 95% of children identified with special health care needs and disabilities had health insurance, 82% reported receiving needed services, and 89% reported having a personal doctor or nurse. Conversely, these statistics revealed that 470,000 children did *not* have insurance, nearly 1.7 million reported *not* receiving all the services they required, and more than 1 million did *not* have a personal medical professional.

The problems surrounding children with special health care needs and disabilities as they grow into adulthood—that is, as they make the *transition* to a different health care environment—is one focus of this chapter. This chapter also focuses on the ethical issues that affect these children as they transition into adulthood, including health care decision making, self-determination, facilitation of health care needs, sexuality concerns, and alcohol and substance use. Each of these foci are influenced by state legislation, regulations, and policies, and it is important that adolescents with special health care needs and disabilities and/or their family members become knowledgeable about how these state practices can and will affect them.

HEALTH CARE TRANSITION ISSUES

The Need for Transition

In 2002, The American Academy of Pediatrics (AAP) together with the American Academy of Family Physicians (AAFP) and the American College of Physicians-American Society of Internal Medicine (ACP-ASIM) published *A Consensus Statement on Health Care Transition for Young Adults with Special Health Care Needs* (hereafter referred to as *Consensus Statement*) outlining the issues and critical needs in health care transition for adolescents with special health care needs and disabilities. The problem for adolescents transitioning to adult health systems of care was outlined in the consensus statement this way:

> Most young people with special health care needs are able to find their way into and negotiate through adult systems of care. However, many adolescents and young adults with severe medical conditions and disabilities that limit their ability to function and result in complicating social, emotional, or behavioral sequelae experience difficulty transitioning from child to adult health care. There is a substantial number whose success depends on more deliberate guidance. (AAP, AAFP, & ACP-ASIM, 2002, p. 1304)

In addition, *Healthy People 2010* included a goal for the provision of a medical home for children and adolescents (see AAP, 2002) that includes not only ongoing health care but also assistance in various life transitions:

> Continuous care assures that the same primary pediatric health care professionals are available from infancy through adolescence and provides assistance with transitions [to home, school, and adult services]. (Department of Health and Human Services [DHHS], 2000, pp. 16–22).

Unfortunately, because of various, complex social structures, not the least of which are insurance and government programs, the health care services accessible to adolescents with special health care needs and disabilities are quite different than those accessible to them as adults. Adolescents growing up within family units have access to a complex array of services beyond health care (e.g., social services, vocational training, even recreational services through educational facilities) that offer support and increased access to their communities. Access to health care for adolescents is often made possible by either commercial insurance

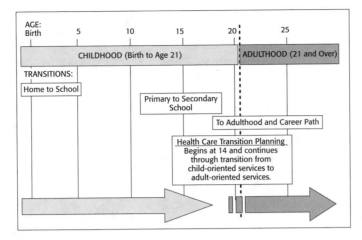

Figure 2.1.   Childhood and adolescent transitions.

covering the family or through special publicly-funded programs if family-based insurance is not available. In this latter category are programs such as the Medicaid State Children's Health Insurance Program (SCHIP), which allows Medicaid authorities to provide health care to adolescents who do not have access, or the Medicaid Early Periodic Screening and Diagnostic Testing (EPSDT) program, which assures comprehensive diagnostic and treatment services for adolescents with special health care needs and disabilities. (For more information on health insurance programs, refer to Chapter 3.) A schematic diagram of childhood and adolescent transitions is shown in Figure 2.1.

These types of specialized programs, however, are no longer accessible to individuals once they reach the age of adulthood—the so-called "aging-out" phenomenon. Nonetheless, adolescents with special health care needs and disabilities do not change in ways that remove the continuing need for assertive, comprehensive health care. Young adults, in other words, are likely to require the same level of care that they received as children and adolescents. Yet, nearly all of the social structures providing access to services are *categorical* in nature, employing bureaucratic definitions, typically age, to determine eligibility.

The problems in accessing health care and other services for adults with special health care needs and disabilities have long been understood (Garrard, 1982; Kastner, 1991). However, even with the publication of *Healthy People 2010* (DHHS, 2000) and the multiorganizational *Consensus Statement* (AAP, AAFP, & ACP-ASIM, 2002), these concerns have not yet coalesced into an easily-identifiable or widely understood need with respect to the provision of health care. It is critical that individuals working in health care systems understand the issues involved in transitioning from a child- and/or adolescent-oriented health care system to an adult-oriented system. Equally critical is that individuals within both systems know how and when to facilitate such transitions.

Overview of Health Care Transition Planning

A person's overall health and well-being, especially for an adolescent, arises when sufficient supports and opportunities are available to meet the developmental needs of that person. During periods of developmental transition, it is especially important that adequate supports and opportunities abound. With regard to health care transition from a child-oriented to an adult-oriented system, there is no set age or clear-cut developmental signal for the optimal time to actually make the transition. Therefore, *health care transition* as used in this chapter refers not to an obvious developmental milestone, but rather to a process consisting of planned and interlocking events that lead the individual from one health care system to another. This is not unlike many of the other "transitions" of adolescence, such as relationship transitions, educational or career transitions, or lifestyle transitions. That is, each of these comprises a set of linked events that, taken together, form a process that produces a developmental change in the person.

A healthy transition between child- and adult-oriented services for adolescents with special health care needs and disabilities is best characterized as a dynamic process that

1.   Meets individualized needs and is person-centered

2.   Maximizes individual functioning and potential

3.   Optimizes the individual's ability to assume adult roles

4.   Involves health services that are flexible, responsive, continuous, comprehensive, and coordinated (AAP, AAFP, & ACP-ASIM, 2002)

As such, the transition process likely will be different for each individual. Depending on their individual needs, some adolescents will be transferred to adult health care providers while others will maintain relationships with their pediatric care providers; some individuals will continue to require specialized care throughout adulthood while others will flourish in generic health care systems.

SERVICE SYSTEM ISSUES

The Medical Home

Families caring for children and adolescents with special health care needs and disabilities or caring for children whose health depends on complex technologies often experience increased parenting stress (Baker et al., 2003; Ricci & Hodapp, 2003; Warfield, Krauss, Hauser-Cram, Upshur, & Shonkoff, 1999) and have questions and concerns that simply do not arise in the general health care of typically developing children and adolescents. To address these concerns, children and adolescents with special health care needs and disabilities and their family members need a reliable source of information and services that is welcoming and supportive—in short they need a "medical home." The MCHB and the Division of Children with Special Needs provide funding to the AAP for the Medical Home initiative, which construes a medical home "not as a building, house, or hospital, but rather an approach to providing health care services in a high-quality and cost-effective manner" (AAP, 2006). Regardless of the location in which health care is rendered, the concept of the medical home requires that the care be accessible, family-centered, continuous, comprehensive, coordinated, compassionate, and culturally effective. Ideally, the source of the medical home is a primary care practitioner who is well-known to the child or adolescent and his or her family.

An adolescent's medical home certainly will have an important bearing on whether and how a transition to adult providers is carried out. Ideally, the values that underlie the medical home suggest that transition is best carried out when it involves movement to an adult system that is also imbued with the values inherent in the medical home approach (Kastner & Walsh, 2006). For additional information on the medical home approach, refer to Chapter 5.

Barriers to Health Care

Large health care systems have difficulty providing the necessary access and competency to effectively serve all adolescents with special health care needs and disabilities. There are several *barriers* to health care that affect this population, including 1) those related to the status or condition of the person (e.g., inability to communicate symptoms, lack of medical history, more complexity in presentation than is typical), 2) those related to the training and experience level of the health care provider, and 3) those related to the health care delivery system overall (e.g., access, insurance, program eligibility) (Kastner & Walsh, 2006).

For example, while the MCHB provides program funds directed toward training pediatric specialists in the care of children and adolescents with special health care needs and disabilities, there is no comparable training infrastructure for providers who eventually will be caring for these patients as adults. Nor is there a similar funding mechanism for any other discipline, such as nursing, that cares for children and adolescents. Children and adolescents who receive health care services over the course of their childhood—often including Medicaid's Early and Periodic Screening, Diagnostic, and Treatment services—are typically no longer eligible for these services after they transition into adulthood. In addition, there are more general problems that lead to poor access for specialty care, dental care, mental health care, and lead to limits on pharmaceuticals and durable medical equipment.

These types of problems have lead to disparities in care for individuals with special health care needs and disabilities of all ages. The U.S. Surgeon General, in 2001, convened a conference dealing with health care disparities as they affected one such group—individuals with mental retardation. Disparities in health care were highlighted in the report from that conference (U.S. Public Health Service, 2002) as follows:

> Compared with other populations, adults, adolescents, and children with mental retardation experience poorer health and have more difficulty in finding, getting to, and paying for appropriate health care. These challenges are even more daunting for people with mental retardation from minority communities . . . [because] the multiple disorders associated with mental retardation are found disproportionately among low-income communities that experience social and economic disparities when they seek health care. Mental retardation compounds these disparities because many health care providers and institutional sources of care avoid patients with this condition. (p. xii)

To offset such health care barriers, the Surgeon General's Report set forth a national blueprint for improvement, establishing the following six goals for health care services for individuals with mental retardations:

1. Integration of health care services into community environments

2. Increased research knowledge and understanding of the population

3. Improved health care quality

4. Increased training for providers

5. Effective financing

6. Increases in the number of providers and access to them

Because multiple factors can prevent the achievement of each goal, a variety of strategies must be employed simultaneously.

Similar findings for children and adolescents with special health care needs and disabilities were reported in MCHB's 2001 national survey. For example, when asked whether there was a time during the past when their child needed services, more than 50% of parent respondents cited the following four services: 1) prescription medications (87.9%), 2) dental care (78.2%), 3) preventive care (74.4%), and 4) specialist care (51%). Furthermore, the report elucidated striking changes in the types of health care their children needed over time. For example, when examined across three age groupings (birth–5 years, 6–11 years, and 12–17 years), mental health services were needed by 9.2% of the youngest group; this figure more than tripled to 27.6% in the 6–11 years age group, and increased further, to 30.9%, in the oldest age group. It is quite significant in the present context that nearly one third of adolescents with special health care needs and disabilities are in need of mental health services at precisely the time when adult transition activities should begin (AAP, AAFP, & ACP-ASIM, 2002).

All of these disparities are made more problematic because of the complexity of the interface between acute and long-term care systems and the lack of coordination between them. This lack of coordination often renders it difficult to implement competent health care plans as well as transition plans across all of the settings in which the adolescent participates, such as schools, residential settings, camps, foster care, recreation programs, and other activity centers. Additional barriers of this type include a lack of skilled direct care staff who can participate in implementing health care plans and excessive care coordination responsibilities due to inefficiency or redundancy of the human service system (Garrard, 1982; Kastner & Luckhardt, 1990; Kastner, Walsh, & Criscione, 1997). Each of these barriers can be complicated by legal and ethical issues, which will be discussed in the next sections.

LEGAL ISSUES

Issues of consent arise for adolescents with special health care needs and disabilities as they transition into adulthood. As with most legal rights, a person younger than the age of majority does not have the legal right to consent. The age of majority is set by each state, and in most states, this age is 18. However, the *mature minor rule* allows mature adolescents who are younger than the age of majority to consent to medical treatment, even if the adolescent's decision goes against the decision of his or her parents (Holder, 2005). The two goals of this rule are to a) offer treatment to a minor when parental consent may cause intra-family conflict or if the treatment is difficult to obtain, (this criteria is not clear as to what is meant) and b) protect physicians who treat mature minors. The legal privilege granted to such *mature minors* is to allow such a minor, who can understand the nature and consequences of medical treatment, the right to consent to treatment and the protection of the confidential doctor–patient relationship (Schlam & Wood, 2000). A person who is judged to have the power to consent also has the power to refuse treatment. A person who has the power to consent can, however, be treated against his or her wishes if the treatment is deemed a public health concern (Holder, 2005). An example would be if someone has a dangerous infectious disease (e.g., Ebola virus) that can be spread easily.

A person can only become a mature minor after a court hearing in which a judge decides if the minor has overcome the burden of *presumed immaturity* (i.e., the idea that based on age or other factors one is considered to make adult decisions, thus he/she is presumed to be immature). There are no tests or standards by which a judge decides whether a person is a mature minor; it is purely a subjective judgment (Schlam & Wood, 2000). When adolescents with special health care needs and disabilities are judged *not* to be mature minors, they are unable to give their own consent, and the responsibility remains with that of their parents or legal guardians.

If a person with an intellectual disability is an adult (over the age of 18 years in most states) and needs a guardian, a similar procedure as that of the mature minor is done. The person's case is heard before a judge in whom the individual is deemed incapable of handling everyday decisions and making important medical decisions.

ETHICAL ISSUES

Ethical Issues in Autonomy: Health Care Decision Making

Transition plans for adolescents with special health care needs and disabilities should include opportunities for them to exercise autonomy in decision making. Weithorn and Campbell (1982) found that adolescents as young as 14 years of age were capable of understanding and reasoning as well as adults in making health care decisions. Adolescents with special health care needs and disabilities often have extensive experience in the health care system and sometimes portray a level of sophistication about the health care system that their typically developing peers lack. Adolescents with special needs should be involved in decision making, as their capacity permits, especially regarding treatment decisions that will have long-term consequences (e.g., correction of scoliosis). Using methods for assessing capacity to consent might be useful for clinicians working with adolescents with special health care needs and disabilities.

Grisso and Appelbaum (1998a) identified the following four components to decision-making capacity: 1) understanding, 2) appreciation, 3) reasoning, and 4) expressing a choice. That is, a person must have an understanding of the factual information, the options, and the decision to be made; the person must have an appreciation of the effect different treatment options may have on his or her life; the person must be able to reason through the consequences of his or her decision (e.g., "If I chose Treatment A, what could happen? If I chose Treatment B, what could happen? If I chose neither option, what could happen?"); and the person must have the ability to express his or her choice. An adolescent's understanding, appreciation, reasoning, and choice can be assessed using this approach, and can serve as a starting point for discussions among the adolescent, his or her parents, and any health care providers in making health care decisions. Grisso and Appelbaum (1998b) developed the MacArthur Competency Assessment Tool for Treatment (MacCAT-T), which is a guide for assessing capacity to consent for treatment. It should also be useful for obtaining assent. (The interviewer should be mindful, however, that assent should be sought only if a refusal will be honored. One should not seek assent if the procedure or intervention will be performed despite refusal.)

Interviewers using the MacCAT-T should gather information prior to the conversation with the person from whom consent (or assent) is being sought. What is the decision to be made, and what are the important factors, for example, with health care decisions, diagnosis, prognosis, options for treatment, risks and benefits of each option, alternatives to treatment, and the time in which the decision must be made? The interviewer must always explain the purpose of the conversation (decision to be made) before beginning the interview process. The interviewer must consider the pace of the conversation and literacy level and gear the interview to the person's intellectual level, decision-making experience, and current emotional well-being.

Grisso and Appelbaum (1998b) recommended the following four-step process for interviewers using the MacCAT-T: 1) disclose information, 2) inquire to assess understanding, 3) probe for further clarification or demonstration of thorough understanding, and 4) redisclose and reinquire. The person's responses are rated 0, 1, or 2, according to the degree of understanding, appreciation, reasoning, and expressing a choice. The scores are added together and divided by the number of subscales for the summary rating. There is no description given by the authors of what constitutes a passing score which is similar to other capacity assessment instruments. Clinicians should use the information to augment other relevant data regarding the person's decision-making capacity.

The MacCAT-T requires that the interviewer use clinical judgment in deciding the threshold for determining capacity. The threshold varies, depending upon the nature of the decision and the degree of risk or harm. The higher the risk of the decision, the higher the threshold should be. For an adolescent contemplating scoliosis surgery, the risks of surgery, complications, or using nonsurgical interventions are high, so the threshold for demonstrating capacity to consent should also be high. Deciding whether to take a medication in liquid or pill form requires a lower threshold of capacity compared to the scoliosis decision. Although parents retain legal authority until age of consent, it is a valuable experience in health care decision making to have adolescents with special health care needs and disabilities participate in the decision-making process.

For decisions regarding end-of-life (EOL) care, McCabe, Rushton, Glover, Murray, and Leikin (1996) offered suggestions for involving the adolescent in advance care planning. If the adolescent has a life-limiting condition, advance care planning should include the adolescent if he or she is capable and willing to be involved. Although the adolescent is not legally recognized as the decision maker, the adolescent may want to share the decision making about EOL care with his or her parents. McCabe and colleagues (1996) recommended a health care provider with an established relationship assess the adolescent for the desire and capacity to be involved in EOL decisions. First, however, the health care provider should meet with the parents to ascertain their wishes in involving their child and to what extent they are willing to honor their child's wishes. With parental agreement, the health care provider can approach and assess the adolescent. McCabe and colleagues did not specify a particular approach in assessing capacity but recommended the assessment occur when the adolescent's condition is stable and there is no pressing time constraint. The adolescent may defer all decision making to his or her parents or may wish to be involved. It is also possible that the adolescent's desire to participate in decisions may change as his or her clinical condition changes. If disagreements over treatment preferences arise between the parents and child, the health care team should work toward reconciliation. It is often useful to have experienced pediatric counselors, such as social workers or psychologists, to aid in discussions on advance care planning with parents and adolescents.

While it is ideal to include adolescents with special health care needs and disabilities in their health care decision making, some adolescents will not have the capacity to give consent or to be involved in advance care planning. Adolescents with intellectual disabilities, for example, may not be able to understand, appreciate, and reason, and they often rely on their parents to make decisions in their best interests. To the extent that the adolescent can be involved, the health care providers and parents should include the adolescent in the decisions, or at a minimum, keep them informed at a level they can comprehend. Teaching adolescents with special health care needs and disabilities to ask questions to improve their understanding is the beginning step to self-advocacy.

Self-Determination

The developmental progression to independence has sometimes been elusive for adolescents with special health care needs and disabilities, as parents and society tend to protect an adolescent, even when the adolescent becomes an adult. Living apart from parents, finding a companion, or having a family may appear to be unreachable, inappropriate goals. The concepts of interdependence and circle of support, however, make the goals more realistic. The Center for Self-Determination identified "principles of self-determination" as:

1. Freedom to live a meaningful life in the community

2. Authority over dollars needed for support

3. Support to organize resources in ways that are life enhancing and meaningful

4. Responsibility for the wise use of public dollars

5. Confirmation of the important leadership that self-advocates must hold in a newly designed system (Center for Self-Determination, 2005)

Self-determination allows adolescents and young adults with special health care needs and disabilities to pursue goals that in the past would have been unattainable. And for many, independence is not possible; yet, in reality, hardly anyone lives independently where they do not depend on others for something. *Interdependence* is a more appropriate concept in that individuals with special health care needs and disabilities can direct their own care to get the necessary assistance they need (e.g., in performing activities of daily living). Adolescents and young adults with special health care needs and disabilities may defer decisions to a trusted individual or a trusted circle of support, including a network of friends, family, and professionals who commit their time and energy when needed. As the adolescent has more opportunities for making decisions, he or she may defer to others less frequently; however, the circle of support that respects the adolescent's self-determination remains and evolves with the person. When the adolescent needs to make a decision, he or she may call on some or all of the people in the circle of support to advise and assist in decision making.

Deference, as defined by O'Brien and O'Brien (1999), is the "reciprocal of self-determination" (p. 23). Deference means that one relies on others to interpret, clarify, and direct a decision in a given situation while keeping the person's values and wishes of utmost importance in the decision. As there is a circle of support, so there may be a "zone of deference" (O'Brien & O'Brien, 1999, p. 24) that permits a person to live as independently as possible. For example, a member of an adolescent's circle of support may make sure that videos are rented on Friday nights because the adolescent likes to watch movies, or the member may make sure to take the adolescent out to eat at his or her favorite restaurant twice a month. If possible, these decisions should be made mutually with members of the circle of support and the adolescent, or a "trial and error" approach can be taken with common activities to identify what the adolescent likes.

Although self-determination seems eminently respectful, it is revolutionary in its application. Self-determination takes more time to foster in adolescents with intellectual disabilities. Most adolescents are permitted to make their own decisions in certain situations such as choosing friends and leisure pursuits, and are permitted to learn by the outcomes whether or not they made a good decision or used a good decision-making process. In other words, typically developing adolescents learn by their mistakes. Adolescents with special health care needs and disabilities, however, are often not given the opportunity to make a mistake in their choices, so they may not benefit from the decision-making experience. Permitting and facilitating self-determination involves exposure to risks, but there is dignity in facing risks. Individuals risk failure, rejection, and heartbreak when they engage in employment, interactions with others, and relationships with others (Nerney, 1999). Self-determination is possible with a circle of support and strategies such as deference.

Ally is a 20-year-old with Down syndrome and is completing her last year in high school. She has identified for her goals upon graduation to live in her own apartment and support herself. Her individual transition plan (ITP) lists those goals and the skills required to achieve the goals, including job-seeking and employment-retention skills, money management, transportation navigation, and housekeeping skills. Through the transition program at her high school, Ally has arranged to apply for jobs and go apartment hunting. Her circle of support consists of her parents, one teacher, her high school counselor, the nurse in her pediatrician's office, and her best friend, who recently graduated from the same special education program.

Ally applied for a job in the cafeteria at the local hospital and is scheduled for a job interview. She talks with her teacher and counselor, and they both work with her to prepare for the job interview. She has also found an apartment through a newspaper ad and has called to see the apartment. For moral support, she invites her best friend to accompany her to the job interview. They take public transportation to and from the interview. After the interview, Ally described what happened to her parents, her teacher, and her counselor, and asks their advice on whether or not she should accept the job. She is able to identify, with probing, what she likes about the job and why she thinks she should take it, as well as what she may not like about the job and why she wouldn't want to take it. With input from her circle of support, she decides that she will wait and continue to search for a job that has more "pros" than "cons."

When Ally goes to see the apartment, she asks her parents to accompany her. She looks in all the rooms, asks a few questions, and then asks her parents what else she should ask about the apartment. The landlord directs all of his questions to Ally's parents, and says that he will require them to co-sign a lease since Ally does not have established credit. Ally is intimidated by the process of finding an apartment and decides that she is not ready to begin her search. She again consults with her circle of support and decides to revise her goals and objectives in her ITP. She believes that she should find a roommate, like her best friend, who can help her in finding an apartment and managing the responsibilities.

The same process would apply to a health-related concern. Ally has a fever and chills. She has learned how to take her temperature and after checking how high her fever is, she calls her parents for advice. They discuss her options and decide that she will take an over-the-counter medication that reduces fever to see if that helps. She will call her parents back after four hours and tell them how she feels and then they will decide what to do next.

Ethical Issues in Planning and Reaching Life Goals: Facilitation of Health Needs

Health Maintenance

As part of self-determination, adolescents with special health care needs and disabilities should learn the skills required to manage their health care; learn what preventive health care measures they should employ, including screening tests and immunizations; and learn what specialty care they need. Oftentimes, pediatricians and other pediatric primary care providers coordinate care for adolescents with special health care needs and disabilities between the pediatric subspecialists. Teaching adolescents with special needs how to coordinate their care or seek assistance to do so is an important step in helping them make the transition to adult health care, and which requires adults to coordinate for themselves their care between the primary physician and specialists. Involving parents in the transition process is critical in terms of supporting adolescents with special health care needs and disabilities, assisting with accessing resources, and so forth. For more information on locating adult providers, refer to Chapter 5. For more information on health maintenance, refer to Chapter 4.

Sexuality

Besides the transition to adult health care, sexuality is an important issue to discuss. Geenen, Powers, and Sells (2003) found that parents' priorities in the transition to adult care differ from the health care providers' priorities. The coordination of health care was the highest priority of the parents, with attention to sexuality, substance abuse, and mental health problems ranked lowest. The authors concluded that open discussion among parents and health care providers should occur to identify what assistance the parents want from health care providers. Parents, however, do not always adequately educate their children on issues of sexuality, substance abuse, and mental health.

Most parents find it difficult to address issues of sexuality with their adolescents, and for adolescents with special health care needs and disabilities, sexuality may not be a priority for parents' attention. A number of studies reveal that adolescents with chronic conditions and disabilities are as sexually active as their typically developing peers (Berman et al., 1999; Blum, 1997; Cheng & Udry,

2002); yet, adolescents with special needs usually are not as well informed. As emerging adults, adolescents with special health care needs and disabilities have the same reproductive rights as their typically developing peers. Transition programs should include life skills such as socialization, establishing and maintaining relationships, sex education, marriage, and parenting. Bass (as cited in Blum, 1997, p. e4) identified several key points in providing sex education:

- Assume that youth with disabilities experience significant social isolation

- Assume that they will have poorer judgment and fewer social skills than peers

- Sexual development may be delayed or inhibited

- Severe disabilities may make marriage unlikely

- Affected persons must know the genetic risks to their offspring

- Information must be simple, clear, and repeated often

Blum (1997) adds,

- The privacy of the individual must be respected

- Be clear about the values being transmitted, because there is no such thing as values-free education

- Do not assume that the person is heterosexual

- Do not assume that parents or other health professionals will have provided ample or accurate information

Depending upon the adolescent's medical condition, contraceptive methods should be tailored to achieve long-term goals, such as preserving fertility, if desired.

Having an intellectual disability does not mean that consent for sexual activity cannot be given. There is a tension between respecting the person's right to explore this aspect of the human experience and protecting the person from abuse, exploitation, sexually transmitted infections, or unwanted pregnancy. Kennedy and Niederbuhl (2001) developed criteria for capacity for sexual consent from people with intellectual disabilities, which could be part of the educational process in preparing the adolescent for sexual activity. They conducted a survey of 305 psychologists who ranked a 56-item questionnaire on the importance each item had in relation to capacity to consent to sexual activity. Through factor analysis, they identified the following five factors:

- Factor 1 was consequences of sexual activity (e.g., pregnancy, sexually transmitted infections)

- Factor 2 was basic and essential sexual knowledge (e.g., differences between the sexes, sexual conduct in terms of time and place)

- Factor 3 was unessential sexual knowledge (e.g., anatomical names, understanding a tubal ligation)

- Factor 4 was safety for self and others (e.g., how to protect oneself or not harm others)

- Factor 5 was basic safety skills (e.g., can say "no," can resist coercion, can recognize a dangerous situation)

Psychologists believe that items in Factor 5 and Factor 1 were essential criteria in determining the capacity to consent to sexual activity, based on their ratings of importance, with items from Factor 2 being rated somewhat important. Educators can work with the parents to incorporate these items in their teaching plans. Parents' attitudes and values toward sexuality are conveyed in the educational process.

Recognizing an adolescent's sexual interests and maturity does not mean, however, that parents should permit sexual activity. Readiness is a combination of education, maturity, opportunity, and choice. Other criteria, such as a committed, monogamous relationship and/or marriage, may be consistent with the family's values.

Alcohol and Substance Use

Education regarding alcohol and other substance use is also important. Leisure activity for adolescents sometimes involves using illegal substances. Parents can teach and advise their children, but they often do not share the same perspective of living with a disability that their children need. Peer mentors and adults with special health care needs and disabilities may be able to provide that unique perspective, as many have remarked that they wished they had role models who had similar needs, or had an opportunity to discuss issues that they were reluctant to discuss with their parents, such as dating, sexuality, and marriage (Klein & Kemp, 2004).

SUMMARY

We have made gains in understanding the needs of adolescents with special health care needs and disabilities who are transitioning to the adult health care system; however, several barriers still exist. It behooves us to confront these barriers and work to their resolution. Tackling these barriers will include providing a successful medical home; considering ethical issues with regard to autonomy in health care decision making, self-determination, and health maintenance; and addressing topics such as sexuality and alcohol and substance use as adolescents with special health care needs and disabilities transition to adulthood and, in many cases, increased independence.

REFERENCES

American Academy of Pediatrics. (2002). The medical home. *Pediatrics, 110,* 184–186.

American Academy of Pediatrics. (2006). *What's a medical home?* Retrieved August 8, 2005, from http://www.medicalhomeinfo.org

American Academy of Pediatrics, American Association of Family Physicians, & American College of Physicians-American Society of Internal Medicine. (2002). A consensus statement on health care transitions for young adults with special health care needs. *Pediatrics, 110*(Suppl. 6), 1304–1305.

Baker, B.L., McIntyre, L.L., Blacher, J., Cronic, K., Edelbrock, C., & Low, C. (2003). Preschool children with and without developmental delay: Behaviour problems and parenting stress over time. *Journal of Intellectual Disability Research, 47,* 217–230.

Berman, H., Harris, D., Enright, R., Gilpin, M., Cathers, T., & Bukovy, G. (1999). Sexuality and the adolescent with a physical disability: Understandings and misunderstandings. *Issues in Comprehensive Pediatric Nursing, 22,* 183–196.

Blum, R.W. (1997). Sexual health contraceptive needs of adolescents with chronic conditions. *Archives in Pediatrics & Adolescent Medicine, 151*(3), 290–296.

Center for Self-Determination. (2005). *Principles of self-determination.* Retrieved October 11, 2005, from http://www.self-determination.com

Cheng, M.M., & Udry, J.R. (2002). Sexual behaviors of physically disabled adolescents in the United States. *Journal of Adolescent Health, 31,* 48–58.

Garrard, S.D. (1982). Health services for mentally retarded people in community residences: Problems and questions. *American Journal of Public Health, 72,* 1226–1228.

Geenen, S.J., Powers, L.E., & Sells, W. (2003). Understanding the role of health care providers during the transition of adolescents with disabilities and special health care needs. *Journal of Adolescent Health, 32,* 225–233.

Grisso, T., & Appelbaum, P.S. (1998a). *Assessing competence to consent to treatment: A guide for physicians and other health professionals.* New York: Oxford University Press.

Grisso, T., & Appelbaum, P.S. (1998b). *MacArthur Competence Assessment Tool for Treatment (MacCAT-T).* Sarasota, FL: Professional Resources Press.

Holder, A.R. (2005). Special categories of consent: Minors and handicapped newborns. In M. Capron & I. M. Birnbaum (Eds.), *Treatise on health care law* (Vol. 3, pp. 1–118). Dayton, OH: Matthew Bender & Company, Inc.

Kastner T. (1991). Who cares for the young adult with mental retardation? *Journal of Developmental Behavioral Pediatrics, 12,* 196–198.

Kastner, T., & Luckhardt, J. (1990). Medical services for the developmental disabled. *New Jersey Medicine, 87*(10), 819–822.

Kastner, T.A., & Walsh, K.K. (2006). A Medicaid managed care model of primary care and health care management for individuals with developmental disabilities. *Mental Retardation, 44,* 41–55.

Kastner, T.A., Walsh, K.K., & Criscione, T. (1997). Overview and implications of Medicaid managed care for people with developmental disabilities. *Mental Retardation, 35,* 257–269.

Kennedy, C.H., & Niederbuhl, J. (2001). Establishing criteria for sexual consent capacity. *American Journal on Mental Retardation, 106,* 503–510.

Klein, S., & Kemp, J. (2004). *Reflections from a different journey: What adults with disabilities wish all parents knew.* New York: McGraw-Hill.

Maternal and Child Health Bureau. (2001). *The national survey of children with special health care needs.* Maternal and Child Health Bureau, Health Resources and Services Administration, U.S. Department of Health and Human Services. Retrieved August 8, 2005, from http://mchb.hrsa.gov/chscn/pages/intro.htm

McCabe, M.A., Rushton, C.H., Glover, J., Murray, M.G., & Leikin, S. (1996). Implications of the Patient Self-Determination Act: Guidelines for involving adolescents in medical decision making. *Journal of Adolescent Health, 19,* 319–324.

McPherson, M., Arango, P., Fox, H., Lauver, C., McManus, M., Newacheck, P., et al. (1998). A new definition of children with special health care needs. *Pediatrics, 102,* 137–140.

Nerney, T. (1999). *Lost lives: Why we need a new approach to quality.* Retrieved October 11, 2005, from: http://www.self-determination.com/lost_lives.pdf

Newacheck, P.W., & Taylor, W.R. (1994). Childhood chronic illness: Prevalence, severity, and impact. *American Journal of Public Health, 82,* 364–371.

O'Brien, J., & O'Brien, C.L. (1999). *Walking toward freedom: One family's journey into self-determination.* Retrieved October 11, 2005, from: http://thechp.syr.edu/Sheri.pdf

Reiss, J., & Gibson, R. (2002). Health care transition: Destination unknown. *Pediatrics, 111* (6, Pt. 2), 1307–1314.

Ricci, L.A., & Hodapp, R.M. (2003). Fathers of children with Down Syndrome versus other types of intellectual disability: Perceptions, stress and involvement. *Journal of Intellectual Disability Research, 47,* 273–284.

Schlam, L., & Wood, J.P. (2000). Informed consent to the medical treatment of minors: Law and practice. *Health Matrix: Journal of Law-Medicine, 10,* 141–174.

U.S. Department of Health and Human Services. (2000). *Healthy People 2010.* Washington, DC: Author. Retrieved August 8, 2005, from http://www.healthypeople.gov/document/html/volume2/16mich.htm

U.S. Public Health Service. (2002). *Closing the gap: A national blueprint for improving the health of individuals with mental retardation. Report of the Surgeon General's conference on health disparities and mental retardation.* Washington, DC: Author.

van Dyck, P.C., Kogan, M.D., McPherson, M.G., Weissman, G.R., & Newacheck, P.W. (2004). Prevalence and characteristics of children with special health care needs. *Archives of Pediatrics & Adolescent Medicine, 158*(9), 884–890.

Warfield, M.E., Krauss, M.W., Hauser-Cram, P., Upshur, C.C., & Shonkoff, J.P. (1999). Adaptation during early childhood among mothers of children with disabilities. *Journal of Developmental and Behavioral Pediatrics, 20,* 9–16.

Weithorn, L.A., & Campbell, S.B. (1982). The competency of children and adolescents to make informed treatment decisions. *Child Development, 53,* 1589–1598.

CHAPTER 3

Health Insurance Options for Transition-Age Adolescents and Young Adults

KATHRYN SMITH AND NICOLE GARRO

Youth with special health care needs and disabilities and their families face numerous challenges related to health insurance as they transition into adulthood. There are three basic vehicles by which individuals can acquire health insurance in our current health care system. The first vehicle is a commercial group plan, often employer-sponsored, which may also include college health insurance plans, special state-run purchasing cooperatives for high-risk individuals, and group plans through organizations such as the American Association of Retired Persons (AARP). The second vehicle is a publicly funded insurance program, such as Medicaid, Medicare, the State Children's Health Insurance Program (SCHIP), the State Title V Children with Special Health Care Needs (CSHCN) Program, or state-specific disease programs. The third vehicle is an individual insurance policy that can be purchased to cover a single individual or a family.

In addition to health care funding sources such as traditional insurance, "wrap-around services" may provide limited support for needed supplies, care coordination and/or transportation. Sometimes these services are provided through not-for-profit specialty organizations, such as the American Cancer Society. Other examples of such programs are found in hospitals that have charitable care programs, such as those offered at Shriners Hospitals for Children or St. Jude Children's Research Hospital. In addition, individual states may fund services for specialized populations through the developmental disabilities, mental health, or foster care systems. This chapter will discuss each of these insurance options, as well as issues that youth and their families face as they negotiate the health care financing system as they transition into adulthood.

COMMERCIAL GROUP PLANS

Employer-Sponsored Health Insurance

The majority of people in the United States obtain their health insurance through employer-sponsored insurance, either through their own employer or through a family member's employer. Employer-sponsored insurance covered 174 million people, or 59.8% of the population, in 2004 (U.S. Department of Health and

Human Services, Office of the Assistant Secretary of Planning and Evaluation [DHHS, ASPE], 2005).

In general, employer-sponsored insurance is offered to employees and their dependents; however, employees usually have to bear a greater financial burden in order to add dependents to their policies. Each year, an employer has "open-enrollment" in which employees can enroll in their health insurance plans. The specific plan offered by employers can take many forms, including health maintenance organizations (HMOs), preferred provider organizations (PPOs), or other options, although some employers may offer only one option. If there is a choice, reviewing the covered benefits of each option will help inform decision making about which option will best meet an adolescent or young adult's special needs. For example, certain plans may have limits on therapy services, durable medical equipment, or other ancillary services. In addition, many adolescents and their families wish to see the same provider over a period of time. Thus, it is important for adolescents and their families to review their policies to be sure that their providers contract with the plan they choose, especially if they are planning to change plans during open enrollment. For more information on appropriate benefits to look for, families may refer to *Evaluating Managed Care Plans for Children with Special Health Care Needs: A Purchaser's Tool* (McManus, n.d.).

As adolescents transition from childhood to adulthood, their eligibility as a dependent on their parents' insurance policies may change. There are often age limits on policies for dependent children, although some allow continuous coverage while a child attends school, or if a child has a permanent disability and dependence on the family. The employer's human resources or benefits department should be able to provide additional information about an individual's health care policy. It is best to attempt to get policy information from both the employer's human resources or benefits department and the health insurance company, as inaccurate information could result in an individual with special health care needs and disability losing valuable coverage.

According to the U.S. Census Bureau (2004), the unemployment rate for people with disabilities who are 16 years and older is 14.3%, as compared with 7.2% for the general population. While not all youth with special health care needs and disabilities are considered disabled, unemployment has serious implications in terms of health insurance availability, necessitating the need to stay on a parent's policy for as long as possible or establishing eligibility for the state's Medicaid program.

In addition, some youth may reach the limits of their family's employer-sponsored coverage. Expensive conditions, such as hemophilia or those requiring organ transplants, may result in the youth reaching the maximum benefit level, and no longer being eligible for coverage. To use an example from the author's experience, an adolescent with an inborn error of metabolism requiring expensive infusion therapy first reached the limits on his mother's employer-sponsored coverage, then reached the limits on his stepfather's coverage. When he went to college, he applied for the college health insurance plan but was concerned that the coverage would not be sufficient for the duration of his stay in college. He hopes to find a job upon graduation and be eligible for his own insurance; however, the problem of reaching the limits of the policy will remain with him and may affect his choice of a plan that would cover him.

College Health Insurance

Colleges and universities often require health insurance of their enrollees, and most schools offer health insurance to incoming students. The premiums for this coverage are usually lower than one would expect to pay for individual insurance. Benefit packages vary depending on the school. In addition, school-sponsored insurance policies often require the use of student health services for primary care, and the levels of specialty care coverage vary by school. Students and their families should consult with their school's admissions department or student health services to learn more about and apply for school-sponsored insurance.

Special State-Run Purchasing Cooperatives

Some states have special purchasing cooperatives for individuals who are not otherwise able to obtain insurance in the individual insurance market. For example, there is a program in California called the Major Risk Medical Insurance Program (MRMIP). For 36 months, the state subsidizes health insurance premiums for the participants in the individual insurance market. At the end of the program, participants are unenrolled and then guaranteed coverage from one of the plans participating in the MRMIP (Managed Risk Medical Insurance Board, 2006). This program is funded by tobacco taxes.

Group Plans Through Organizations

In some cases, organizations may offer group health insurance plans. For example, professional associations or other trade organizations, such as the American Nurses Association, may offer group health insurance programs to their members. Much like employer-based insurance, youth with special health care needs and disabilities should consider the benefits offered, the cost incurred by the individual, and the limits on coverage when making a decision about these group plans.

PUBLICLY FUNDED PROGRAMS

Medicaid

Medicaid is an entitlement program authorized by Title XIX of the Social Security Act. As an entitlement program, it must pay for medical care for specific individuals who meet federally mandated eligibility requirements. Medicaid is jointly funded by the federal and state governments. There are broad requirements at the federal level, while each state is responsible for developing their eligibility standards, scope of services, method of service delivery, payment for services, and administration of the program (DHHS, Centers for Medicare and Medicaid Services, 2005a).

Eligibility Standards

Eligibility for Medicaid may vary widely among states, however there are certain mandatory groups, deemed "categorically needy" for which federal matching funds are provided to each state. Given the variability of state guidelines, a person may be eligible in one state for Medicaid and not in another. These categorically needy groups include the following:

1. Individuals who meet the Temporary Aid to Needy Families (TANF) program (the state's welfare cash assistance program) eligibility requirements that became effective in their state on July 16, 1996

2. Pregnant women and children ages birth through 5 years who live at or below 133% of the federal poverty level

3. Recipients of Supplemental Security Income (SSI)

4. Recipients of foster care assistance (Title IV of the Social Security Act)

5. Special protected groups (usually those who lost cash assistance due to increased earnings but may continue Medicaid for a time)

6. Children between ages 6 and 19, who live at or below 100% of the federal poverty level

7. Specific low-income Medicare beneficiaries (DHHS, Centers for Medicare and Medicaid Services, 2005a)

In addition, states may provide Medicaid coverage to optional "categorically related" groups. In general, these groups share some of the same characteristics as the mandatory "categorically needy" groups but are included under broader guidelines. Examples include certain working people with disabilities who would qualify for SSI if they did not work, or infants (younger than 1 year) and pregnant mothers living at or below the federal poverty level (DHHS, Centers for Medicare and Medicaid Services, 2005b). "Medically needy" individuals fall under this optional category as well. Those who are medically needy would be eligible for Medicaid under either the mandatory or optional groups; however, they fall under the optional category if they have income or resources above the state's eligibility level. Often benefits may be restricted for these medically needy groups, for example, the state may opt to cover prenatal services, delivery, and postpartum care for pregnant women, but no other conditions.

The Ticket to Work Incentives Improvement Act of 1999 authorizes Medicaid coverage for certain working individuals with disabilities. Individuals with higher incomes contribute to premiums for Medicaid coverage on a sliding scale basis (DHHS, Centers for Medicare and Medicaid Services, 2005c). This program encourages employment for those with disabilities, but it allows them to keep Medicaid coverage, even though they receive income from work. Additional information on the Ticket to Work program may be found through the Social Security Administration web site.

Scope of Services

Medicaid provides a generous benefits package; however, states have some flexibility in their plans. Each state's program must offer coverage for a basic package of services to the categorically needy program, funded in part by federal matching funds. In addition, there are 34 optional services that states may offer that are also eligible for matching funds. Examples of optional services include medical transportation services, prescription drugs, and physical therapy.

Method of Service Delivery

Traditionally, Medicaid services have been paid on a fee-for-service basis, in which an individual could go to the Medicaid provider of their choice for care. Increasingly, however, states are providing services through managed care arrangements in which patients choose a health plan and/or a primary care provider who then approves and coordinates all health care services through the plan. States, then, can limit the duration and scope of services within broad federal guidelines.

Payment for Services

States have flexibility in how services are paid for. The federal government imposes upper limits on payments to providers; however, states must pay providers enough to maintain an adequate supply to provide sufficient access to Medicaid beneficiaries. Having a sufficient pool of providers can be a challenge in many states, particularly in those states in which provider reimbursement is low. Medicaid-eligible adolescents with special health care needs and disabilities may have difficulty finding specialty care providers where reimbursement is low, or they may experience long waits for services.

Administration of the Program

Medicaid waivers allow states to administer Medicaid services outside of the federal requirements (this is known as "waiving" the federal requirements). Each state has different waivers that must be approved by the federal government. One type of waiver, the Katie Beckett Waiver, allows states to consider the children's income and assets rather than the parents' income and assets, if the child has a disability. Children who qualify for Medicaid waiver services must be in need of care that would normally be provided in a hospital or nursing home. Otherwise, they receive the same package of services as children who qualify due to their parents' income. The Katie Beckett Waiver allows youth who would otherwise be institutionalized to remain in the community.

Medicare

Although the majority of Medicare recipients are older adults (ages 65 or older), a small group of individuals younger than 65 receive health benefits through the Medicare program due to special health care needs and disabilities. Medicare is funded entirely by the federal government and premiums from individuals. The federal government determines eligibility and regional payment rates.

Eligibility Standards

In addition to older adults, adolescents with end-stage renal disease are eligible for Medicare benefits. Dependent children and youth with end-stage renal disease may be eligible for Medicare if at least one parent has met certain work requirements (earning at least 6 credits in the last three years under Social Security, the Railroad Board, or as a federal government employee), and the child meets certain medical requirements. These requirements include needing regular dialysis or having had a kidney transplant (DHHS, Centers for Medicaid and Medicare Services, 2005b).

Scope of Services

Medicare provides comprehensive health benefits to beneficiaries through three separate parts. Part A covers hospital costs and is provided to all Medicare beneficiaries with no additional premiums. Part B covers outpatient and physician services, but requires monthly premiums; these premiums were $78.20 per month in 2005. Part D, the newest component of Medicare, covers prescription drugs. Part D includes a $250 deductible and then covers 75% of drug costs to a total of $2,250. Individuals are responsible for total drug costs between $2,251 and $5,100. When total drug costs reach $5,100, the prescription drug plans covers 95% of the total drug cost. Individuals may apply for Medicare and SSI (if applicable), at their local Social Security Administration Office (DHHS, Centers for Medicaid and Medicare Services, 2005c).

The State Children's Health Insurance Program

The State Children's Health Insurance Program (SCHIP) was authorized in 1997 under Title XXI of the Social Security Act. Like Medicaid, it is a federal–state partnership, and it provides medical coverage to "targeted low-income children" (DHHS, Centers for Medicaid and Medicare Services, 2005c).

Eligibility Standards

Children who live in families below 200% of the federal poverty level or with family income 50% higher than the state's Medicaid eligibility threshold are eligible for SCHIP. Many states have expanded eligibility beyond this level, and some states cover parents as well. Certain groups, however, are ineligible for SCHIP. These groups include

1. Children currently covered by either a group health plan or through individual insurance

2. Children from families eligible for state employee insurance

3. Children living in institutions

4. Children eligible for Medicaid (DHHS, Centers for Medicaid and Medicare Services, 2005c)

Administration of the Program

Like Medicaid, the state has considerable flexibility in program design and administration. States have three options for program design: a) expanding Medicaid eligibility to children who did not previously qualify, b) designing a separate SCHIP program, or c) combining the Medicaid expansion and separate program options. The federal government provides states with an enhanced match rate for those enrolled in SCHIP, above that of Medicaid.

States may have cost-sharing provisions; however, they cannot require cost sharing for preventive services (well child visits or prenatal care) or immunizations, and cost sharing may not exceed 5% of a family's income. In general, coverage tends to be less comprehensive than Medicaid, although SCHIP must still cover a basic package of services, similar to that of the state employees benefit package, the federal employees benefit package, or the largest health maintenance organization in the state.

Application Process

The process for applying for SCHIP and Medicaid vary by state and are often similar. In some states, individuals may contact their local social services office; in other states, they may contact their local health departments; and in some states, streamlined applications are tied to other services, such as the school lunch program, or can be completed by mail.

While Medicaid and SCHIP are national in scope, states have latitude in establishing program eligibility and determining benefits and payment structures. In addition, state-run programs vary considerably in whom they serve and the services they provide. Therefore, it is critical that providers become familiar with the specific service systems in their states and communities. Providers serving adolescents and young adults should also know basic information about who is served by which program and what services are provided. And since program eligibility and service delivery vary from region to region, providers should not rely on information about the system of care from other locales in which they have previously worked.

Establishing eligibility for a specific program can be a complicated process. For example, in determining financial eligibility, the program may consider some sources of income but not others, and some assets (typically defined as things one owns) may be considered as well. In determining medical eligibility for a program, strict eligibility requirements may make a child eligible for care, while another with the same or similar condition may not be considered if there is a severity criterion applied. Given that eligibility determination can be complex, providers should refer clients to programs that serve youth without making assumptions about eligibility, allowing program staff to determine whether or not the individual can be served.

Title V Children with Special Health Care Needs and Programs

Title V of the Social Security Act authorizes the Maternal Child Health Services Block Grant to provide the funding for a variety of state maternal and child health programs, including services for children with special health care needs and disabilities up to age 21, which is known as the State Title V State Program for Children with Special Health Care Needs (Title V CSHCN Program).

Eligibility Standards

The Title V CSHCN Program aims to provide family-centered, community-based, coordinated care to children with eligible conditions. Because Title V CSHCN Programs are state-run programs, eligible conditions can be defined differently by each state. In general, these eligible conditions are either life threatening or chronic medically complex conditions that require highly specialized care that tends to be costly.

Scope of Services

The Title V Program may fund direct services, function primarily as a coordinator of services through other systems, or do both. For example, some states contract with centers of care to provide highly specialized services to children with complex medical conditions. In other states, mainly wraparound services are provided that supplement other insurance that the children may have. These wrap-around services typically cover services beyond the scope of health insurance, such as additional occupational/physical therapy services, additional visits to mental health providers, transportation assistance, care coordination, and so forth.

Application Process

The application process for Title V varies by state. In some cases, the Medicaid program or SCHIP may refer children and youth to the State Title V CSHCN Program for specialized services. In other cases, families or providers must seek out the program themselves, or be referred by a knowledgeable provider.

Financing of Services

There are various financing arrangements in different states. For example, California's Title V CSHCN Program operates as a carve-out (in most counties) in which the child may have Medicaid or SCHIP for their routine heath care and all services related to their eligible condition will be "carved out" and financed by the Title V CSHCN Program. The Title V CSHCN Program will also work with a commercial insurer to meet unmet needs for those children who are eligible.

State-Specific Disease Programs

Some states have state-specific disease programs that cover a limited number of chronic conditions, often conditions that were previously covered under the State Title V CSHCN Program. For example, in California, the Genetically Handicapped Persons Program (GHPP) provides services through special care centers for individuals with hemophilia, sickle cell disease, thalassemia, Huntington's disease, Friedreich ataxia, Joseph's disease, and selected hereditary metabolic disorders such as phenylketonuria (PKU) and von Hippel-Lindau syndrome. Individuals who are enrolled in these disease-specific programs may or may not have additional insurance, although these programs may not cover a comprehensive set of medical and related services (California Department of Health Services, 2000). The Title V CSHCN Program in a given state may help direct clients to these state-specific programs.

INDIVIDUAL INSURANCE POLICIES

Another insurance option, in addition to commercial group plans and publicly funded insurance programs, is purchasing individual insurance policies. Directly purchased individual insurance policies covered 26.9 million or 9% of the population in 2005 (DHHS, ASPE, 2005). Premiums for these policies generally are higher than those purchased through employer-sponsored plans. Two main reasons account for this increased cost: 1) the individual purchaser must bear the entire burden of the cost of the insurance policy, unlike employer-sponsored health insurance where a portion is paid for by the employer; and 2) when insurance companies underwrite health policies, they consider risk, meaning they account for health status when predicting how much it will cost them to provide care for the people they are insuring. With employer-sponsored insurance, all employees are included in this risk pool, so no one individual is held financially responsible for the cost of their health care. However, if a policy is purchased individually for an adolescent with special health care needs and disabilities, it is likely that the policy premiums will be much higher than they would be for a typically developing adolescent with minimal special health care needs. Individuals may purchase insurance through insurance brokers, or increasingly, they may access information on individual policies at health plan web sites.

OTHER PROVIDERS OF HEALTH RELATED SERVICES/WRAP-AROUND PROGRAMS

State Programs for Children with Developmental Disabilities

The federal Developmental Disabilities and Bill of Rights Act Amendments of 2000 mandates that states have a State Council on Developmental Disabilities and a Protection and Advocacy agency. State Councils on Developmental Disabilities are charged with increasing independence, productivity, inclusion, and community integration for people with developmental disabilities. States organize direct services for people with developmental disabilities in different ways. Some offer care coordination services and may provide or arrange for health services not covered by health insurance or other programs. For example, in California, there are 21 regional centers throughout the state that arrange for services for individuals with developmental disabilities. Each client is assigned to a service coordinator who is responsible for coordinating services that are agreed upon during the client's annual individual program plan (IPP). Other states, including New York, Pennsylvania, Michigan, and Florida, have similar programs.

State and County Mental Health Services

State and county departments of mental health provide mental health services mainly to children who are from low-income families, who are uninsured, or who receive mental health services through special education, generally up to age 21. Depending on the specific state, state and county departments of mental health may also provide services for children served by Medicaid and SCHIP. The level of benefits and eligibility varies by state. As youth transition out of the child-focused mental health system, they will have to reapply and qualify for adult mental health services. Often the eligibility criteria and application procedures differ from the child mental health system. This further complicates the transition process and may lead to decreased access to services for those wishing to continue these services into adulthood.

Foster Care

In addition to the various psychosocial issues faced by children in foster care, many children in foster care also suffer from complex special health care needs and disabilities. Children in foster care are eligible for Medicaid by law; however, they often face delays in needed health care due to slow-moving bureaucracy, transportation issues, caregivers who have little knowledge of the condition or are unaware of the services available, and so forth. As youth in foster care transition to the adult health care system, they face unique challenges in accessing appropriate care. Adolescents transitioning out of foster care may be eligible for employer-sponsored insurance if they are employed or they may seek to enroll in a health plan through their college or university. Many foster children may continue to be eligible for Medicaid if they are able to quality for SSI; however, many will be left without insurance. Early planning for youth in foster care is critical in order to ensure that all options are sufficiently examined for this vulnerable population.

STRATEGIES FOR MAINTAINING COVERAGE FOR ADOLESCENTS AGING OUT OF A CHILD-CENTERED HEALTH CARE SYSTEM

Proactive Planning

It is essential that youth with special health care needs and disabilities and their families begin to think about and discuss health care and related transitions as the youth enters adulthood. As discussed previously, publicly funded health care often ends at 19 years of age, or in the case of the Title V Programs, 21 years of age. Additionally, other factors need to be considered, including locating appropriate health care providers, locating equipment vendors and pharmacists who can supply specialized equipment and medication, and continued educational and vocational planning. (For additional information on locating health care providers and accessing needed supplies, equipment, and community resources, refer to Chapters 4 and 5.)

Current providers can assist families in identifying needed resources. Hospital-based social workers, advanced practice nurses, and case managers who work with adolescents are typically well versed in locating and accessing adult-focused resources. School nurses employed in high schools also may have information about providers in their areas who will work with transitioning youth (see Chapter 10). In addition, the youth's medical home provider (see Chapter 5) may be able to provide a linkage to an appropriate medical home focusing on adults, including those with the youths' unique health considerations. Insurance plan member services departments can help youth with special health care needs and disabilities and their families identify providers within their plan who can take over the youth's care. Ideally, these resources are identified prior to transition so that the youth and his or her family have the opportunity to visit and speak with potential providers and discuss their views on care.

Many youth have access to care coordinators through the various service systems in which they receive services. These professionals can provide needed support and information to youth and their families, and can work together with other professionals to develop a cohesive and comprehensive transition plan. Primary nursing professionals who see the youth are well positioned to invite the youth, his or her family, and key providers and agencies together to plan for the youth's transition. A nurse's educational background in human development, his or her knowledge of the technical nature of the youth's condition, and the availability of community resources all serve as important components in leading the transition team. (For additional information on care coordination, refer to Chapter 14.)

Understanding Relationships within the Service System

A solid knowledge of the relationships of the programs and services available to the youth is of key importance to the youth and his or her family. For instance, eligibility for Medicaid is often linked to eligibility for SSI. Therefore, it is essential for the youth to follow up with all requests related to SSI eligibility in order to maintain Medicaid. Youth who are SSI beneficiaries will need to undergo a re-determination process at age 18 if they want to continue to receive SSI and Medicaid benefits. The developmental disabilities system may only serve as the payer of last resort and may require other sources of funding, such as Medicaid or commercial insurance, to pay for services first, and then provide coverage if needed. Likewise, the Title V CSHCN Program may require that the school system, the developmental disabilities system, or Medicaid pay for services first, before providing benefits.

Key to understanding the services system is paying careful attention to all correspondence that comes from agencies and programs. Both parents and their children, if able, should read all material and become familiar with the content and requirements. Quick responses are important, as deadlines need to be met, and requests for additional paperwork may be required. Programs are often not forgiving when it comes to missed deadlines, sometimes requiring an application to begin again, or sometimes dismissing benefits. Waiting for records from providers can impede the application process for services. Record keeping can be managed by maintaining a notebook with all key materials that relate to the youth's care and copies provided to requesting agencies.

A number of good examples of notebooks are available on the Web, including *All About Me* (n.d.). This tool allows parents and youth to organize materials from various service systems and providers, including diagnostic test results, the individualized educational plan and other service system plans, key contacts, lists of medications, treatments and hospitalizations, and copies of correspondence. This notebook, which allows information to be readily available in one location when consulting with a new provider or completing an application, helps to expedite services. Another important document to be included in the notebook is the *Emergency Information Form for Children with Special Needs*. This form is designed to help children with special needs receive fast and efficient care in case of an emergency by providing necessary information to providers who may be treating them in an emergency situation.

The Importance of Vocational Training in Helping to Maintain Health Insurance

The importance of vocational training as a means to gainful employment and possible employer-sponsored health insurance cannot be understated. As discussed previously, employer-sponsored health insurance is the vehicle by which most Americans receive their health care; however, those with disabilities are underrepresented in this group. While one may not consider the positive affect of vocational training on health, the impact is huge, both in terms of enhanced self-esteem, as well as access to insurance. Vocational training opportunities should be discussed by a provider, teacher, or guidance counselor to youth and their families early in high school, particularly if it appears that the youth will not be attending college. Plans should be made for the youth to transition to a job-training program when high school is complete, with the ultimate goal of entry into the labor market, both for self-sufficiency and access to health care. For additional information on vocational training opportunities, refer to Chapter 12.

SUMMARY

This chapter provides a review of private and public insurance options available for adolescents and young adults with special health care needs and disabilities. Unfortunately, major issues exist that are associated with insurance coverage for adolescents and young adults who age out of the pediatric health insurance coverage, including issues related to inadequate or lack of insurance coverage with employment options.

REFERENCES

All about me. (n.d.) Retrieved December 4, 2006, from http://mchneighborhood.ichp.ufl.edu/medicalhomela

California Department of Health Services. (2000). Genetically handicapped persons program [brochure]. Retrieved November 11, 2005, from http://www.dhs.ca.gov/pcfh/cms/ghpp/pdf/ghppbrochure.pdf

Developmental Disabilities and Bill of Rights Act Amendments of 2000, PL 106-402, 42 U.S.C. §§ 6000 *et seq.*

Managed Risk Medical Insurance Board, California Major Risk Medical Insurance Program. (2006). *2006 application and handbook.* Retrieved February 2, 2006, from http://www.mrmib.ca.gov/MRMIB/MRMIPBRO.pdf

McManus, M. (n.d.). *Evaluating managed care plans for children with special health needs: A purchaser's tool.* Columbus, OH: Children with Special Health Care Needs Continuing Education Institute. Retrieved December 5, 2006, from http://policyweb.ichp.ufl.edu/ichp/purchaser/Default.html

U.S. Census Bureau. (2004). *American community survey: Employment statistics.* Retrieved January 7, 2006, from http://factfinder.census.gov/servlet/STTable?_bm=y&-geo_id=D&-qr_name=ACS_2004_EST_G00_S2301&-ds_name=D&-_lang=en

U.S. Department of Health and Human Services, Administration on Children and Families, Administration on Developmental Disabilities. (2006). *ADD fact sheet.* Retrieved February 7, 2006, from http://www.acf.dhhs.gov/programs/add/factsheet.html

U.S. Department of Health and Human Services, Centers for Medicare & Medicaid Services. (2005a). *Medicaid at-a-glance 2005: A Medicaid information source.* Retrieved November 11, 2005, from http://www.cms.hhs.gov/MedicaidGenInfo/Downloads/MedicaidAtAGlance2005.pdf

U.S. Department of Health and Human Services, Centers for Medicare & Medicaid Services. (2005b). *Medicare for children with chronic kidney disease.* Retrieved January 1, 2006, from http://www.Medicare.gov/Publications/Pubs/pdf/11066.pdf

U.S. Department of Health and Human Services, Centers for Medicaid & Medicare Services. (2005c). *State children's health insurance program summary.* Retrieved February 1, 2006. from http://www.cms.hhs.gov/MedicaidGenInfo/05_SCHIP%20Information.asp#TopOfPage

U.S. Department of Health and Human Services, Office of the Assistant Secretary of Planning and Evaluation. (2005). *Overview of the uninsured in the United States, an analysis of the 2005 Current Population Survey.* Retrieved November 29, 2005, from http://aspe.hhs.gov/health/reports/05/uninsured-cps/

CHAPTER 4

Promoting Health Care Self-Care and Long-Term Disability Management

CECILY L. BETZ AND LIONESS AYRES

The Centers for Disease Control and Prevention (2005a) estimated that 17% of U.S. children and youth have a developmental disability (e.g., autism, cerebral palsy, intellectual disability) that severely impacts their daily living. According to a recent national survey, 12.8% of children and youth have a special health care need (van Dyck, Kogan, McPherson, Weissman, & Newacheck, 2004), and each year 500,000 adolescents with special health care needs become adults. As adolescents transition from pediatric to adult health care services, they also must develop skills in self-care and long-term disability management. Assuming responsibility for one's health by acquiring the knowledge and skills needed to manage one's health care needs is essential to the youth's successful health care transitioning. Possessing the knowledge and skills necessary for self-management will enable the youth to adhere to the recommended treatment regimen to support stability or improvement of his or her condition and prevent or minimize the emergence of complications and/or secondary conditions.

Whether the youth is newly diagnosed with a special health care need or disability, was born with a congenital condition, or was diagnosed between these end points, learning the self-management skills necessary to function as independently as possible is a lifelong endeavor. Children with special health care needs and disabilities who are diagnosed at birth or at an early age will rely primarily on their parents and other caregivers to assume the major responsibilities for their treatment regimen and long-term chronic care needs. The extent to which a child can learn to assume more self-care and long-term disability management responsibilities will be dependent in part on their developmental level of functioning. For example, children with moderate to severe disabilities will have limited self-care and disability management capabilities.

Children and youth whose parents and health care providers teach them to assume more of their self-management responsibilities will require ongoing, periodic updates in their level of knowledge and will require refinement of their current level of skills as their developmental competencies advance and their health literacy increases. Circumstances may change and create new needs for learning, such as the emergence of secondary conditions or complications, the availability of newer treatment modalities and medications, and the life changes that arise such as moving to a new community or getting married.

According to a recent Institute of Medicine report, health literacy refers to "the degree to which individuals can obtain, process, and understand the basic health information and services they need to make appropriate health decisions" (Nielsen-Bohlman, Panzer, & Kindig, 2004). Health literacy is an important component of self-management as it is essential to managing the treatment needs associated with having special health care needs and disabilities, navigating the complex health care system, and communicating with health care professionals (Beckman et al., 2004; U.S. Department of Health and Human Services, 2000). Youth and young adults who have cognitive and physical limitations affecting their ability to read and comprehend problems, visual impairments, or limitations with fine motor skills affecting their ability to hold reading material, are at higher risk for having health literacy problems (Beckman et al., 2004). As research has demonstrated, individuals with low health literacy skills are at a higher risk for poorer health outcomes, limited understanding of their health care needs, using fewer health resources, increased rates of hospitalization, and increased health care costs (Beckman et al., 2004; Hardin, 2005; Williams et al., 1995).

The costs of failure to accomplish self-management affect both youth with special health care needs and disabilities and society. For example, people with physical disabilities are less likely to have health insurance; are less likely to use the health care system, especially for primary preventive care such as mammography or dental care; and have higher rates of preventable secondary conditions such as amputations and fractures (Centers for Disease Control, 2005b). Poor self-management is related to an increased incidence of complications and secondary conditions that lead to higher rates of hospitalization and emergency department visits. Increased hospitalization and emergency care in turn create higher health care costs (Bryden, Dunger, Mayou, Peveler, & Neil, 2003; Collins, Kaslow, Doepke, Eckman, & Johnson, 1998).

Psychosocial outcomes for adolescents with special health care needs and disabilities can be negatively affected as well, resulting in increased school absences, increased mental health problems, lower levels of self-esteem, impaired social relationships, and increased dependency, thereby limiting the prospects of youth and young adults living independently and productively in the community (Bryden et al., 2003; Collins et al., 1998). For example, between 1994 and 1996, children and youth ages 5 to 17 years missed an average of 14 million days of school annually due to asthma (Mannino, Homa, Akinbami, Gwynn, & Redd, 2002). Increased absence decreases the likelihood of success in school. Perhaps as a consequence, people with disabilities have lower rates of formal education and are more likely to be unemployed (National Center on Birth Defects and Developmental Disabilities, 2005).

This chapter focuses on the challenges adolescents with special health care needs and disabilities face when attempting to transition from pediatric and child health programs to adult health care and systems and describes the scope of effort required to support these individuals as they become more independent. This chapter begins with a discussion of pertinent terms and concepts and then continues with a synthesis of research findings on adherence and self-management and a discussion of the factors that influence adherence and self-management. The chapter concludes with practice implications for educators and health care providers who are employed in schools and other community settings, such as work settings.

PERTINENT TERMS AND CONCEPTS

Any discussion of health care self-care, self-management, and long-term disability management should begin with a discussion of the terms *adherence, compliance, self-care,* and *self-management,* as they are not only encountered in the literature but also practiced in community settings.

The terms *adherence* and *compliance* have erroneously been used interchangeably. There is an important difference in meaning between the two terms. Adherence refers to the extent to which an individual's behavior is consistent with the treatment recommendations for sustained home care proposed by his or her health care professional(s). Adherence also refers to the comprehensive array of behaviors associated with an individual's long-term care management, which include assumption of treatment responsibilities, the individual's level of participation in managing his or her chronic condition, and interactions with health care professionals for treatment-related purposes. Treatment regimen adherence is dependent on the individual's input and agreement with the plan (Kyngas, 2000; Kyngas & Rissanen, 2001; Shaw, 2001; World Health Organization [WHO], 2003). Whether an individual adheres to the treatment regimen can be judged on a continuum, rather than in the absolute terms of either *yes* or *no* (Kyngas, 2000). A number of factors, such as developmental competencies, family support, access to resources, and the complexity of the treatment regimen influence an individual's ability to adhere to it. (These factors are described in greater detail in the following section.) The term *compliance* has a similar meaning to adherence but with the important difference that it is the health care professional who prescribes the treatment approach for an individual with the expectation that he or she will comply with the therapeutic plan without necessarily considering the individual's input (WHO, 2003). Judgment of the individual's performance by the health care providers is implicit with both adherence and compliance (Milnes & Callery, 2003; Schilling, Knafl, & Grey, 2006).

Next, the term *self-care* refers to those actions that are undertaken by an individual that are based on the treatment regimen requirements. The individual performs the tasks as prescribed by the treatment plan with the understanding that these actions are necessary to achieve the treatment goals of managing the disease/disability needs, promoting health, and minimizing the potential for secondary conditions and complications (Orem, 2003). Self-care involves a combination of cognitive-behavioral and motor tasks. These tasks may include fine and gross motor behaviors, such as learning to use a walker or wheelchair, learning to use a syringe, or learning to wrap a limb with a dressing. Cognitive-behavioral tasks include learning new pathophysiological concepts about the condition, continuing self-monitoring, and navigating a new system of care (Shegog et al., 2001). Unlike adherence and compliance, self-care refers to a more narrowly defined set of behaviors associated with care responsibilities.

Finally, *self-management* is similar in meaning to self-care and is a term now used more frequently than self-care in the literature and in practice. The focus of self-management and self-care is on the individual's performance of the treatment tasks rather than an assessment of the individual's performance according to predetermined standards established by health care professionals (Harris et al., 2000). According to Schilling, Grey, and Knafl, self-management "both captures the complexity of living with a disease . . . and suggests the need to control the disease in the context of one's life" (2002, p. 88). Thus, for youth with special health care needs and disabilities, self-management includes not only the adolescent, but significant adults who have some degree of responsibility or role in his or her life. These adults include parents or guardians and other adult authorities, such as teachers, school nurses, coaches, physicians, or bus drivers (Milnes & Callery, 2003; Schilling, Knafl, & Grey, 2006).

In addition, self-management for adolescents with special health care needs and disabilities is a process; that is, it changes over time (Schilling et al., 2002). Self-management begins as a parent-dominant process, wherein the parents or primary caregiver assumes the primary responsibility for illness management for youth, ages 11 up to 15 years. The next phase, transitional management, occurs between ages 15 and 17 years when both parent and child share the responsibilities for illness and/or disability care. Adolescent-dominant self-management is characterized by management responsibilities assumed by older children, ages 17 years and beyond (Milnes & Callery, 2003; Schilling, Knafl, & Grey, 2006).

FACTORS THAT INFLUENCE ADHERENCE AND SELF-MANAGEMENT

Estimates of treatment adherence by children and adolescents with special health care needs and disabilities vary widely. Experts offer differing statistics ranging from 4% to 100%, with an average estimate of 50% (Burkhart & Dunbar-Jacob, 2002; Kyngas, 2000; Rapoff, 1999, 2000). Rates of adherence are difficult to determine given the variances associated with treatment regimens and problems associated with the accuracy of self-reports by youth and parents. In addition, the methods used to measure adherence differ greatly among researchers (Burns & Grove, 2005).

The difference between adherence and self-management is more than semantic. Rather, as some experts have suggested, an individual's level of adherence occurs in the context of the daily demands youth and families face, the amount of resources available to manage ongoing treatment needs, youth and families' competencies in modifying the treatment regimen to conform to their lifestyle needs, and their ability to evaluate the effectiveness of their care. Issues associated with treatment adherence are better understood when operationalized in meaningful terms for the adolescent and family members. Ongoing chronic care treatments can interfere substantially with adolescent and family activities of daily living and their quality of life. Adherence is affected by the level of pain, discomfort, inconvenience, intrusiveness, and intensity caused by the treatment regimen itself, as manifested, for example, in dietary restrictions and blood glucose monitoring associated with Type I diabetes, repeated daily self-catheterizations done by youth with spina bifida, home enteral feedings required for infants with short bowel syndrome, or the respiratory regime of aerosolized treatments and postural drainage followed by children and youth with cystic fibrosis.

Required treatments can be painful as evidenced by daily injections, regular blood drawings, bone marrow aspirations, and lumbar punctures required by certain conditions. A study of youth with Type I diabetes revealed that they forewent insulin injections believing that they did not need them, only to discover later more insulin was needed as serum glucose was severely elevated (Kyngas, 2000; Weissberg-Benchell et al., 1995). Similarly, medications can result in significant changes in physical appearances, as demonstrated by the hair loss and weight gain of chemotherapy, and the growth of facial hair and a "puffy" facial appearance due to immunosuppressive agents.

It is no wonder that youth and families will devise approaches to lessen the burden of the ongoing care of the youths' special health care needs and disabilities. This treatment adaptation has been described by a number of researchers using terms such as *adapative noncompliance* (Deaton, 1995), *educated noncompliance* (Koocher, McGrath, & Gudas, 1990), and *adaptive incomplete adherence* (Shaw, 2001; Shaw, Palmer, Hyte, Yorgin, & Sarwal, 2001). Alterations in treatment approaches by youth and their families suggest the need to engage both health care providers and those in need of care to devise a workable and realistic plan of care that meets the needs of the youth and family and corresponds to the youth's ongoing need for care (Shaw et al., 2001).

Therefore, it is important to distinguish between problematic nonadherence and adaptive self-management and assess the extent to which a youth is adherent to the treatment regimen, as there may be any number of reasons why adherence is problematic. Adolescents who use adaptive self-management strategies will alter treatment regimen requirements to meet their lifestyle needs. For example, a youth with epilepsy may choose to ride a bicycle in contradiction to the advice of the pediatrician. An adolescent with exercise-induced asthma may continue to play on the softball team against the recommendations of a doctor (Shaw, 2001). Several factors have been identified as impacting treatment adherence, including developmental characteristics, condition-related factors, lack of developmentally appropriate information, family characteristics, and the systemic barriers associated with the health care system (Strawhacker, 2001).

Developmental Characteristics

Understanding normal and abnormal adolescent development provides insights about the needs and behaviors of adolescents with special health care needs and disabilities. Therefore, a discussion of normal adolescent development, in conjunction with a discussion about development for adolescents with special health care needs and disabilities, is warranted. During adolescence, development takes place physically, cognitively, and psychosocially.

Physical Development During Adolescence

Dramatic physical changes typically occur during adolescence. This period of development is characterized by a bodily transformation, also known as *puberty*, that features observable increases in skeletal growth and weight, acne development, the appearance of secondary sex characteristics (e.g., breasts, pubic hair), and the capacity to reproduce. For girls, puberty development refers to the beginning of menstruation and the redistribution of fat resulting in further development of the hips, legs, stomach, buttocks, and breasts. For boys, puberty development includes the coarsening of facial hair, the deepening of the voice, an increase in muscle mass, testicular growth, and nocturnal emissions. The process of puberty begins approximately 2 years earlier for girls than boys. The onset of puberty, however, varies considerably among adolescents, with a typical age range of 12 to 15 years. Hormonal changes evident during puberty also contribute to mood swings and highly emotional behavior (American Academy of Pediatrics, nd; Green & Palfrey, 2002; Katchadourian, 1978; McCarthy, 2000; Tanner, 1962).

For youth with special health care needs and disabilities, the typical physical changes associated with puberty can be affected by the youth's chronic condition or its treatments. A youth's condition may have a visible effect on his or her physical appearance or functioning, as with the youth with cystic fibrosis whose chest circumference becomes barrel-shaped and whose height is below the developmental norm (Betz & Sowden, 2003).

Treatment for youth with special health care needs and disabilities may have temporary or long-term effects on physical development. For example, treatment effects youth with cancer may have to endure include alopecia (hair loss) and cushingoid features (puffy reddened facial appearance) due to chemotherapeutic agents, skin discoloration due to radiation, and, in some cases, amputation (Betz & Sowden, 2003; Keene, 2003). Youth with epilepsy who take antiepileptic medications may be subjected to the unwanted side effects of weight gain and hyperplasia of the gums (Marin, 2005).

Cognitive Development During Adolescence

Cognitive development during adolescence includes the development of *formal operations,* in which an adolescent's thinking typically evolves from the concrete approach in learning and interacting with his or her world to thinking in more abstract or symbolic terms. This shift in thinking—from the concrete, grounded style of needing graphic representations and illustrative explanations to conceptualizing the "what ifs," the less obvious, and the subtle nuances of more complex reasoning—will develop at different rates in adolescents. The differences in cognitive development depend on previous life experiences, innate capabilities, and the quality of environment stimulation and supports within which the adolescent was raised (Piaget, 2001; Piaget & Inhelder, 1958).

Youth with special health care needs and disabilities often have challenges acquiring the cognitive capacities of this developmental stage or applying the cognitive abilities they have to the situations they confront during puberty. For example, younger adolescents with cognitive limitations are likely to manifest thinking characteristic of *concrete operations* (Piaget & Inhelder, 1958). Developmentally, the younger adolescent is more focused on the present, and learning is dependent on concrete representation of concepts, such as explanations of disease symptomology and treatments. Therefore, it is difficult for younger adolescents with special health care needs and disabilities to project the effects of long-term consequences of nonadherence, and they may have difficulties fully realizing concepts related to delayed gratification. In addition, younger adolescents require further assistance with adherence behavior, as their behavior repertoire is limited (Piaget, 2001). Older adolescents with special health care needs and disabilities typically are capable of comprehending more abstract explanations as well as understanding the meaning of behavioral consequences. Adolescents also engage in what Elkind (1967) has described as adolescent egocentrism, meaning that the adolescent is unable to conceive perspectives of others or their own vulnerabilities. The adolescent may not believe that consequences of not taking medication or not monitoring behavior applies to him or herself based on their egocentric belief (Elkind, 1967; Feinstein et al., 2005).

Interestingly, contrary to developmental theory, a number of studies have reported that adherence levels are lower for adolescents as compared with younger children (Matsui, 2000; Quittner et al., 1996). Explanations for these unexpected findings indicate that parents may have supervised younger children more closely, or that parents assumed primary responsibility for their child's treatment regimen. Differences in treatment adherence also have been found between adolescent boys and girls. A study of adolescent boys and girls with Type I diabetes found that most of the girls had assumed responsibility for their insulin injections and were less inhibited about injecting themselves in public. In contrast, boys were more reliant on their mothers for assistance in managing their diabetes and were resistant to injecting themselves in public for fear of disclosure. Researchers suggest that the differences may be attributable to socialization and perceived gender roles (Williams, 1999, 2000).

Psychosocial Development During Adolescence

According to Erikson (1963, 1968, 1978, 1980), the major developmental task, during the stage of young adulthood, known as *Intimacy vs. Isolation*, is to develop meaningful and intimate relationships with others. The ability to achieve both personal and sexual intimacy with others is predicated on successful identity development. The nature of an individual's relationships will vary depending on whether the individual is a same or opposite-sex friend, spouse, or child. The essence of intimacy with others is the ability to be responsive and sensitive to their needs, to learn to love and trust, and to engage in reciprocal communication of feelings (Johnson, 2004). By this cognitive stage of development, biologic maturity typically is complete; however, the psychosocial maturity normally expected with this stage may yet to be realized in youth with special health care needs and disabilities (Katchadourian, 1978). For example, young adults with special health care needs and disabilities are at a higher risk for social isolation and loneliness, as their physical limitations may make it more difficult to socialize with friends. As a result, they may have inadequate social skills due to restricted social contacts (D'Auria, Christian, Henderson, & Haynes, 2000).

Gould (1978), an adult developmentalist, asserted that young adulthood was a pivotal stage of development, as it was a period of life reorientation. During the preadult stage of *Leaving Our Parents' World*, the young adult reexamines the childhood assumptions of parental protection and dependency that are no longer relevant. The young adult begins to emotionally address the paradox of parental dependency and personal independence and autonomy. Young adults with special health care needs and disabilities, however, are at higher risk for not successfully achieving this task and the other young adulthood (ages 18 to 35 years) tasks proposed by Havighurst (1953).

Developmental Tasks of Early Adulthood

Selecting a mate

Learning to live with a significant other, partner, spouse

Beginning a family

Raising children

Maintaining a residence

Beginning to work in an occupation/profession

Becoming involved in community/civic activities

Creating a network/circle of friends

As data on adult outcomes demonstrate, adults with special health care needs and disabilities have higher rates of unemployment, lower rates of participation in postsecondary programs, fewer friends, and less active social lives (National Council on Disability, 1996; Presidential Task Force on the Employment of Adults with Disabilities, 1998; Wagner, Newman, Cameto, & Levine, 2005).

Identity development is a paramount developmental task of adolescence. Youth struggle with the conflicts associated with becoming independent, learning to be more socially engaged with peers, dealing with the changing societal expectations of becoming an adult, and changing bodily appearance, shape, and functioning (Erikson, 1963, 1968, 1978). Motivating youth to be adherent to their treatment regimen is a challenge, particularly if it involves complicated, time-consuming procedures or taking medications that cause undesirable side effects such as weight gain, increased facial hair, and nausea and vomiting (Anarella, Roohan, Balistreri, & Gesten, 2004; Scarfone, Zorc, & Capraro, 2001; Shaw, 2001). It is difficult for adolescents with special health care needs and disabilities to have to deal with unpleasant, painful, and time-consuming procedures when their typically developing peers are engaging actively in the usual activities of someone in this stage of development (Woodgate, 2005). Youth with cancer, for instance, reported that during periods of illness, they experienced "life as a klutz, life as a prisoner, life as an invalid, as an alien, life as a zombie and life as a kid" (Woodgate, 1998, p.10). In other words, the effects of their illness and treatments created feelings of alienation with their body.

Adolescents may resist treatment adherence as it poses a way of rebelling against the frustration of having a disease that marks them as being different from their peers and the limitations imposed on them at a time when they want to be more independent and "grown up." Others have suggested that nonadherence may be a result of adolescent–parent conflict, given that separation and individuation is a major developmental challenge for adolescents, or a way to manipulate parents (Anderson, Brackett, Ho, & Laffel, 2000; Shaw, 2001, Shaw et al., 2001). Youth may insist that they are adhering to the prescribed treatment regimen even with empirical evidence demonstrating the opposite is true (Lask, 1994). Other youth may be unwilling or not prepared to assume more responsibility for their self-management and leave that responsibility with their parents (Velsor-Friedrich, Vlasses, Moberley, & Coover, 2004).

Condition-Related Factors

An adolescent's chronic condition—whether it be a developmental disability, such as an intellectual disability, a special health care need, or a mental health condition—can adversely affect the level of treatment regimen adherence. Based on the particular condition or treatment-related effects, the youth may be limited in fully comprehending and understanding illness-related explanations provided and in fully assuming self-management responsibilities. For example, youth with intellectual disabilities (i.e., mental retardation) and other neurological conditions such as hydrocephalus and seizure disorders will encounter challenges in learning the complicated requirements of a treatment regimen unless it can be operationalized in understandable terms. Other condition-related limitations include those associated with restricted movement and visual or auditory impairments. Youth who have encountered frequent school absences and prolonged periods of disruptions with school attendance due to their illness or disability may not be functioning on a grade level comparable to their typically developing peers (Caldwell & Sirvis, 1991; Fowler, Johnson, & Atkinson, 1985; Loveland et al., 1994; Newacheck, McManus, & Fox, 1991; Shaw, 2001; Shaw et al., 2001; Velsor-Friedrich et al., 2004).

A psychiatric co-morbidity can negatively influence the youth's self-management behavior. Having a mental health problem can adversely affect the youth in many ways. The youth may not be able to learn a new skill for performing a treatment or the youth may not be adherent if he or she is not ready to perform a treatment independently. The youth may feel depressed and overwhelmed with the requirements of the daily treatment regimen and may be unable to perform the task requirements. In other circumstances, the youth's emotional problems may interfere with the ability to communicate adequately or the ability to express emotions (Shaw et al., 2001).

Lack of Developmentally Appropriate Information

Studies of children, youth, and adults demonstrate that all groups need updated and developmentally appropriate instruction about their chronic condition, especially information that they could use to become better consumers of health care and informed and responsible managers of their own health (Collins et al., 1998; Nehring & Faux, 2006). If youth do not have sufficient information to manage their conditions—such as how to avoid additional problems associated with their condition (e.g., preventing skin breakdown from prolonged sitting in a wheelchair) or how to perform a treatment task (e.g., testing their blood for glucose)—then their ability to adhere to the treatment is compromised (Delamater, 2000). Health care researchers have reported that personalized feedback enhances an individual's level of adherence (Onyirimba et al., 2003; Strawhacker, 2001). Providing youth with disease/condition-specific information can assist them in realizing the consequences of learning or not learning self-management skills to control their conditions, which can lead to improvements in coping and adjusting to their conditions (Collins et al., 1998).

Other studies have examined the relationship between self-management knowledge of children and youth with special health care needs and their health outcomes. Research studies have demonstrated that children and youth lacked basic information about their own chronic health problem, which prevented them from being proactive when their symptoms worsened. A study of 32 school-age and preadolescent children found that they had little knowledge of the triggers or situations that would precipitate an asthmatic attack (Pradel, Hartzema, & Bush, 2001, as cited in Wilkerson, 2002). A meta-analysis of studies examining the effects of asthma self-management instruction for children and youth (between 2 and 18 years of age) found they had fewer days of school absences and restricted activity, fewer disrupted nights of sleep, and fewer visits to emergency departments. In addition, this group of children and youth demonstrated improved lung functioning and reported higher levels of self-control (Guevara, Wolf, Grum, & Clark, 2003; Wolf, Guevara, Grum, Clark, & Cates, 2005).

As the evidence reveals, efforts to foster self-management competencies in children and youth with special health care needs have been associated with improved clinical outcomes. These outcomes include improvements in clinical status, prevention of secondary conditions and complications, and improvements in overall level of daily functioning (Collins et al., 1998; Delamater, 2000).

Family Characteristics

A number of family-related factors have been identified as being associated with decreased youth self-management. These characteristics include parental overprotectiveness, lack of parental support, parental posttraumatic stress disorder (PTSD), family socioeconomic status, and other factors such as lifestyle and family conflict.

Parental Overprotectiveness

Some parents respond to their children's chronic conditions by becoming overprotective. This reaction is predicated by the anxieties that their children may be overtaxed by activities beyond their abilities; their children need additional protection to safeguard them from potential harm, hurt, or duress; or their children do not have the functional abilities comparable to their typically developing peers that could create feelings of disappointment, inadequacy, and shame in their children (Holmbeck et al., 2002; Mador & Smith, 1989; Manuel, Balkrishnan, Camacho, Smith, & Koman, 2003; Shah, 2002).

Lack of Parental Support

Researchers have found that positive parental approaches, such as providing encouragement and joint planning of self-care activities, were associated with improved levels of compliance as compared with parental insistence the youth assume self-care responsibilities (Kyngas, Hentinen, & Barlow, 1998; Kyngas & Rissanen, 2001). Researchers have also reported that strategies to foster parent–adolescent interdependence involving the reorganization of responsibilities between the parent and youth resulted in improved levels of adherence (Anderson et al., 2000). Efforts to improve the quality of communication between parents and youth with cystic fibrosis were found to improve treatment adherence (Quittner et al., 2000).

Parental Posttraumatic Stress Disorder

Some researchers have suggested that parents can experience PTSD as a result of their children's condition that negatively affects their interactions with their children (Shaw, 2001). For example, PTSD symptoms were related to lower rates of adherence in a sample of children who had liver transplants (Shemesh et al., 2000). Additional research is needed to explore the relationship between parental PTSD and level of adherence.

Family Socioeconomic Status

Family socioeconomic status is another important factor affecting adherence levels. The economic impact on a family raising a child with a chronic condition is immense, especially for families with limited funds (Lukemeyer, Meyers, & Smeeding, 2000). Families with finite resources face difficult choices in allocating funds as it may mean other family members go without certain things to enable the treatment needs of the adolescent with special health care needs to be met.

Other Factors

Other factors associated with lower levels of self-management include lifestyle of the youth and family, such as those associated with overly permissive/neglectful parental oversight, limited family resources, poverty (Milnes & Callery, 2003), parental and family conflict, and single parenting, as the youth was expected to assume more responsibility than he or she was capable of performing (Buford, 2004; Burkhart, Dunbar-Jacob, & Rohay, 2001; Hurtado, 1995; Schilling, Grey & Knafl, 2006; Shaw, 2001; Strawhacker, 2001). Studies conducted with families of children with intellectual disabilities demonstrate similar findings. Findings revealed that children had less access to health care services and had poorer health care status (Hogan, Rogers, & Msall, 2000). Studies on family impact found mothers often were unable to work due to the child's caretaking requirements and had higher rates of work absenteeism, and families' organizational patterns were significantly altered (Curran, Sharples, White, & Knapp, 2001; Rehm & Bradley, 2005).

Systematic Barriers Associated with the Health Care System

A number of barriers to self-management instructional programs have been identified in terms of promoting the learning of self-management knowledge and skills by youth. One of the major barriers to self-management is the inadequacy of the instructional programs developed by health care providers for targeted children and youth. Problems with these programs include lack of developmentally appropriate curriculums, use of teaching approaches that were not age-appropriate, unrealistic expectations for learning that were not sensitive to the burden of time and resources needed, and inadequate assessment of needs. Other problems include lack of appropriate supplemental instructional materials, lack of documentation of training, and no formalized evaluation process (Krishna et al., 2003).

Health care providers also may not be knowledgeable about instructional design methodology or about the health literacy of youth learners. For example, in a study of 433 children and youth seen in the emergency department for treatment of an acute asthmatic attack, researchers found that home management instruction details received from the primary care provider varied from nearly 40% to 80% according to predetermined guidelines (Scarfone et al., 2001). In addition, health care professionals are typically not reimbursed for patient education, nor are their responsibilities for patient education a priority in terms of their position responsibilities, which can make them less interested in providing client education (Cabana et al., 2001; Krishna et al., 2003; Scarfone et al., 2001). Similarly, the lack of time that health care providers have in providing patient education can result in haphazard approaches to teaching. Kyngas (2000) found that health care provider support was positively associated with higher levels of adherence among youth with special health care needs and disabilities, with nursing support being the strongest predictor of good adherence. A study of the treatment adherence perceptions of French physicians and youth with Type I diabetes revealed differences. French youth rated themselves higher on adherence than their physicians, as the physicians relied more heavily on HbA1c levels and equated these levels with adherence, suggesting that physicians used limited criteria to assess adherence (DuPasquier-Fediaevsky & Tubiana-Rufi, 1999).

There are a number of factors that can affect a youth's self-management of his or her condition and adherence to the treatment regimen. The extent to which these factors affect youth with special health care needs and disabilities and their treatment adherence will require systematic assessment. Identification of the factors affecting self-management and treatment adherence needs to be addressed in an individualized plan of care to facilitate the acquisition of these competencies.

It is important to note that there are limitations associated with the research on adherence and self-management of youth with special health care needs and disabilities. Currently, most of the research has been conducted with populations of children and youth with asthma and diabetes mellitus. Little is known about the adherence issues and self-management needs of other populations of youth with chronic conditions. In most instances, study samples were composed of a broad age range of children and youth with differing cognitive and psychosocial capacities. Prescreening of children and youth pertaining to their cognitive level of functioning was rarely conducted. As mentioned previously, adherence and self-management have been defined and operationalized differently by researchers, making analysis of study findings difficult and conclusions limited (Toelle & Ram, 2005). Given these limitations, more research is needed to better understand the issues associated with adherence and self-management with this population. However, there is an evolving body of evidence that can be applied in providing the services and programs needed to facilitate self-management and treatment adherence in youth with special health care needs and disabilities, as is described in the remaining portions of this chapter.

PRACTICE IMPLICATIONS

This section on practice implications will be separated into two main areas of discussion. First, content on the development of an individualized plan for self-management, with an application to educational settings will be presented. This section will include recommendations for including self-management instruction into a 504 plan and individualized education program (IEP). Next, a brief overview of instructional programs for self-management that demonstrate promise for clinical application will be described.

Self-Management Planning and Implementation

Although there is increasing realization of the importance of integrating health care and related service needs into IEPs and 504 plans, there have been few resources available to assist health care professionals and educational personnel to bridge the boundaries of practice to collaborate effectively and to engage in joint transition planning. As mentioned in Chapter 1, best practice principles have been formulated to provide guidance to all interdisciplinary professionals who are involved with health care transition planning.

Initiating the Process

Ideally, the self-management needs of youth with special health care needs and disabilities who are returning to the school setting involves coordination between the school and members of the youth's specialized health care team. Before communication and coordination can be initiated between both settings, signatures must be obtained on consent and assent forms enabling disclosure of the youth's private information. If the youth is younger than 18 years of age, parents are responsible for signing the consent form; youth 18 years and older may sign their own consent. Youth who have not yet reached the age of majority should be consulted as to their willingness to release private information, and they should sign assent forms as their parents sign consent forms. In selected circumstances, youth younger than 18 years of age may obtain legal consent via the mature minor rule. For additional information on legal aspects pertaining to consent, refer to Chapter 2.

Initial Contact

The collaboration between health care providers and educational personnel can begin following the signing of necessary consent and assent forms. Several discussion points need to be highlighted during the initial conversation, including: 1) a process for jointly identifying comprehensive care needs for home/long-term management; 2) a process for jointly identifying the youth's self-management needs/skills and the extent to which the youth is independent in these skills; 3) a process for discussing the self-management knowledge/skills that will require monitoring and reinforcement in the school setting; 4) a discharge report/status report of youth's special health care needs and/or disabilities, including a summary of hospitalizations, ongoing needs for treatment and follow-up care, and prognosis; 5) contact information, including name, position, e-mail address, and phone and fax number; 6) a preferred mode of communication (e.g., via e-mail, phone); and 7) the availability to participate in IEP and/or 504 planning and team meetings.

Depending on the school setting, the responsibilities for serving as the school contact may be assigned to the school counselor, the school nurse, the youth's teacher, or the vice-principal for academic affairs. For further information on other components of comprehensive transition planning, refer to Chapters 8, 9, and 10.

Assessment of Health Care and Self-Management Needs

Coordination among educational personnel and health care providers will be a valuable asset in determining the youth's and family's continued needs for management of special health care needs and/or disabilities in the school setting. First, the youth's health care providers need to share with educational personnel the youth's disease/disability status and ongoing treatment needs, which will provide important contextual information for better understanding the youth's current health status. For example, health care providers can communicate information about the disease symptomology that indicates an exacerbation, untoward reaction to a treatment, or the development of complications. Other information health care providers should share with educational personnel include side effects of medications, anticipated scheduling of outpatient visits, forthcoming surgeries, or other illness-related needs for hospitalizations.

After baseline/diagnostic information has been shared, the implications for ongoing services on the school campus can be identified and discussed in a preliminary fashion, as more in-depth planning should be conducted when the youth and family are present. Joint planning may require creative approaches given the time constraints and divergent professional responsibilities between both settings and with the youth and his or her family. Conference calls, video streaming, and Internet conferencing are just some of the options available when the planning team cannot all be in the same place at the same time. In circumstances in which technology resources are limited, other flexible arrangements can be made, such as emailing, sequencing meetings according to a predetermined schedule of activities, and having the youth and his or her family serve as liaisons between settings. An ideal planning meeting would be a face-to-face meeting with all parties involved to hash out the planning activities. The logistics of assessing the youth's needs can be determined before the transition planning assessment process begins.

Health care providers and educational personnel can jointly assess the youth's health care transition needs to identify the range of needs the student has for services, supports, and self-management instruction/monitoring in the school setting. This assessment can be conducted using standardized tools that have been developed specifically to assess transition health care self-management needs. Some of these tools, (e.g., *CAHRTW Transition Health Care Assessment Tool, Massachusetts Provider Transition Checklist and Timeline, Transitioning to Adulthood: How Ready Are You* and *Transition Developmental Checklist*) were designed using a generic format that can be used with youth who have special healthcare needs or disabilities (see Figure 4.1). Other assessment tools available are disease-specific and provide pertinent and detailed information about the treatment-related needs and skills the youth with disease-specific conditions currently possesses (Harris et al., 2000). An example of a disease-specific tool is the *Diabetes Self-Management Profile* (DSMP). This tool has been tested with 105 youth with Type I diabetes ages 6 to nearly 16 years of age. The 50 item semistructured interview assesses diabetes management in six areas: exercise, blood glucose management, insulin administration, insulin dose adjustment, dietary restrictions, and hypoglycemic management (Harris et al., 2000). It is likely that the health care provider on the youth's specialized health care team has a copy of the disease-specific health care transition tool that he or she can share with educational personnel.

All of these tools identify areas of need that can be used as the basis for identifying which needs can be delegated to the youth as part of learning self-management knowledge/skills and which needs require professional coordination, services, supports, and referrals. It is important to carefully review tools as the questionnaire items may not be reflective of current practice standards (Harris et al., 2000). It is also important to remember that assessment of needs

Transition Health Care Assessment

For each question, please circle one: Yes, No, N/A (not applicable), or W/A (with assistance).

Do you know about your health condition and how to take care of yourself?

1. Do you understand what caused your medical condition?   Yes   No   N/A   W/A

2. Do you understand the changes/symptoms caused by your medical condition?   Yes   No   N/A   W/A

3. Do you manage your daily treatment needs?   Yes   No   N/A   W/A

4. Do you have any problems with your daily treatment needs?   Yes   No   N/A   W/A

5. Do you understand the action of the medications you take?   Yes   No   N/A   W/A

6. Do you have an understanding of the laboratory and diagnostic tests you have?   Yes   No   N/A   W/A

What do you do to keep healthy?

1. Do you have a primary care physician (PCP) that you see regularly?   Yes   No   N/A   W/A

2. Are you up-to-date with immunizations and health care screenings?   Yes   No   N/A   W/A

3. Do you use alcohol, cigarettes or drugs, or engage in unprotected sex?   Yes   No   N/A   W/A

4. Do you use self-protection devices such as wearing orthotics/helmet?   Yes   No   N/A   W/A

5. Do you wear a Medi-Alert bracelet/necklace?   Yes   No   N/A   W/A

6. Do you exercise regularly?   Yes   No   N/A   W/A

7. Do you see a dentist on a regular basis?   Yes   No   N/A   W/A

8. Do you brush and floss your teeth?   Yes   No   N/A   W/A

9. Do you know when you're getting sick, such as getting a cold or urinary tract infection?   Yes   No   N/A   W/A

(continued)

Figure 4.1. Transition health care assessment. Reprinted from *Nursing Clinics of North America*, Vol. 39, C.L. Betz, Adolescents in transition of adult care: Why the concern? pp. 681–713, copyright 2004, with permission from Elsevier.

Figure 4.1.   *(continued)*

What do you do in an emergency?

1.	Do you have a phone to use in case of an emergency?	Yes	No	N/A	W/A
2.	Do you have the phone numbers of family and friends to call in emergencies?	Yes	No	N/A	W/A
3.	Do you have the phone numbers of health and non-health emergency services, and the poison control center?	Yes	No	N/A	W/A
4.	Do you know where the closest emergency room is?	Yes	No	N/A	W/A
5.	Have you notified the fire department of your special needs and developed an emergency evacuation plan?	Yes	No	N/A	W/A
6.	Have you notified the gas/electric companies of your additional service needs?	Yes	No	N/A	W/A

Have you needed environmental modifications/accommodations?

1.	Do you have the needed electrical modifications or other durable equipment?	Yes	No	N/A	W/A
2.	Do you have storage space for your supplies and equipment?	Yes	No	N/A	W/A
3.	Does your home have wheelchair ramps and other modifications (e.g., doors, tubs)?	Yes	No	N/A	W/A
4.	Are you able to properly and safely dispose of supplies (e.g., needles)?	Yes	No	N/A	W/A

Do you know how to monitor special health care needs?

1.	Do you know when to see the doctor?	Yes	No	N/A	W/A
2.	Can you recognize when you're getting ill?	Yes	No	N/A	W/A
3.	Do you know what situations (e.g., increased elevations, large crowds, airport scanners) to avoid for health reasons?	Yes	No	N/A	W/A

Do you know how to manage your special health care needs?

1. Are you responsible for making appointments with specialty care provider(s)?   Yes No N/A W/A

2. Are you responsible for refilling medications and supplies?   Yes No N/A W/A

3. Do you know when to replace durable equipment?   Yes No N/A W/A

4. Do you have extra/backup supplies or equipment?   Yes No N/A W/A

5. Do you have an attendant, home health aide, school aide, interpreter(s)?   Yes No N/A W/A

6. Are you responsible for their supervision?   Yes No N/A W/A

7. Do you hire the personal attendants/ assistants that you need?   Yes No N/A W/A

Do you know how to communicate effectively?

1. Do you seek answers to health related concerns?   Yes No N/A W/A

2. Are you able to ask questions of providers?   Yes No N/A W/A

3. Are you able to obtain appropriate communication devices/systems as needed?   Yes No N/A W/A

4. Do you make contact with teen/ young adult support groups/camps?   Yes No N/A W/A

Do you know how to use community resources?

1. Do you know how to get services in your area?   Yes No N/A W/A

2. Have you used services in your community?   Yes No N/A W/A

3. Are you able to use community transportation when you need it?   Yes No N/A W/A

4. Do you have an individualized health plan developed by the school nurse that is used at your school?   Yes No N/A W/A

(continued)

Figure 4.1.   *(continued)*

Do you demonstrate responsible sexual activity?

1. Are you able to avoid dangerous situations (e.g., exploitation, victimization)?   Yes   No   N/A   W/A

2. Are you able to provide a reliable sexual history?   Yes   No   N/A   W/A

3. Do you know what a sexually transmitted disease (STD) is and how it can affect you?   Yes   No   N/A   W/A

4. Do you have enough information about contraception and ways to prevent STDs?   Yes   No   N/A   W/A

Do you obtain information and reproductive counseling when needed?

1. Do you know when to seek reproductive counseling?   Yes   No   N/A   W/A

2. Do you understand the problems associated with teenage/unplanned pregnancy?   Yes   No   N/A   W/A

3. Do you think you understand the responsibilities with being a parent?   Yes   No   N/A   W/A

Do you keep track of health records?

1. Do you have a copy of your health records?   Yes   No   N/A   W/A

2. Does your doctor/therapist have a copy of your health records?   Yes   No   N/A   W/A

3. Do you have an insurance card or copy of it?   Yes   No   N/A   W/A

4. Do you have a method for keeping track of your health care appointments?   Yes   No   N/A   W/A

Do you have knowledge of health insurance concerns and issues?

1. Do you know what are the eligibility requirements for your health insurance?   Yes   No   N/A   W/A

2. Have you applied for income assistance (SSI) and other public services?   Yes   No   N/A   W/A

Do you demonstrate knowledge of rights and protections?

1. Do you have the school/work setting accommodations that you need?   Yes   No   N/A   W/A

2. Have you contacted the college/university Office of Disabled Students?   Yes   No   N/A   W/A

3. Do you understand the rights you have because of the Americans with Disabilities Act?   Yes   No   N/A   W/A

4. Have you applied for other public services (social services, vocational rehabilitation)?   Yes   No   N/A   W/A

Do you use transportation safely?

1. Do you have a driver's license?   Yes   No   N/A   W/A

2. Do you use buses, trains, or other types of public transportation?   Yes   No   N/A   W/A

3. Do you use bus or other travel schedules for getting rides?   Yes   No   N/A   W/A

4. Do you have the money you need to get bus passes/use your car?   Yes   No   N/A   W/A

5. Do you have any problems in getting to your travel destinations?   Yes   No   N/A   W/A

6. Do you know etiquette according to the mode of transportation (e.g., waiting one's turn, getting up for elderly)   Yes   No   N/A   W/A

7. Do you use Dial-A-Ride or Access Van?   Yes   No   N/A   W/A

8. Do you feel safe taking the bus or van or driving?   Yes   No   N/A   W/A

9. Do you usually arrive and leave on time?   Yes   No   N/A   W/A

10. Do you avoid sitting next to passengers with colds or a cough?   Yes   No   N/A   W/A

11. Do you know how you should interact with strangers when traveling/using public transportation?   Yes   No   N/A   W/A

12. Do you carry the phone number of friends/family when you travel/use transportation?   Yes   No   N/A   W/A

13. Do you let others know when you take trips or leave the house?   Yes   No   N/A   W/A

is an ongoing process that will require periodic reassessment to determine the extent to which the youth has, has not, or is continuing to work on achieving self-management objectives.

Developing the Transition Plan and Addressing Self-Management Needs

Following the assessment of health care and self-management needs, the youth, his or her family, educational personnel, and health care providers need to jointly prioritize the youth's needs. It is during this process that the team creates an effective self-management plan with a clear understanding of what are desirable and/or achievable objectives. Clarity as to perceptions of what constitutes successful achievement of health care transition goals and objectives has been shown to vary between the parents, youth, and health care providers. What may be considered to be acceptable to the parent or school nurse may not be the case for the adolescent (Milnes & Callery, 2003). For example, hair loss or weight gained due to chemotherapy is more difficult for the youth to accept than for an adult, given the extreme pressure youth feel from their peers and their desire to "fit in" with their friends. Also the use of terminology used to describe physical symptoms or treatments will have different meaning depending on the individual's perspective whether it be the youth, parent, health professional or non-health professional (Cane, Ranganathan, & McKenzie, 2000; Milnes & Callery, 2003). This is a youth-centered process, and it should be driven by the youth's needs, interests, strengths, and preferences. Consultation between educational personnel and health care providers will provide additional insights and recommendations that may not have been considered if this planning had been done without collaboration.

Development of Transition Plan Objectives

Once the youth's needs are prioritized, an individualized plan is developed to address instructional needs the youth requires and constant monitoring of the youth's ability to manage treatment requirements as independently as possible that are imposed by their special health care needs/disability. The objectives—the skills or knowledge to be obtained—need to be clearly defined and measurable. Objectives related to self-management in the health care transition plan include the following components: a) the skill or knowledge to be achieved in behavioral terminology, b) the time frame for achievement of the objective, and c) conditions under which the objective should be met. Examples of behavioral objectives for a health care transition plan related to self-management skills are listed under these health care self-care objectives.

1. The student will independently test blood glucose.

2. The student will perform self-catheterization every 4 hours in the school nurse's office.

3. The student will report to her teacher episodes of lightheadedness.

4. The student will wear his Medi-Alert bracelet when in school.

5. The student will self-administer medication at prescribed times.

6. The student will notify her teacher of absences due to scheduled outpatient appointments.

7. The student will notify the teacher of the need for rest periods in the school nurse's office.

8. The student will enroll in adaptive PE classes.

9. The student will sit in the front of the class.

10. The student will inform his teacher of need for homework accommodations.

11. The student will be excused from attending school during periods of high communicability.

12. The student will notify her teacher of the need for testing accommodations.

13. The student will be allowed to be excused from class for restroom breaks without raising hand to inform teacher.

14. The student will not be disciplined for walking on campus while class is in session.

Identification and Description of Instructional Activities Needed to Achieve the Objectives

Coordination among educational personnel and health care providers will facilitate the identification of instructional activities needed for the youth to acquire the self-management knowledge and skills specified in the objectives. Based on their previous experiences in working with the youth, both the educational personnel and health care providers can specify instructional strategies that can be jointly undertaken. It may be, for example, that a skill such as glucose monitoring is initiated in the clinical setting with reinforcement and monitoring conducted in the school setting. In another example, the school nurse may take the lead in monitoring the youth's rehabilitation progress as treatment is obtained through the onsite physical therapy clinic supported by the State Title V Program for children with special health care needs. The youth and members of his or her IEP team may agree that a course on human sexuality offered at the high school might be the optimal choice for learning information about human sexuality and reproductive concerns. Reinforcement of information and answering additional questions can be done during clinic visits with the physician or another member of the youth's specialized health care team. The arrangements for instructional activities are dependent upon the coordination efforts of the educational personnel and health care providers.

The instructional strategies will need to reflect each youth's individualized needs for learning self-management knowledge and skills. For example, taking medication could be simplified by using terminology and concepts appropriate to the youth's cognitive level by describing pills by their color or shape, linking administration time to a daily event such as a meal, and depicting the number of pills to take with pictures of the number of pills on a display board. Instruction on self-care needs may be paced differently and content may need to be provided in different formats. Based on a youth's developmental level, his or her understanding of the concepts of illness and health can vary. For example, a youth with asthma may try to "hold on" and delay alerting parents of his or her worsening asthma condition hoping to avoid a hospitalization (Velsor-Friedrich et al., 2004). The adolescent with an organ transplant may take "drug holidays" until signs of acute rejection are evident (Feinstein et al., 2005). Therefore, explanations have to be based on the individual's cognitive level (Milnes & Callery, 2003). As the child develops the capacity for learning and understanding more abstract concepts, disease and treatment related information will need to be updated as appropriate to the child's cognitive level of functioning (Oeffinger, 2002; Shaw et al., 2001). Adolescents who possess more abstract levels of thinking benefit from hearing about the positive effects of their treatment, as they are capable of better understanding long-term consequences of treatment effects that are not necessarily immediately apparent (Shaw et al., 2001).

Monitoring and Evaluation of the Self-Management Plan

Both educational personnel and health care providers will provide input based on observations of behavior in their respective environments that may have not been obvious in the other's setting. Furthermore, professionals can offer each other descriptions of significant events (e.g., vacation, new course of treatment, untoward reaction to medication), behaviors (e.g., behavior problems, adherence problems, academic challenges) changes in disease course (e.g., relapse, remission, forthcoming surgery), and self-management instruction (e.g., reinforcement of new skill, instruction on equipment modification) that will facilitate the coordination of efforts between settings related to self-management training. The frequency of contacts among educational personnel and health care providers will depend on the youth's circumstances. In some situations, for example, a weekly discussion may be necessary; in others, professionals may meet more infrequently, as in quarterly or semi-annual meetings. They can offer guidance to each other as a means of information cross-training to ensure the youth obtains needed services, supports, and accommodations. For example, the school nurse may request a letter from the physician indicating the need for frequent school absences for follow-up health care visits, or the health care provider may confer with educational personnel about ensuring health-related accommodations are included in the 504 plan. (For additional information on school and workplace accommodations, refer to Chapter 6.) Problems noted with the youth's achievement of his or her self-management objectives on the youth's plan require collaboration among health care providers and educational personnel. The collective input of professionals from divergent settings who provide services to the youth will enhance both the identification of the problems and the needed revisions to the plan. These revisions may include possibly revised objectives for achievement, timeline, and instructional approaches.

INSTRUCTIONAL PROGRAMS FOR SELF-MANAGEMENT

A number of effective and evidence-based instructional models to teach youth self-management strategies have been developed and tested. Some of these programs can be integrated into health care transition planning. A brief overview of these programs is presented in this chapter.

STRATEGIES FOR SUPPORTING
YOUTH TO LEARN SELF-MANAGEMENT

Care Coordination

Care partners refers to resource experts, whether it be in a community setting such as a school or during a hospitalization, who work closely with the youth to facilitate learning of skills necessary for long-term management. Using this model, a designated expert is responsible for coordinating the instructional plan beginning with instructing the youth on the particular skill with the expectation that the youth will eventually assume responsibility once the skill has been achieved. Other members in the setting are continually apprised as to the extent they are expected to reinforce instruction, observe youth demonstration of the skill and correction, and shape skill enactment as needed (Sterner-Allison, 1999).

A critical component of this approach is the clearly defined behavioral expectations of the task to be learned. For example, if the youth is to learn how to prevent the development of reddened or open areas on bony prominences while sitting for prolonged times in a wheelchair, then the youth needs to demonstrate both the behavior as well as articulating the rationale for shifting of body position every 10–15 minutes. A care partner functions similarly to a case manager or coordinator except that the individual is not necessarily paid for this position. Any number of professionals or trained lay persons can assume this role.

Technology-Inspired Programs and Devices

Using a personal digital assistant (PDA) has been suggested as a method for increasing adherence to treatment regimens. It is a device that would enable adolescents to email their nurse or other health care team members questions about treatments concerns, set up appointments, conduct electronic monitoring, and/or store their health and health care information. The costs are a worthwhile investment of a few hundred dollars as compared with an emergency department visit or hospitalization (Chang, Omery, & Mayo, 2003).

Other technology inspired programs have been demonstrated as effective for instructional purposes. A web-based interactive educational program with a nursing "webmaster" titled *Healthy Buddy* was found to be effective in teaching youth to manage their asthma. Youths ages 8 to 16 years old enrolled in the "Healthy Buddy" program (*n* = 66 youth) learned self-management skills (environmental controls to decrease triggers and medication administration and adjustment) and to seek the consultation of the respiratory nursing specialist when problems or questions arose. Both the control and treatment group received the usual asthma instruction from the specialty nurse. Children in the *Healthy Buddy* program reported less coughing and wheezing and fewer days of activity limitation as compared with youth in the control (Guendelman et al., 2002).

Interactive Multimedia Programs

Although its use has been reported primarily with children and youth with asthma, interactive multimedia programs show promise as supplemental resources for instructing youth in self-management of their chronic condition. In a randomized control trial, researchers demonstrated that 228 children and youth, from birth to 17 years who were enrolled in an Internet-enabled program, *Interactive Multimedia Asthma Education Program* (IMPACT), had significantly improved health outcomes as compared to those who received asthma education as part of their usual care. Children and youth exposed to the IMPACT program had significantly increased asthma knowledge, fewer asthma symptom days, fewer visits to the emergency department, and lower daily doses of inhaled corticosteroids. School-age children and adolescents had fewer physician visits and used medications less. In addition, those in the IMPACT program had significantly greater reduction of school absences (5.4 days) compared with the control group (1.6 days) (Krishna et al., 2003). Lastly, the IMPACT resulted in $615.70 cost savings per child as compared with the control group.

In a randomized control trial, 76 children and youth with asthma ages 9 to 13 years participated in a study to test the effectiveness of a computer assisted program titled *Watch, Discover, Think and Act* (WDTA). Those in the WDTA group had significantly higher asthma knowledge scores and self-efficacy scores as compared with participants in the control group (Shegog et al., 2001).

In another example of educational technology, a Super Nintendo asthma video game—as part of an asthma protocol that included nursing case management, access to specialty medical care, and a hotline staffed by pediatric nurses—was examined in a study of 119 children ages 5 to 12 years old from low-income families with moderate to severe asthma. Findings revealed that children in the intervention group scored higher in asthma knowledge and quality of life as compared to the control group. Although not significant, there was a trend in findings toward reductions in asthma morbidity (Shames et al., 2004).

Using interactive multimedia programs is advantageous because they are flexible and can be used in any number of settings. A program could be integrated at school, in the home, and in the clinic setting (Shames et al., 2004). An Internet program could be accessible to many school sites and downloaded for minimal costs if the costs could be shared by many programs. In addition, training can be more easily standardized, as it can be replicated in numerous environments while minimizing the idiosyncratic problems associated with trainers. Evaluation of training can be standardized as well and particularly useful for between-group comparisons (Christopher, Nangle, & Hansen, 1993).

Social Skills Training

Social skills interventions, although used primarily to teach skills for developing and/or improving social interactions for high-risk, at-risk, and vulnerable youth populations—such as those with developmental disabilities or substance abuse, behavioral, and severe emotional problems—can be used for youth with special health care needs and disabilities (Bielecki & Swender, 2004; Weiss & Harris, 2001). Social skills training would be appropriate for instructing youth to learn skills for promoting interpersonal competence in dealing with health care providers. Training content would include learning conversational skills to use in provider–youth interactions, such as posing questions, disclosing symptoms appropriately, and verifying information communicated. Other content would include self-management strategies, use of problem-solving skills, and learning how to initiate, sustain, and terminate social interactions in health care settings. A number of different instructional methods could be used such as role playing, cognitive rehearsal, role modeling, use of multimedia, and peer-group discussions.

Support/Self-Help Groups

Support/self-help groups are an atypical mechanism for instructing youth and young adults on learning self-management skills. However, this type of learning venue lends itself for use with adolescents and young adults, as peers are a predominant source of social support. Support/self-help groups provide an opportunity for youth to recognize that others have similar and very unique life experiences (Velsor-Friedrich et al., 2004).

Parental Supervision

Fostering parental supervision of the youth's self-management is a somewhat paradoxical strategy. The goal of continued parental involvement in the monitoring or supervising of the youth is to foster self-reliance and independence. Experts have suggested that this strategy can be effective in promoting treatment adherence (Weissberg-Benchell et al., 1995).

Motivational Interviewing Interventions

Motivational interviewing (MI) involves a series of brief adolescent-directed sessions that are approximately 15 minutes in length. This psychoeducational approach has been used primarily with adults; however, its use with adolescents shows promise, although its application has been limited to adolescents with Type I diabetes (Channon, Huws-Thomas, Gregory, & Rollnick, 2005). A graphic depicting the issues of immediate concern to the adolescent serves as the tool for setting the agenda for discussion. Youth are also asked to specify a typical day, which helps the adolescent to clearly articulate the ramifications of having a chronic illness on daily activities. MI is used to review the positives and negatives about living with diabetes and the changes required, which is designed to provide structure, raise awareness, and elicit thoughts and feelings about behavior. Another MI strategy used is called the "journey of change" wherein the adolescent is asked to recall a previous change and how he or she managed that change, not how it might be applied to a new situation of dealing with diabetes (Channon et al., 2005).

SUMMARY

Youth with special health care needs and disabilities face many challenges in learning self-management skills as they transition from child health pediatric care to adult health care. Many factors affect a youth's learning of self-management skills and adherence to his or her treatment regime.

My Story   Ed Flores

For 7 years now I have legally been able to sign my own consents for my medical procedures. But on more than one occasion I was in no condition to give my consent for these very important procedures. In times in which my condition was so bad that I should not have been making these decisions it would have been nice to know about my right to have someone else make my medical decisions for me. I was 23 years old before I ever knew about those rights. From August 2003 to May 2004, I went through a life-threatening experience, and it was only then that I learned about power of attorney. During this time I had to have nine surgeries in nine months. For a few of these procedures I should not have been signing my own consents for surgery. The doctors could not give any information to my parents about my condition because they legally did not have a right to know about my condition. Just because I was legally able to sign my life away does not mean they should have let me sign for those procedures. The doctors never took into account my emotional and mental status and did not care whether or not I understood what was going on. They need to explain things to patients in greater detail in a way that the patient can fully understand their rights. That never happened that way with me.

REFERENCES

American Academy of Pediatrics. (n.d.). *Puberty information for boys and girls.* Retrieved October 24, 2005, from http://www.aap.org/family/puberty.htm

Anarella, J., Roohan, P., Balistreri, E., & Gesten, F. (2004). A survey of Medicaid recipients with asthma: Perceptions of self-management, access, and care. *Chest, 125,* 1359–1367. Retrieved July 15, 2005, from http://www.chestjournal.org/cgi/content/full/125/4/1359

Anderson, B.J., Brackett, J., Ho, J., & Laffel, L.M.B. (2000). An intervention to promote family teamwork in diabetes management tasks: Relationships among parental involvement, adherence to blood glucose monitoring, and glycemic control in young adolescents with Type I diabetes. In D. Drotar (Ed), *Promoting adherence to medical treatment in chronic childhood illness: Concepts, methods, and interventions* (pp. 347–365). Mahwah, NJ: Lawrence Erlbaum Associates.

Beckman, N.D., DeWalt, D.A., Pignone, M.P., Sheridan, S.L., Lohr, K.N., Lux, L., et al. (2004). *Literacy and health outcomes. Evidence report/technology assessment no. 87* (Prepared by RTI International-University of North Carolina Evidence-Based Practice Center under Contract no. 290-02-0016). AHRQ Publication No. 04-E007-2. Rockville, MD: Agency for Healthcare Research and Quality.

Betz, C.L. (1998a). Adolescent transitions: A nursing concern. *Pediatric Nursing, 24,* 23–30.

Betz, C.L. (1998b). Facilitating the transition of adolescents with chronic conditions from pediatric to adult health care and community settings. *Issues in Comprehensive Pediatric Nursing, 21,* 97–115.

Betz, C.L., Hunsberger, M., & Wright, S. (1989). *Family-centered nursing care of children* (2nd ed.). Philadelphia: W.B. Saunders.

Betz, C.L., & Sowden, L. (2003). *Mosby's pediatric nursing reference* (5th ed.). St. Louis: Mosby Yearbook.

Bielecki, J., & Swender, S. (2004). The assessment of social functioning in individuals with mental retardation: A review. *Behavior Modification, 28*(5), 694–708.

Bryden, K.S., Dunger, D.B., Mayou, R.A., Peveler, R.C., & Neil, H.A. (2003). Poor prognosis of young adults with Type I diabetes. *Diabetes Care, 26,* 1052–1057.

Buford, T.A. (2004). Transfer of asthma management responsibility from parents to their school-age children. *Journal of Pediatric Nursing: Nursing Care of Children and Families, 19*(1), 3–12.

Burkhart, P., & Dunbar-Jacob, J. (2002). Adherence research in the pediatric and adolescent populations: A decade in review. In L. Hayman, M. Mahom, & R. Turner (Eds.), *Chronic illness in children: An evidence-based approach* (pp. 199–229). New York: Springer.

Burkhart, P.V., Dunbar-Jacob, J.M., & Rohay, J.M. (2001). Accuracy of children's self-reported adherence to treatment. *Journal of Nursing Scholarship, 33,* 27–32.

Burns, N., & Grove, S.K. (2005). *The practice of nursing research: Conduct, critique, and utilization,* (5th ed.). St. Louis: Elsevier Saunders.

Cabana, M.D., Ebel, B.E., Cooper-Patrick, L., Powe, N.R., Rubin, H.R., & Rand, C.S. (2000). Barriers pediatricians face when using asthma practice guidelines. *Archives of Pediatric and Adolescent Medicine, 154*, 685–693.

Caldwell, T., & Sirvis, B. (1991). Students with special health conditions: An emerging population presents new challenges. *Preventing School Failure, 35*(3), 13–18.

Cane, R.S., Ranganathan, S.C., & McKenzie, S.A. (2000). What do parents of wheezy children understand by 'wheeze'? *Archives of Disease in Childhood, 82*, 327–332.

Centers for Disease Control and Prevention. (2005a). *Trends in diabetes prevalence among American Indian and Alaska Native children, adolescents, and young adults—1990–1998.* (Fact Sheet). Retrieved August 16, 2005, from http://www.cdc.gov/diabetes/pubs/factsheets/aian.htm

Centers for Disease Control and Prevention. (2005b). *How common are Autism Spectrum Disorders?* Retrieved August 16, 2005, from http://www.cdc.gov/ncbddd/autism/asd_common.htm

Chang, R.L., Omery, A., & Mayo, A. (2003). Use of personal digital assistants by adolescents with severe asthma: Can they enhance patient outcomes? *AACN Clinical Issues, 14*(3), 379–391.

Channon, S., Huws-Thomas, M., Gregory, J.W., & Rollnick, S. (2005). Motivational interviewing with teenagers with diabetes. *Clinical Child Psychology and Psychiatry, 10*, 43–51.

Christopher, J.S., Nangle, D.W., & Hansen, D.J. (1993). Social-skills interventions with adolescents. *Behavior Modification, 17*, 316–338.

Collins, M., Kaslow, N., Doepke, K., Eckman, J., & Johnson, M. (1998). Psychosocial interventions for children and adolescents with sickle cell disease (SCD). *Journal of Black Psychology, 24*, 432–454.

Curran, A.L., Sharples, P.M., White, C., & Knapp, M. (2001). Time costs of caring for children with severe disabilities compared with caring for children without disabilities. *Developmental Medicine and Child Neurology, 43*(8), 529–533.

D'Auria, J.P., Christian, B.J., Henderson, Z.G., & Haynes, B. (2000). The company they keep: The influence of peer relationships on adjustment to cystic fibrosis during adolescence. *Journal of Pediatric Nursing: Nursing Care of Children and Families, 15*(3), 175–182.

Delamater, A.M. (2000). Critical issues in the assessment of regimen adherence in children with diabetes. In D. Drotar (Ed.), *Promoting adherence to medical treatment in chronic childhood illness: Concepts, methods, and interventions* (pp. 173–195). Mahwah, NJ: Lawrence Erlbaum Associates.

DuPasquier-Fediaevsky, L., & Tubian-Rufi, N. (1999). Discordance between physician and adolescent assessments of adherence to treatment. *Diabetes Care, 22*(9), 1445–1449.

Elkind, D. (1967). Egocentrism in adolescence. *Child Development, 38*, 1025–1034.

Erikson, E.H. (1963). *Childhood and society.* New York: W.W. Norton.

Erikson, E.H. (1968). *Identity youth and crisis.* New York: W.W. Norton.

Erikson, E.H. (Ed.). (1978). *Adulthood.* New York: W.W. Norton.

Erikson, E.H. (1980). *Identity and the life cycle.* New York: W.W. Norton.

Feinstein, S., Keich, R., Becker-Cohne, R., Rinat, C., Schwartz, S.B., & Frishberg, Y. (2005). Is noncompliance among adolescent renal transplant recipients inevitable? *Pediatrics, 115*, 969–973.

Fowler, M.G., Johnson, M.P., & Atkinson, S.S. (1985). School achievement and absence in children with chronic health conditions. *Journal of Pediatrics, 106*(4), 683–687.

Gould, R.L. (1978). *Transformation: Growth and change in adult life.* New York: Simon and Schuster.

Green, M., & Palfrey, J.S. (Eds.). (2002). *Bright futures: Guidelines for health supervision of infants, children, and adolescents* (2nd ed., rev.). Arlington, VA: National Center for Education in Maternal and Child Health.

Guevara, J.P., Wolf, F.M., Grum, C.M., & Clark, N.M. (2003). Effects of educational interventions for self-management of asthma in children and adolescents: Systematic review and meta-analysis. *British Medical Journal, 326*, 1308–1309. Retrieved July 29, 2005, from http://bmj.com/cgi/content/full/326/7402/1308

Hardin, R. (2005). Counseling patients with low health literacy. *American Journal of Health Systems Pharmacy, 62*, 364–365.

Harris, M.A., Wysocki, T., Sadler, M., Wilkinson, K., Harvey, L.M., Buckloh, L.M., et al. (2001). Validation of a structured interview for the assessment of diabetes self-management. *Diabetes Care, 23*, 1301–1304.

Havighurst, R. (1953). *Human development and education.* New York: Longmans, Green.

Holmbeck, G.N., Johnson, S.Z., Wills, K.E., McKernon, W. Rose, B., Erklin, S., et al. (2002). Observed and perceived parental overprotection in relation to psychosocial adjustment in preadolescents with a physical disability: The medicational role of behavioral autonomy. *Journal of Consulting & Clinical Psychology, 70,* 96–110.

Hurtado, A.M. (1995). Childhood asthma prevalence among Puerto Ricans and Mexican Americans: Implications for behavioral intervention research. *Hispanic Journal of Behavioral Sciences, 17*(3), 362–374.

Johnson, D. (2004). Gender, grade, relationship differences, in emotional closeness with adolescent relationships. *Adolescence.* Retrieved March 22, 2006, from http://www.findarticles.com/p/articles/mi_m2248/is_154_39/ai_n6364174

Katchadourian, H. (1978). Medical perspectives on adulthood. In E.H. Erikson (Ed.), *Adulthood* (pp. 33–60). New York: Norton.

Keene, N. (2003) *Educating the child with cancer: A guide for parents and teachers.* Kensington, MD: Candlelighters Childhood Cancer Foundation.

Koocher, G.P., McGrath, M.L., & Gudas, L.J. (1990). Typologies of nonadherence in cystic fibrosis. *Journal of Developmental and Behavioral Pediatrics, 11,* 353–358.

Krishna, S., Francisco, B.D., Balas, E.A., König, P., Graff, G.R., & Madsen, R.W. (2003). Internet-enabled interactive multimedia asthma education program: A randomized trial. *Pediatrics, 111,* 503–510.

Kyngas, H. (2000). Compliance of adolescents with chronic disease. *Journal of Clinical Nursing, 9*(4), 549–566.

Kyngas H., Hentinen M., & Barlow, J. (1998). Adolescents' perceptions of physicians, nurses, parents and friends: Help or hindrance in compliance with diabetes self-care. *Journal of Advanced Nursing 27,* 760–769.

Kyngas, H., & Rissanen, M. (2001). Support as a crucial predictor of good compliance of adolescents with a chronic disease. *Journal of Clinical Nursing, 10*(6), 767–773.

Lask, B. (1994). Non-adherence to treatment in cystic fibrosis. *Journal of the Royal Society of Medicine, 87*(Suppl.) 25–27.

Loveland, K., Stehbens, J., Contant, C., Bordeaus, J., Sirois, P., Bell, T., et al. (1994). Hemophilia growth and development study: Baseline neurodevelopmental findings. *Journal of Pediatric Psychology, 19*(2), 223–239.

Lukemeyer, A., Meyers, M.K., & Smeeding, T. (2000). Expensive children in poor families: Out-of-pocket expenditures for the care of disabled and chronically ill children in welfare families. *Journal of Marriage and the Family, 62,* 399–415.

Mador, J., & Smith, D. (1989). The psychosocial adaptation of adolescents with cystic fibrosis. *Journal of Adolescent Health Care, 10*(2), 136–142.

Mannino, D.M., Homa, D.M., Akinbami, L.J., Moorman, J.E., Gwynn, C., & Redd, S.C. (2002). Surveillance for asthma. *MMWR Surveillance, 51,* 1–13.

Manuel, J.C., Balkrishnan, R., Camacho, F., Smith, B.P., & Koman, L.A. (2003). Factors associated with self-esteem in pre-adolescents and adolescents with cerebral palsy. *Journal of Adolescent Health, 32*(6), 456–458.

Marin, S. (2005). The impact of epilepsy on the adolescent. *Maternal Child Nursing Journal, 30*(5), 321–326.

Matsui, D.M. (2000). Children's adherence to medication treatment. In D. Drotar (Ed.), *Promoting adherence to medical treatment in chronic childhood illness: Concepts, methods, and interventions* (pp. 135–152). Mahwah, NJ: Lawerence Erlbaum Associates.

McCarthy, A.R. (2000). *Healthy teens: Facing the challenges of young lives* (3rd ed.). Birmingham, MI: Bridge Communications.

Milnes, L.J., & Callery, P. (2003). The adaptation of written self-management plans for children with asthma. *Journal of Advanced Nursing, 41,* 444–453.

National Center on Birth Defects and Developmental Disabilities. (2005). *Disability and health in 2005: Promoting the health and well-being of people with disabilities.* Atlanta, GA: Author. Retrieved on August 20, 2006, from http://www.cdc.gov/ncbdd/factsheets/Disability_Health_AtAGlance.pdf

National Council on Disability. (1996, July). *Achieving independence: The challenge for the 21st century: A decade of progress in disability policy setting an agenda for the future.* Washington, DC: Author.

Nehring, W.M., & Faux, S.A. (2006). Transitional and health issues of adults with neural tube defects. *Journal of Nursing Scholarship, 38,* 63–70.

Newacheck, P., McManus, M., & Fox, H. (1991). Prevalence and impact of chronic illness among adolescents. *American Journal of Diseases in Children, 145,* 1367–1373.

Nielsen-Bohlman, L., Panzer, A.M., & Kindig, D.A. (Eds). (2004). *Health literacy: A prescription to end confusion.* Washington, DC: The National Academies Press.

Oeffinger, K.C. (2002). *Longitudinal cancer-related health care for adult survivors of childhood cancer.* National Cancer Policy Board Commissioned Paper, Institute of Medicine. Retrieved March 23, 2006, from http://www.iom.edu/Object.File/Master/15/242/Survivors-20%Cancer20%Health%20Care.pdf

Onyirimba, F., Apter, A., Reisine, S., Litt, M., McCusker, C., Connors, M., et al. (2003). Direct clinician-to-patient feedback discussion of inhaled steroid use: Its effect on adherence. *Annals of Allergy, Asthma, & Immunology, 90,* 411–415.

Orem, D. (2003). Self-care and health promotion: Understanding self-care. In K.M. Renpenning & S.G. Taylor (Eds.), *Self-care theory in nursing: Selected papers of Dorothea Orem* (pp. 212–222). New York: Springer Publishing.

Piaget, J. (2001). *Psychology of intelligence.* New York: Routledge Classics.

Piaget, J., & Inhelder, B. (1958). *The growth of logical thinking from children to adolescence.* New York: Basic Books.

Presidential Task Force on Employment of Adults with Disabilities. (1998). *A report of the Presidential Task Force on Employment of Adults with Disabilities.* Washington, DC: Author.

Quittner, A.L., Drotar, D., Ievers-landis, C., Slocum, N., Seidner, D., & Jacobsen, J., (2000). Adherence to medical treatments in adolescents with cystic fibrosis: The development and evaluation of family-based interventions. In D. Drotar (Ed.), *Promoting adherence to medical treatment in chronic childhood illness: Concepts, methods, and interventions* (pp. 383–407). Mahwah, NJ: Lawrence Erlbaum Associates.

Quittner, A.L., Tolbert, V.E., Regoli, M.J., Orenstein, D., Hollingsworth, J.L., & Eigen, J. (1996). Development of the Role-Play Inventory of Situations and Coping Strategies for parents of children with cystic fibrosis. *Journal of Pediatric Psychology, 21,* 209–235.

Rapoff, M.A. (1999). *Adherence to pediatric medical regimens.* New York: Plenum.

Rapoff, M.A. (2000). Facilitating adherence to medical regimens for pediatric rheumatic diseases: Primary, secondary, and tertiary prevention. In D. Drotar (Ed.), *Promoting adherence to medical treatment in chronic childhood illness: Concepts, Methods, and Interventions* (pp. 329–345). Mahwah, NJ: Lawrence Erlbaum Associates.

Rehm, R.S., & Bradley, J.F. (2005). Normalization in families raising a child who is medically fragile/technology dependent and developmentally delayed. *Qualitative Health Research, 15*(6), 807–822.

Scarfone, R.J., Zorc, J.J., & Capraro, G.A. (2001). Patient self-management of acute asthma: Adherence to national guidelines a decade later. *Pediatrics, 108,* 1332–1338. Retrieved July 31, 2005, from http://www.pediatrics.org/cgi/content/full/108/6/1332

Schilling, L.S., Grey, M., & Knafl., K.A. (2002). The concept of self-management of type 1 diabetes in children and adolescents: An evolutionary concept analysis. *Journal of Advanced Nursing, 37,* 87–99.

Schilling, L.S., Knafl, K.A., & Grey, M. (2006). Changing patterns in self-management in youth with Type I diabetes. *Journal of Pediatric Nursing, 21*(6), 412–424.

Shah, P. (2002). Psychosocial aspects of epilepsy. *Journal of the Indian Medical Association, 100*(5), 295–298.

Shames, R.S., Sharek, P., Mayer, M., Robinson, T.N., Hoyte, E.G., Gonzalez-Hensley, F., et al. (2004). Effectiveness of a multicompenent self-management program in at-risk, school-aged children with asthma. *Annals of Allergy, Asthma, & Immunology, 92,* 611–618.

Shaw, R.J. (2001). Treatment adherence in adolescents: Development and psychopathology, *Clinical Child Psychology and Psychiatry, 6,* 137–150.

Shaw, R.J., Palmer, L., Hyte, H., Yorgin, P., & Sarwal, M. (2001). Case study: Treatment adherence in a 13-year-old deaf adolescent male. *Clinical Child Psychology and Psychiatry, 6,* 551–562.

Shegog, R., Bartholomew, L.K., Parcel, G.S., Sockrider, M.M., Mass, L., & Abramson, S.L. (2001). Impact of a computer-assisted education program on factors related to asthma self-management behavior. *Journal of American Medical Informatics Association, 8,* 49–61.

Shemesh, E., Lurie, S., Stuber, M.L., Emre, S., Patel, Y., Vohra, P., et al. (2000). A pilot study of posttraumatic stress and nonadherence in pediatric liver transplant recipients. *Pediatrics, 105*, E29.

Sterner-Allison, J.L. (1999). Management of adolescent and adult inpatients with cystic fibrosis. *American Journal of Health-System Pharmacy, 56*(2), 158–160.

Strawhacker, M.T. (2001). Multidisciplinary teaming to promote effective management for type 1 diabetes for adolescents. *Journal of School Health, 71*, 213–217.

Tanner, J.M. (1962). *Growth at adolescence.* Oxford: Blackwell Scientific Publications.

Toelle, B.G., & Ram, F.S.F. (2005). Written individualized management plans for asthma in children and adults. *The Cochran Database of Systematic Reviews.*

U.S. Department of Health and Human Services. (2000). *Healthy People 2010: Understanding and improving health* (2nd ed.). Washington, DC: U.S. Government Printing Office.

van Dyck, P.C., Kogan, M.D., McPherson, M.G., Weissman, G.R., & Newacheck, P.W. (2004). Prevalence and characteristics of children with special health care needs. *Archives of Pediatrics & Adolescent Medicine, 158*(9), 884–890.

Velsor-Friedrich, B., Vlasses, F., Moberley, J., & Coover, L. (2004). Talking with teens about asthma management. *The Journal of School Nursing, 20*, 140–148.

Wagner, J., Newman, L., Cameto, R., & Levine, P. (2005). *National Longitudinal Transition Study 2: Changes over time in the early post-school outcomes of youth with disabilities: A report of the findings from the National Longitudinal Transition Study and National Longitudinal Study 2.* Menlo Park, CA: SRI International.

Weiss, M.F., & Harris, S.L. (2001). Teaching social skills to people with Autism. *Behavior Modification, 25*, 785–802.

Weissberg-Benchell, J., Glasgow, A.M., Tynan, W.D., Wirtz, P., Turek, J., & Ward, J. (1995). Adolescent diabetes management and mismanagement. *Diabetes Care, 18*, 77–82.

Wilkerson, R.R. (2002). Younger and older children had different experiences of asthma and its management. *Evidence Based Nursing Online, 5*, 123. Retrieved July 29, 2005, from http://ebn.bmjjournals.com/cgi/content/full/5/4/123

Williams, C. (1999). Gender, adolescence, and the management of diabetes. *Journal of Advanced Nursing, 30*, 160–166.

Williams, C. (2000). Doing health, doing gender: Teenagers, diabetes, and asthma. *Social Science & Medicine, 50*, 387–396.

Williams, M.V., Parker, R.M., Baker, D.W., Parikh, N.S., Pitkin, K., Coates, W.C., et al. (1995). Inadequate functional health literacy among patients at two public hospitals. *Journal of the American Medical Association, 274*, 1677–1682.

Wolf, F.M., Guevara, J.P., Grum, C.M., Clark, N.M., & Cates, C.J. (2005). Educational interventions for asthma in children. *Cochrane Database of Systematic Reviews 1*, CD000326.

Woodgate, R.L. (1998). Adolescents' perspective of chronic illness: 'It's hard'. *Journal of Pediatric Nursing, 13*, 210–223.

Woodgate, R.L. (2005). A different way of being: Adolescents' experiences with cancer. *Cancer Nursing, 28*, 8–15.

World Health Organization (WHO). (2003). *Adherence to long-term therapies: Evidence for action.* Geneva, Switzerland: Author.

CHAPTER 5

Strategies for Locating Adult Primary and Specialty Physicians

DEBRA S. LOTSTEIN

All youth with special health care needs and disabilities will eventually need to transition into some aspect of the adult-oriented medical service system. This transition will be necessary because some aspect of a youth's current care is likely to be unavailable when he or she becomes an adult, either one or more of the youth's health care providers will not see adult patients, and/or his or her public or private payment or service program will be limited to children. Transition is a good idea, as youth with special health care needs and disabilities, like their typically developing peers, should continue to get age-appropriate care as they grow into adulthood. Guideline statements from a number of medical societies emphasize that youth with special health care needs and disabilities should transfer to adult-oriented providers (American Academy of Pediatrics, American Academy of Family Physicians, and American College of Physicians-American Society of Internal Medicine, 2002; Baldassano et al., 2002; Cystic Fibrosis Foundation, 1998; Smith, 2001; Webb & Williams, 2001). Yet for youth with special health care needs and disabilities, changing between the two systems is complicated by the differences between the pediatric and adult medical systems with regard to treating chronic conditions. While some of these differences support the need for transition, others can make transitioning to age-appropriate care difficult.

This chapter discusses the differences between pediatric and adult service systems and provides a series of strategies that can help youth with special health care needs and disabilities, their families, and the health professionals serving them as they seek high-quality, accessible medical care in the adult health care system.

DIFFERENCES BETWEEN PEDIATRIC AND ADULT MEDICAL PROVIDERS

Some terminology commonly used by pediatric providers may be unfamiliar to adult providers. For example, the terms *special health care needs* and *developmental delay* may be unfamiliar to adult providers who would be more likely refer to a *chronic condition* or a *cognitive impairment*. These differences in terminology might lead to miscommunication between providers during the transition process. In addition to terminology, other differences between pediatric and adult medical

Table 5.1. Differences between pediatric and adult providers and systems of care for youth with special health care needs and disabilities

Categories	Pediatric	Adult
Knowledge of the youth's personal medical history	Intimate knowledge	Unfamiliar
Pediatric disease knowledge	Common knowledge	Unfamiliar
Common co-morbidities seen	Primary viral infection	Cancer, diabetes, atherosclerosis
Provider–patient interactions	Dependency More family-centered	Autonomy More disease specific
Extent of community-based/ publicly funded service system	More extensive	More limited

providers include knowledge of an individual's personal medical history, pediatric disease knowledge, comorbidities common to the population the provider serves, provider–patient interactions, and the extent of the community-based/publicly funded service system. Table 5.1 summarizes these differences between pediatric and adult providers.

Knowledge of Personal Medical History

If a child and pediatric provider have had an ongoing relationship, the pediatric provider will have an intimate knowledge of the child's personal medical history. For example, the provider will know which treatments have worked for the child and which have failed or had untoward side effects, as well as the psychosocial elements of the child and his or her family that might influence care processes. A new provider will have no knowledge of an individual's past history, so the pediatric provider will need to summarize this information and transfer it to the new provider. An individual's personal medical history must be comprehensive and include a family history, the youth's medical and physical examination history, growth patterns, results of developmental testing, family pedigree, history of medications and allergies, salient lab work and x-rays, and a current health problem list.

Pediatric Disease Knowledge

Adult health care providers may be unfamiliar with childhood-onset conditions, especially those that previously had limited survival to adulthood. In addition, they may have little knowledge of the trajectory of chronic childhood conditions across the lifespan. Other conditions that occur in both children and adults, such as diabetes and end-stage renal disease, may have unique manifestations in developing children and young adults that may be unfamiliar to adult-oriented providers.

Changes in Common Comorbidities

Along with the typical morbidities that accompany aging, comorbidities of chronic childhood conditions may change with age. For example, among those who are immunocompromised, primary viral infections are a common issue, while cancer, atherosclerosis, and diabetes are more common in adults (and at a younger age than in the general population). Thus, the index of suspicion for various conditions and screening tests used will differ with the age of the population. Little is known about how adults with chronic childhood conditions are affected by typical morbidities that come with aging. For example, females with Down syndrome experience menopause earlier than women without Down syndrome (Seltzer, Schupf, & Wu, 2001), but the life experiences or symptomatology of women with Down syndrome undergoing menopause is unknown. Moreover, youth with special health care needs and disabilities and their pediatric providers may not be comfortable discussing more common "adult" issues (e.g., sexual health, drug use), especially if they have known each other for many years in a relationship that is more like a parent–child relationship (Britto et al., 1999). These differences support the need for changing to age-appropriate providers.

Provider–Patient Interactions

There are differences in the typical interactions between providers and patients that can be attributed to the age/developmental level of the patient. For example, discussion of more personal issues requires autonomy, which may not have existed in the pediatric model (except in the adolescent model in which that is the norm). A relationship that is more like a parent–child relationship may exist with pediatric providers in contrast to adult medical providers, in part arising from the dependent status of most children as they rely on others for arranging and ensuring their care (e.g., scheduling follow-up appointments, making arrangements for referrals and outside tests as needed). It is important for pediatric providers to help children and youth with special health care needs and disabilities become their own health advocates so that once they transition to adult services, they have the skills to advocate for their own health care needs.

In addition, family-centered care is emphasized in pediatrics via the use of multidisciplinary teams including physicians, nurses, therapists, social workers, nutritionists, and psychological service providers. This type of care is consistent with the "medical home" model developed and supported by the American Academy of Pediatrics (AAP, Committee on Disability, 2005; Cooley, 2004). This model is based on the premise that ideal pediatric care is coordinated, comprehensive, continuous, accessible, family centered, culturally competent, and compassionate (For more information on the medical home, refer to Chapter 2.). While not all pediatric providers are able to establish a medical home, just over half of children with special health care needs and disabilities receive the kind of care that meets criteria established by the Maternal and Child Health Bureau (MCHB) for a medical home (Strickland et al., 2004).

Although the idea of patient-centered and coordinated care is not new in adult-oriented medical care, the implementation of this kind of care has not been widespread. Young adults switching to adult care often note the loss of a personal feeling to their care (Reiss, Gibson, & Walker, 2005). Recent initiatives of two major physician groups mark the expansion of the "medical home" beyond pediatrics. The American Academy of Family Physicians formally endorsed the medical home concept in 2004, and in January 2006, the American College of Physicians (the association of internists) put forward a similar model of an "advanced medical home" (American College of Physicians, 2006; Future of Family Medicine Project Leadership Committee, 2004). In addition, national efforts to implement the Chronic Care Model offer promise in improving care for adults with chronic childhood conditions along with other adults (Bodenheimer, Wagner, & Grumbach, 2002). This model lays a framework of six components that together can improve the quality and patient-centeredness of care received by people with chronic illnesses. The six components include: linkages to community resources, leadership of the health care organization towards chronic care, disease self-management support, delivery system design, decision support (or the integration of evidence-based guidelines into daily practice), and computerized clinical information systems, including patient registries (Bodenheimer et al., 2002).

Also, as will be discussed later in the chapter, adult-oriented care is typically more disease specific. Adolescents receiving care only from subspecialists for their chronic condition will also need a primary care provider after moving into the adult medical system.

Extent of Community-Based, Publicly Funded Service System

The public service system is more comprehensive for children than it is for young and nonelderly adults, as demonstrated by the work of the MCHB and the Title V Children with Special Health Care Needs (CSHCN) Program it oversees, the Individuals with Disabilities Education Act, and relatively generous Medicaid eligibility for children (For more information on health insurance options for transition-age adolescents and adults, refer to Chapter 3). The lack of comparable systems of care for adults with complex medical conditions and disabilities can cause serious limitations in access to care for youth with special health care needs and disabilities when they age out of the pediatric service system.

In moving between the pediatric and adult health care systems, there is the potential for young adults with chronic childhood conditions to lose access to the services they need, including medical care, insurance coverage, and other services, such as home health assistance and durable medical equipment needs. Connecting to high-quality adult-oriented care can prevent this potentially disastrous outcome. High-quality adult-oriented medical services means having a provider (and often a team of providers) who:

- Is comfortable caring for a young adult with a chronic childhood condition and/or with a developmental disability

- Is easily accessible to the family

- Has condition-specific knowledge and/or is willing to collaborate with other physicians who have this knowledge

- Is able to effectively communicate with the patient and his or her family so that their questions are answered and their concerns are addressed

- Is able to provide age-appropriate preventive care

- Can make accommodations as needed (e.g., using appropriate equipment for physical examinations, providing more time for visits)

- Has an understanding of the young adult's past treatment and psychosocial history so that ineffective treatments can be avoided, effective treatment continued, and ongoing issues addressed

STRATEGIES TO ACCESS ADULT MEDICAL CARE

The process of seeking adult services includes a) assessing the current medical service needs of the youth with special health care needs and disabilities, b) determining which available models of medical care for adults with childhood onset conditions in the community are appropriate, and c) determining which adult insurance options are appropriate and available.

Assessing Medical Service Needs

A comprehensive medical services needs assessment includes assessing which services the youth is currently using and identifying the services he or she is likely to need in the foreseeable future. This process also involves determining whether there are age limitations associated with the various providers and services currently used, so that age-related transfers can be planned to avoid gaps in care. Also, anticipated changes in the youth's living situation (e.g., moving from home to independent housing, moving to another geographic area) should be discussed to identify needs that these changes might bring about, such as the need to find a provider who is closer to their new home. Other important elements of the transition needs assessment process include understanding the youth's mental health, work, and social needs. Also, health care providers will need to take into consideration how a family's cultural background might have an impact on how the youth and his or her family views adulthood and independence, which will in turn influence transition planning. For more information on these elements of transition preparation and planning, refer to Chapters 8, 12, and 13.

A medical service needs assessment is an essential first step in understanding a family's needs and resources for accessing adult medical services. As many families of youth with special health care needs and disabilities lack comprehensive professional care coordination, there may be no one outside of the family who is aware of all the services a youth is receiving (McPherson et al., 2004). As of 2006, no standardized needs assessment process is widely used (Lotstein, McPherson, Strickland, & Newacheck, 2005). The assessment is often performed in piecemeal fashion by different service providers who might help families make plans within their own realm of available services, with the family left to fill in the gaps that may result from the fragmentation. For example, a specialty provider might help the family find an adult specialist but may not address other changes in primary care or educational realms due to lack of time and knowledge of resources and referrals. Ideally, the medical services needs assessment process would be done comprehensively, taking into account all aspects of the youth's life. The ideal person to do this would be a health care provider who understands both the pediatric and adult health service systems well. This person may be the youth's physician, nurse, social worker, or occupational or physical therapist. In other situations, a team of adult- and pediatric-oriented providers from different disciplines and service sectors might be best able to assess current and future needs. Three main domains should be assessed during this process, including the youth's current medical provider need, insurance coverage, and community services used (see Chapter 7).

Current Medical Providers

All of the medical providers who currently are working with the youth should be determined. This includes primary and specialty care providers, along with the health care providers who render medically-related therapies and treatments (e.g., occupational therapist, community vendors). While many youth with special health care needs and disabilities may get all of their care from primary care providers, others may receive the majority of their care from specialists (Perrin, Kuhlthau, Gortmaker, Beal, & Ferris, 2002).

The following questions should be addressed for each provider the youth currently sees:

- Does this provider limit their practice to patients younger than a certain age?

- Does the youth still need services from this provider, or has that particular issue been resolved?

- Does the provider have a comprehensive list of subspecialists to whom he or she typically refers the youth?

- Will the provider be able to see the youth if there is a change in type of insurance coverage?

Often the youth and his or her family will not be able to answer these questions without first consulting with their health care providers. Written reminders and forms including these questions can help the youth and family in collecting this information.

If it is determined during the medical needs assessment that the youth will need a new type of provider (either primary or specialty care), a provider should be identified who will follow the youth at least through older adolescence/young adulthood (if not longer). This will help minimize the number of transfers of care and assure continuity in care if some transfers must happen sooner than others. The importance of assuring a source of primary care will be discussed in more detail later in this chapter.

Current Insurance Coverage

Medical care insurance is another domain to explore during the medical services needs assessment. It should be determined what sources of health insurance coverage the youth currently has, and the age limits for that particular policy (White, 2002). Again, this information might not be available without further investigation into a particular plan (especially for private health plans). Families may need assistance in determining this information. Families should be encouraged to contact either the employee health benefits representative at their place of employment or a Medicaid benefits counselor in their community, depending on what type of insurance their child has. For families whose child is enrolled in the Medicaid or State Child Health Insurance Program, they can also access information via the Internet at http://www.cms.hhs.gov/medicaid/. Finally, professionals should help the family determine what types of health insurance options they might be eligible for once their child ages out of their current coverage. (See discussion later in this chapter and see Chapter 3 for more information on this topic)

Current Community Services

Other nonmedical services that the youth receives (or might be eligible for) should be explored. The importance of these various services in preparing the youth with special health care needs and disabilities for adulthood will be discussed in Chapters 13 and 14, but these agencies can also be important sources of information about adult-oriented services as well. Examples of these types of services include community-based disability agencies and independent living centers, which serve populations of adults with disabilities, including developmental disabilities. Other community-based services include special education services through the schools, specialized programs at community colleges, and vocational rehabilitation services. See Chapters 11 and 13 for a further discussion of these services.

Determining Appropriate Model of Adult Medical Care

The next component of seeking adult-oriented medical services is to determine which available models of medical care for adults with childhood onset conditions are appropriate, including primary and specialty care.

The Changing Importance of Primary Care versus Specialty Care

While primary care is important to individuals of all ages, it assumes a new level of importance for youth with special health care needs and disabilities. First, they need care professionals who can provide holistic, patient-centered care (rather than disease-specific care), and there is evidence that suggests most adult subspecialty physicians do not provide this type of care. For example, one study of Medicare beneficiaries found that relatively few ambulatory visits to medical specialists included care for conditions outside of the specialist's traditional domain (Rosenblatt et al., 1998). Similarly, compared with those who received the majority of their care from adult-oriented primary care providers, those mostly seeing adult medical specialists were less likely to have received an influenza vaccination—a marker of having received basic primary care services (Rosenblatt et al., 1998). Shea and colleagues (1999) found that adult-oriented physicians who identified as subspecialists reported a low likelihood of coordinating care among physicians and providing primary care.

   With aging, the number of comorbid conditions experienced by an individual may expand, increasing the need for additional care from multiple providers and, in turn, the need for a primary care provider who can coordinate this care. The "ideal" adult medical home provider is a physician or nurse practitioner who is comfortable caring for young adults and individuals with multiple special health care needs and disabilities (see discussion on interviewing providers later in this chapter). An adult medical home physician might have training in internal medicine, combined pediatrics and internal medicine, or family medicine, while a nurse practitioner might have preparation in adult, family, and/or women's health, either alone or in combination with pediatrics, public health, and mental health.

   Furthermore, some childhood conditions may require more or less subspecialty care in adulthood. This may be because of changes in disease severity level, comorbidities, and provider comfort level with treating a given condition. For example, many general pediatricians refer patients with diabetes to pediatric endocrinologists, as they are generally less familiar with treating diabetes than an adult primary care provider (as diabetes is less common in children compared to adults). There may be less of a need for an endocrinology specialist once a young adult with diabetes changes to adult-oriented primary care.

Models of Specialty Care

A number of specialty care models for adults with chronic childhood conditions exist, including adult clinics for conditions of childhood onset, ongoing care from a pediatric specialty care center, and transfer to adult specialty care.

Adult Clinics for Conditions of Childhood Onset
With the increase in adult survival rates, there has been an emergence of adult specialty clinics for historically "pediatric" diseases of relatively high prevalence. This includes, but is not limited to, adult cystic fibrosis, Down syndrome, congenital heart disease, spina bifida, and sickle cell disease centers. Each of these conditions had been under the purview of pediatrics subspecialists, as in the past affected children did not typically survive into adulthood. As a result, training for the adult counterparts of these specialists did not usually include education in these diseases. With improvements in therapies and systems of care, survival has improved, creating a demand for these adult-oriented clinics.

First, in the case of cystic fibrosis, the number of youth living into adulthood has increased significantly. In 1990, 30% of individuals in the cystic fibrosis registry were older than 18 years old, while in 2004, more than 41% of the individuals were adults, with the median age of survival at 35 years old (Cystic Fibrosis Foundation, 2005). In order to best meet the needs of this growing population, the Cystic Fibrosis Foundation has encouraged the establishment of adult-oriented specialty clinics, along with improved support for the transition process (Cystic Fibrosis Foundation, 1998).

Second, there also are a number of clinics dedicated to caring for adults with Down syndrome. For example, the Adult Down Syndrome Center at the Advocate Lutheran General Hospital in Park Ridge, Illinois was founded in 1992, at the request of an organization of parents of young adults with Down syndrome (Chicoine, McGuire, Hebein, & Gilly, 1994). The clinic is multidisciplinary so that patients are evaluated by a family physician, a social worker, a nutritionist, and an audiologist. Other commonly used health care services (e.g., occupational and physical therapy) are available through a referral network. This clinic uses standardized checklists for recommended screening tests and standardized evaluations for physical, emotional, and developmental needs (Smith, 2001).

Third, as approximately 85% of individuals with congenital heart disease will survive into adulthood, there has been a growing demand for adult congenital heart disease providers. In response to this population trend, the American College of Cardiology (ACC) has developed guidelines that outline appropriate levels of care for adults with congenital heart disease (Webb & Williams, 2001). While the exact number of adult congenital heart disease centers in the United States is unclear, the ACC recommends at least 30–50 centers nationally, far more of the current reality (Webb & Williams, 2001). Increased training is needed to have enough practitioners to staff this model of care for adults with congenital heart disease.

Fourth, a number of clinical centers for adults with sickle cell disease have now been established across the United States. In the past 40 years, there has been an increase in the need for adult-oriented providers educated in the care of individuals with sickle cell disease. Historically, most individuals suffering from sickle cell disease did not live beyond 15 years old, but individuals with this condition are now living well into their 40s on average (Platt et al., 1994).

While multidisciplinary clinics composed of physical and occupational therapy, primary care, and other medical specialties (i.e., neurology, physical medicine and rehabilitation, and urology) have been fairly commonplace for children with neurologic and muscular conditions like cerebral palsy and spina bifida, having similar multidisciplinary clinics for adults with childhood-onset conditions is a newer development. An exemplary model of this type of clinic is the Gillette Lifetime Specialty Healthcare clinic in Minnesota. This clinic was founded in 2001, to meet the needs of former pediatric patients who were experiencing gaps in their care after becoming adults. The clinic currently provides services for patients who are diagnosed with cerebral palsy, spinal cord injury, and spina bifida. Services provided include transition planning and care coordination, occupational and physical therapy, urology, neurology, physical medicine and rehabilitation, and primary care (Gillette Children's Specialty Healthcare, 2006). In addition, this clinic was built to be accessible for individuals in wheel chairs, with lifts and other modifications usually not seen in adult medical clinics. It is unclear exactly how many other similar adult-oriented clinics currently exist, but the number is probably small.

Ongoing Care from a Pediatric Specialty Care Center

Ongoing Care from a Pediatric Specialty Care Center   Another model of medical care for adults with chronic childhood conditions continues to be the pediatric specialty center. Most often, ongoing adult care is provided from the centers adults visited as youth. This model may work best for very low-prevalence conditions in which there is not enough of an adult population to have a separate clinic, as found with adults with rare genetic and immunologic conditions. In addition, some providers such as rheumatologists and surgical subspecialists who treat youth with special health care needs and disabilities also treat adults. This model does provide a viable option for continuous care but relies on young adults having ongoing insurance in order to access the adult-oriented services. Young adults who continue to receive care from a pediatric specialty center should seek out an adult-oriented primary care provider who can communicate with the specialists, coordinate care, and provide adult primary care.

Transfer to Adult Specialty Care

Transfer to Adult Specialty Care   A final, and possibly the most common, model for medical care for adults with chronic childhood conditions is the transition directly to traditional adult specialty care providers. This model of care typically works best when the disease process is similar or the same in adults and children, as in populations with asthma, diabetes mellitus, or organ transplantation. However, problems may arise when there are unique disease-specific issues that adult providers are less familiar with, as demonstrated with common pediatric causes of organ failure than can recur in transplanted organs and yet are rare in adults. Another area of potential difficulty with this model is related to the developmental aspects of the care that young adults receive from adult providers. As mentioned previously, the service approach varies in many ways from pediatric services. The developmental issues associated with adolescence and young adulthood, such as pubertal changes, cognitive level of functioning, and psychosocial characteristics, may be unfamiliar to adult specialists caring mostly for older adults (Reiss et al., 2005).

Determining Appropriate Adult Insurance Options

At least in the United States, health insurance coverage is fairly central to the options a youth will have in their choice of health care providers. Making the best arrangements with the most ideal adult provider will come to nothing if the youth has no way to pay to see the provider. As mentioned previously, it is especially important that individuals counseling youth and their families are familiar with the landscape of adult insurance options, as they are different from those offered in the pediatric system. For a more in-depth discussion on specific health insurance options for youth with special health care needs and disabilities, refer to Chapter 3.

Insurance coverage rates are relatively high among youth with special health care needs and disabilities (McPherson et al., 2004). Those who are younger than 18 years old are generally covered by their parent's private insurance or the relatively generous Medicaid policies for children from low-income families. Young adults (ages 21 to 35) in the general population, however, have the highest rates of being uninsured of any age group (Callahan & Cooper, 2005; Fishman, 2001). While longitudinal data are not available, information that is available suggests that young adults with disabilities have higher uninsurance rates compared with youth with special health care needs and disabilities (Callahan & Cooper, 2006; Fishman, 2001).

While some young adults in the general population may choose not to buy health insurance as they feel it is unnecessary, the majority lack insurance because they have not worked long enough in full-time jobs that offer health insurance benefits (Collins, Schoen, Tenney, Doty, & Ho, 2005). Young adults with chronic childhood conditions may be even less likely to work full-time in jobs with health benefits, as they typically enter entry-level jobs with low pay and low skills. However, there are other ways that this population is partially protected from the overall low insurance coverage rate, mainly by meeting federal criteria for being "disabled."

Young adults who qualify as "disabled" based on Supplemental Security Income (SSI) guidelines will be eligible for various forms of health insurance coverage (White, 2002). If their income is lower than their state's eligibility limits, they will qualify for Medicaid. This situation puts some individuals in the position of choosing between earning more salary and keeping their publicly funded insurance coverage. While there are programs to encourage individuals with disabilities to work and maintain their Medicaid coverage, these programs are generally underutilized (Fishman, 2001). If officially disabled, these young adults may continue to qualify for ongoing coverage from their parents' private coverage, which otherwise ends after one is no longer a full-time student or by age 25 for most plans (White, 2002). In addition, if a disabled individual is the child of a Medicare-eligible parent (who is retired, deceased, or disabled), the young adult could be covered by Medicare.

There are categorical programs that cover groups of adults with specific chronic conditions, many of which begin in childhood. Some states have programs that are similar to the Title V CSHCN Program for adults with certain conditions (e.g., the Genetically Handicapped Persons Program in California). Nationally, there are programs for adults with HIV/AIDS (e.g., the Ryan White Act) and Medicare coverage for those on dialysis.

As an alternative to public coverage and employer-sponsored coverage, the individual private insurance market is not a realistic option for most young adults with chronic childhood conditions. The majority of young adults would be eliminated based on their preexisting conditions. Even where there are state-sponsored high-risk pools to protect against this, the policies typically are prohibitively expensive. It is unclear what effect the newer low cost–high deductible plans might have on this population, although the issue of preexisting conditions may still be a barrier to enrollment. If young adults with special health care needs and disabilities were able to enroll, prior research suggests that the young adults in these types of plans might forgo needed care (including preventive care) due to higher cost-sharing premiums (Fuchs, 2002).

Youth with special health care needs and disabilities who are not U.S. citizens face additional challenges in accessing insurance. While they may have had access to care as children through programs such as the Title V CSHCN Program, they may not be eligible for public coverage as adults (Rehm, 2003). Also, non–U.S. citizens are less likely to have employer-based coverage, because often they are ineligibile for legal working arrangements or they are unable to secure jobs that offer health benefits. One option for this population available in California, for example, is the provision for individuals with disabling conditions who are "permanently residing in the U.S. under the color of the law". Non–U.S. citizens generally need much assistance in accessing this type of program, especially given the frequent language and cultural differences between these families and the general health care system.

For individuals without any insurance coverage options in adulthood, finding adult-oriented services can be especially challenging. Professionals assisting families and youth should be aware of, and develop relationships with, free clinics and safety net hospital programs. Informal arrangements of consultation with pediatric and adult specialists might be arranged to help individuals being cared for in less-specialized environments.

SUGGESTIONS TO IMPROVE TRANSITION INTO ADULT ORIENTED MEDICAL SERVICES

A comprehensive medical service needs assessment and knowledge of local adult-oriented medical providers and insurance status will go a long way to ensure that youth with special health care needs and disabilities have continuous access to needed health care and services. However, other strategies, at both the clinical and policy levels, are needed to achieve even greater success toward the goal of high-quality adult-oriented care for all youth with special health care needs and disabilities.

Using Referral Networks Outside of the Medical System

Given the lack of established networks for transitioning youth with special health care needs and disabilities to adult providers, especially in the areas of mental health and dentistry, youth and their families may have to be creative in finding sources of needed medical care. Any organization that serves adults with chronic childhood conditions is likely to be aware of providers who are willing and able to see this population of adults. Oftentimes, these agencies have supplemental funding or other special arrangements to improve access to providers for adults, given the limitations of public insurance financing in most states. For example, developmental centers care for relatively large numbers of adults with intellectual disabilities who also often have other co-morbid medical conditions. Over time these centers may have developed networks of providers who are experienced and willing to care for this population of adults. Similarly, independent living centers and vocational rehabilitation centers could be another source for recommendations. Agencies that serve mostly children and youth with special health care needs and disabilities, such as Title V CSHCN agencies and parent support centers, are also potential resources for recommendations for medical and health-related providers. Finally, youth and their families could turn to disease-specific support networks, parent groups, and peer groups for recommendations and advice from others who have been down the road before them. Often these support groups have web pages with valuable information on a variety of topics and may include a chat-room or discussion board that allows individuals and/or families to talk to each other over the Internet.

Youth and Family Preparation

Preparing youth with special health care needs and disabilities for the adult medical environment is an important aspect of the preparation for the transition to adult services (Reiss & Gibson, 2002). Setting appropriate expectations without biasing or instilling fear is a key aspect of preparing for the adult clinical experience. For example the "feeling" of an adult-oriented clinic or office may be very different from a pediatric office, with shorter visit times and less interaction with multidisciplinary staff. Other patients sitting in the waiting room might be off-putting to the young adult with special health care needs and disabilities, especially when the majority of adults with a particular disease come from a different demographic than the pediatric population, such as individuals with HIV/AIDS, cardiac disease, or end-stage renal disease. Interactions with providers may be different, particularly when compared with the longstanding relationships with pediatric providers. In particular, providers who typically treat only adults may have less experience working with individuals who have intellectual disabilities, and may be less accustomed to dealing with an individual's family and caregivers. In addition, as discussed previously, adult subspecialists may be less willing to address primary care needs, and so the importance of finding primary care providers should be stressed.

Interviewing New Providers

Assessing transition needs with youth and their families far in advance from an actual transfer date will allow families time to interview with potential new providers. During this interview process, the young adult and his or her family will want to assess the provider based on the aspects of quality care listed at the start of this chapter in addition to any other personal criteria the family may have, including willingness to coordinate care and accessibility (see Figure 5.1).

Services provided

1. What types of providers would I be able to see as a patient here?

2. Is there easy access to social work, nutrition, physical and occupational therapy, and other providers that I might need?

Provider knowledge and comfort with condition

1. Have you treated other adults with the same or similar conditions?

2. Are you willing to learn more about my condition? (If the provider is unfamiliar with the condition)

3. Are you willing/able to communicate with my previous health care providers about my past medical history?

4. Are you willing/able to consult with/coordinate my care with my other providers, such as my other subspecialty physicians, and those from outside agencies?

5. Are you willing to consider the number of required medications needed so that this number can be minimized and that no medications adversely interact with each other?

Accessibility

1. Is the office wheelchair accessible?

2. Is equipment available for individuals needing accommodations for conducting the physical examination?

3. Are there lifts for use with scales and examining tables?

4. What languages are spoken by the provider and the office staff? Are translators available?

5. Is the office convenient to public transportation?

6. Does the office accept the insurance I have now and/or the type I am likely to have in the future?

Figure 5.1. Questions for potential adult-oriented medical providers.

They will want to ask about the experience the provider has had with other young adults with the same or similar conditions. During these meetings, it is important that the youth and his or her family get a sense of whether the provider will appreciate that they are the experts in what it means to live with the condition, and whether the provider will treat them with respect. Ideally, providers will also respect the active involvement of family in the life of young adults with special health care needs and disabilities while at the same time promoting independence to the fullest extent possible.

Interprovider Communication

Improving communication between pediatric and adult providers has the potential to help ensure better continuity of care. Formal, comprehensive patient summaries can help ensure that youth with special health care needs and disabilities will continue to receive high-quality care from new providers. These summaries can be used as a kind of youth-held "health passport" that would accompany the individual to new providers. In addition, expansion of electronic health records that are easily accessible by providers and patients could facilitate this kind of information transfer.

Locally, formal and informal conferences between pediatric and adult providers to discuss individual patients and/or general transition issues could also facilitate quality care for youth in transition. At a broader level, national and international organizations of health care providers can work to create care guidelines, ideally evidence-based when possible, that would outline best practices for optimizing the health of youth with special health care needs and disabilities across the lifespan (see, e.g., guidelines for Down syndrome [Smith, 2001; Webb & Williams, 2001]). The widespread dissemination of these guidelines could help to support adult-oriented providers with less personal experience caring for adults with chronic childhood conditions.

Networks of Providers

Efforts should be made to create networks of providers to facilitate the transfer of care. Having established networks of medical and health-related providers will help to make the process of finding new providers for youth with special health care needs and disabilities more routine. This can be done at the local level where pediatric providers can seek relationships with nearby adult-oriented providers. In addition, national organizations of physicians and disease-specific organizations (see, e.g., the Cystic Fibrosis Foundation, 1998) can work towards developing connections that bridge the pediatric and adult medical systems and would assist physicians locally. Finally, payers such as Title V CSHCN agencies and health plans should also facilitate connections by helping to create referral networks of providers.

Increase the Number of Adult Providers Educated in the Care of Young Adults with Chronic Childhood Conditions

Expanding the number of adult providers with education in historically pediatric conditions will increase the available pool of physicians and other providers who are able to provide high-quality care to adults with childhood onset conditions. For example, there is a recognized need for more adult-oriented specialists in congenital heart disease and cystic fibrosis (Cystic Fibrosis Foundation, 1998; Webb & Williams, 2001). This need for enhanced education of health professionals is emphasized more broadly in the "Surgeon General's Call to Action to Improve the Health and Wellness of Persons with Disabilities," which states that "health care providers (should) have the knowledge and tools to screen, diagnose and treat the whole person with a disability with dignity" (U.S. Department of Health and Human Services, 2005, p.10).

More research in how to improve long-term outcomes in youth with special health care needs and disabilities will also help inform the education needed for providers in order to improve care during the transition period. Finally, beyond the unique disease-specific issues, raising awareness of the comprehensive needs of young adult survivors with chronic conditions among adult-oriented providers will also help improve the quality of care received.

Improve Insurance Coverage for Young Adults

State and national policy efforts are needed to improve insurance coverage available to young adults in the United States. As discussed previously, lack of coverage is a significant barrier to care for young adults generally and in particular for those with chronic childhood conditions (Callahan & Cooper, 2006; White, 2002). Promising policy solutions to this include expanding eligibility for child-oriented public programs to age 25, and possibly Medicaid waivers that allow ongoing eligibility for the program for young adults with special health care needs and disabilities (Collins et al., 2005; Fishman, 2001). More radically, health insurance reform that removes the heavy reliance on employer-based coverage would likely improve coverage options for young adults with chronic childhood conditions.

Support for Transition Preparation Services

Sustained incentives, including financial support, are needed for the transition needs assessment and care coordination described in this chapter. Prior funding available for transition programs primarily via demonstration grants from the MCHB is no longer available. In addition, many adult clinics, primarily condition-specific, housed in children's hospitals have lost funding and are no longer in existence. Ongoing support from federal and state agencies, such as Title V CSHCN, for these services is needed and may require legislative action. Reimbursement from public and private payers for individual transition services would also help to ensure the availability of transition assistance for youth with special health care needs and disabilities and their families.

Areas for Future Research

Further research examining the transition from pediatric to adult services for youth with special health care needs and disabilities is needed to understand which factors are associated with a successful transition into adult health care. Also, research toward understanding the best ways to prepare youth and their families for the adult health care system can help to prevent discontinuities in care. Exploring ways to improve communication between adult and pediatric providers centered on the handoffs in care will also help ensure high-quality, continuous care for young adults with special health care needs. For example, a standardized, comprehensive transition needs assessment form could help to accomplish this goal.

SUMMARY

In the transition to adult-oriented health care, youth with special health care needs and disabilities face a number of challenges associated with changing between various providers and different systems of care. Strategies outlined in this chapter can help youth with special health care needs and disabilities access high-quality, family-centered, age-appropriate care. Increasing efforts towards improving communications and networks at the provider level in addition to local and national policy changes are needed to improve the transition to adult health care systems for youth with special health care needs and disabilities.

REFERENCES

American Academy of Pediatrics, Committee on Disability. (2005). Care coordination in the medical home: Integrating health and related systems of care for children with special health care needs. *Pediatrics, 116,* 1238–1244.

American Academy of Pediatrics, American Academy of Family Physicians, & American College of Physicians-American Society of Internal Medicine. (2002). A consensus statement on health care transitions for young adults with special health care needs. *Pediatrics, 110*(6), 1304–1306.

American College of Physicians. (2006). *Advanced medical home: A policy monograph.* Retrieved September 18, 2006, from http://www.acponline.org/hpp/adv_med.pdf

Baldassano, R., Ferry, G., Griffiths, A., Mack, D., Markowitz, J., & Winter, H.R. (2002). Transition of the patient with inflammatory bowel disease from pediatric to adult care: Recommendations of the North American Society for Pediatric Gastroenterology, Hepatology and Nutrition. *Journal of Pediatric Gastroenterology and Nutrition, 34*(3), 245–248.

Bodenheimer, T., Wagner, E.H., & Grumbach, K. (2002). Improving primary care for patients with chronic illness. *Journal of the American Medical Association, 288*(14), 1775–1779.

Britto, M.T., Garrett, J.M., Dugliss, M.A., Johnson, C.A., Majure, J.M., & Leigh, M.W. (1999). Preventive services received by adolescents with cystic fibrosis and sickle cell disease. *Archives of Pediatric and Adolescent Medicine, 153*(1), 27–32.

Callahan, S.T., & Cooper, W.O. (2005). Uninsurance and health care access among young adults in the United States. *Pediatrics, 116*(1), 88–95.

Callahan, S.T., & Cooper, W.O. (2006). Access to health care for young adults with disabling chronic conditions. *Archives of Pediatric and Adolescent Medicine, 160*(2), 178–182.

Chicoine, B., McGuire, D., Hebein, S., & Gilly, D. (1994). Development of a clinic for adults with Down syndrome. *Mental Retardation, 32*(2), 100–106.

Collins, S.R., Schoen, C., Tenney, K., Doty, M.M., & Ho, A. (2005). Rite of passage? Why young adults become uninsured and how new policies can help. *Commonwealth Fund Issue Brief, 649,* 1–12.

Cooley, W.C. (2004). Redefining primary pediatric care for children with special health care needs: The primary care medical home. *Current Opinion in Pediatrics, 16,* 689–692.

Cystic Fibrosis Foundation. (1998). *Guidelines for the implementation of adult CF programs.* Bethesda, MD: Author.

Cystic Fibrosis Foundation. (2005). *Patient Registry 2004 annual report.* Bethesda, Maryland. Retrieved September 18, 2006, from www.cff.org/uploadfiles/publications/files/2004%20patient%20registry%20report.pdf.

Fishman, E. (2001). Aging out of coverage: Young adults with special health needs. *Health Affairs, 20,* 254-266.

Fuchs, V.R. (2002). What's ahead for health insurance in the United States? *New England Journal of Medicine, 346,* 1822–1824.

Future of Family Medicine Project Leadership Committee. (2004). The future of family medicine: A collaborative project of the family medicine community. *Annals of Family Medicine, 2*(Suppl. 1), S3–32.

Gillette Children's Specialty Health Care. (2006). *Gillette lifetime specialty healthcare.* Retrieved December 8, 2006, from http://www.gillettechildrens.org/fileupload/All%About%20Gillette.pdf

Lotstein, D.S., McPherson, M., Strickland, B., & Newacheck, P.W. (2005). Transition planning for youth with special health care needs: Results from the National Survey of Children with Special Health Care Needs. *Pediatrics, 115,* 1562–1568.

McPherson, M., Weissman, G., Strickland, B.B., van Dyck, P.C., Blumberg, S.J., & Newacheck, P.W. (2004). Implementing community-based systems of services for children and youths with special health care needs: How well are we doing? *Pediatrics, 113*(Suppl. 5), 1538–1544.

Perrin, J.M., Kuhlthau, K.A., Gortmaker, S.L., Beal, A.C., & Ferris, T.G. (2002). Generalist and subspecialist care for children with chronic conditions. *Ambulatory Pediatrics, 2,* 462–469.

Platt, O.S., Brambilla, D.J., Rosse, W.F., Milner, P.F., Castro, O., Steinberg, M.H., et al. (1994). Mortality in sickle cell disease. Life expectancy and risk factors for early death. *New England Journal of Medicine, 330,* 1639–1644.

Rehm, R.S. (2003). Legal, financial, and ethical ambiguities for Mexican American families: Caring for children with chronic conditions. *Qualitative Health Research, 13,* 689–702.

Reiss, J., & Gibson, R. (2002). Health care transition: Destinations unknown. *Pediatrics, 110*(6 Pt. 2), 1307–1314.

Reiss, J.G., Gibson, R.W., & Walker, L.R. (2005). Health care transition: Youth, family, and provider perspectives. *Pediatrics, 115,* 112–120.

Rosenblatt, R.A., Hart, L.G., Baldwin, L.M., Chan, L., & Schneeweiss, R. (1998). The generalist role of specialty physicians: Is there a hidden system of primary care? *Journal of the American Medical Association, 279,* 1364–1370.

Seltzer, G.B., Schupf, N., & Wu, H.S. (2001). A prospective study of menopause in women with Down syndrome. *Journal of Intellectual Disability Research, 45*(Pt 1), 1–7.

Shea, J.A., Kletke, P.R., Wozniak, G.D., Polsky, D., & Escarce, J.J. (1999). Self-reported physician specialties and the primary care content of medical practice: A study of the American Medical Association physician masterfile. *Medical Care, 37,* 333–338.

Smith, D.S. (2001). Health care management of adults with Down syndrome. *American Family Physician, 64,* 1031–1038.

Strickland, B., McPherson, M., Weissman, G., van Dyck, P., Huang, Z.J., & Newacheck, P. (2004). Access to the medical home: Results of the National Survey of Children with Special Health Care Needs. *Pediatrics, 3*(Suppl. 5), 1485–1492.

United States Department of Health and Human Services. (2005). *The Surgeon General's call to action to improve the health and wellness of persons with disabilities.* Retrieved February 28, 2006, from http://www.surgeongeneral.gov/library/disabilities/calltoaction/future.html

Webb, G.D., & Williams, R.G. (2001). Care of the adult with congenital heart disease: Introduction. *Journal of the American College of Cardiology, 37,* 1166.

White, P.H. (2002). Access to health care: health insurance considerations for young adults with special health care needs/disability. *Pediatrics, 110*(6 Pt. 2), 1328–1335.

CHAPTER 6

Accommodations for School and Work

WENDY M. NEHRING

It is essential that every youth and adult with special health care needs and disabilities have the consideration and opportunity to experience their optimal quality of life. For many individuals with disabilities, this will involve the use of accommodations for either a short- or long-term period of time and for either part or all of their day. Accommodations can either assist an individual to live his or her life optimally or eliminate barriers prohibiting that individual from his or her optimal quality of life. A number of federal laws address the process and types of accommodations acceptable for school and work settings. This chapter opens with a discussion of these laws as they apply to accommodations. This chapter then describes the national and international organizations that address the issue of accommodations, with a focus on the model of supports published by the American Association on Mental Retardation, now the American Association on Intellectual and Developmental Disabilities (AAIDD; Luckasson et al., 2002). Next, the chapter details possible accommodations and their provisions by functional area and systems. This section is followed by a discussion of the process of requesting and receiving accommodations in both the school and work setting. This chapter concludes with a vignette.

FEDERAL LAWS ADDRESSING ACCOMMODATIONS

Three federal laws directly discuss accommodations for individuals with disabilities. The Individuals with Disabilities Education Improvement Act of 2004 (IDEA 2004; PL 108-446) is specific to elementary and secondary school settings. Section 504 of the Rehabilitation Act of 1973 (PL 93-112), and the Americans with Disabilities Act (ADA) of 1990 (PL 101-336) describe accommodations in all settings. In addition, the Assistive Technology Act Amendments of 2004 (PL 108-364) discusses the use of technology by individuals with disabilities and is included in this discussion because technical assistive devices and services may be used as accommodations. Each of these federal acts provide guidelines and/or information regarding accommodations that can be of assistance to individuals with disabilities as they work with their families and outside agencies, including school and/or work, to enhance the quality of their lives.

A special thank you is extended to Sally Colatarci, RN, M.S., Director of Nursing at Matheny Medical and Educational Center, for her assistance in obtaining the photographs for this chapter.

The Individuals with Disabilities Education Improvement Act of 2004

In IDEA 2004, accommodations are discussed as they apply to classroom and standardized testing situations. Reasonable accommodations must be made so that students can have the best opportunity to perform well in testing situations. In the case of a student with severe intellectual and developmental disabilities, alternative assessments might take place. The assessment process is a case in which accommodations would not provide an optimal and successful environment; instead, the youth is assessed using alternative methods to evaluate their learning (e.g., a portfolio of their work). The revision of IDEA in 2004 requires the local school district or the state educational agency to publicly report the number of youth with intellectual and other related disabilities who participated in the standardized testing with no assistance and the number who participated with accommodations. If the numbers of youth can be statistically measured, the performance of these youth in the two groups must be documented. For youth who need alternative assessment, the individualized education program (IEP) team must provide a rationale for why the youth could not participate in the standardized assessment with or without accommodations. A rationale should also be given for the choice of alternative assessment (IDEA 2004; Silverstein, 2005).

A definition of accommodations is not given in IDEA 2004. Definitions are, however, provided for an assistive technology device and an assistive technology service. An *assistive technology device* is "any item, piece of equipment, or product system, whether acquired commercially off the shelf, modified, or customized, that is used to increase, maintain, or improve functional capabilities of a child with a disability" (IDEA 2004, §§ 60). A communication board is an example of an assistive technology device. An *assistive technology service* basically helps to assist the youth in selecting, acquiring, and/or using the best assistive device(s) for his or her needs. Such devices can be realized as accommodations. Examples of such services would include a formal evaluation of the youth's needs in the home, school and/or work setting; the fitting and customization of a wheelchair; and the provision of training for the youth and/or family on how to use a technology device.

IDEA 2004 also describes technology development and the need for emerging technologies to be used in practice in order to provide optimal environments for youth with disabilities. The law further provides support for the use of web-based communication strategies for youth with intellectual and developmental disabilities.

Section 504 of the Rehabilitation Act of 1973

In contrast with IDEA 2004, Section 504 of the Rehabilitation Act of 1973 covers accommodations for school and work settings in great depth. Related aids and services are included in the definition of *appropriate education* provided in this Act as part of ensuring such education. Accommodations are considered a related aid or service and may involve devices, educational strategies, attendants, technology, and/or agencies (American Academy of Pediatrics, Committee on Children with Disabilities, 2000; Schulzinger, 1999).

Section 504 discusses the need for accommodations to provide an optimal learning environment. Such provisions are often available for youth who do not qualify for IDEA provisions. The law provides the use of accommodations for

1) students who miss school on a frequent basis or over a long period of time due to health conditions, 2) students who experience pain, anxiety, and/or fatigue due to their health conditions that result in concentration problems, 3) students who experience side effects or other untoward effects of their medications, 4) students who need assistive technology to function, 5) students who need medical technology, 6) students who come back to school after an extended health-related condition such as an injury or serious illness, and 7) students who may have a disability, substance abuse habit, or a chronic illness (Betz, 2001; Schulzinger, 1999).

The Americans with Disabilities Act of 1990

The Americans with Disabilities Act (ADA) of 1990 discusses accommodations for employees in the first Title of the Act. Employers are required to provide reasonable accommodations if they do not result in "undue hardship" to the employer or substantially alter the manner in which the business of the employer is carried out (National Council on Disability, 2005). Examples of undue hardship to an employer would include an accommodation that would affect the safety of others in the room, would be too expensive, or would significantly alter the job responsibilities.

Assistive Technology Act Amendments of 2004

The Assistive Technology Act Amendments of 2004 were written so that statewide technology assistance programs could be developed and supported in order to provide technical assistance devices and services to individuals with disabilities. Such devices and services can be considered accommodations.

SYSTEMS OF SUPPORT FOR INDIVIDUALS WITH INTELLECTUAL DISABILITIES

In 1992, the AAIDD (then AAMR) published the 9th edition of *Mental Retardation: Definition, Classification, and Systems of Support* (Luckasson et al.). In this edition, the authors substantially changed the focus to include the concept of supports and a description of a system of supports. The definition of *supports* is similar to that of an accommodation in that "supports are resources and strategies that aim to promote the development, education, interests, and personal well-being of a person and that enhance individual functioning" (Luckasson et al., 1992, p. 145). This focus has been expanded in the 10th edition of the book (Luckasson et al., 2002) so that five dimensions of supports are listed, including intellectual abilities; adaptive behavior; context; health; and participation, interactions, and social roles. The supports model is illustrated in Figure 6.1 and can be applied to all individuals with disabilities regardless of age and condition.

Inherent in this model are the concepts of *person-centered planning, person-environmental interactions, quality of life, inclusion and equity,* and *supports in the natural environment.* Many factors must be identified and considered before planning for supports. These include the person's capabilities and adaptive skills, their natural environments, their informal and formal supports already in place, and any risk and/or protective factors that affect the quality of their lives. It is also assumed that an individual's supports are fluid and change over time. Sources of support can be self, others (formal and informal), services, or technology related.

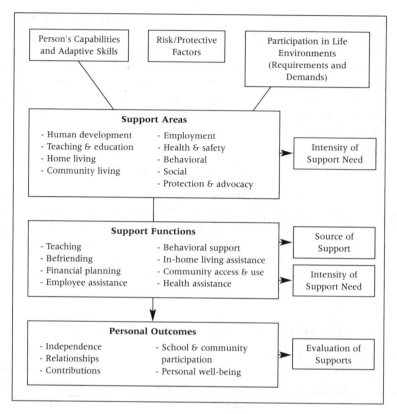

Figure 6.1. Supports model for people with mental retardation (Reprinted with permission from the American Association on Intellectual and Developmental Disabilities).

The needed intensity of the supports is important to consider and can be a) intermittent, b) limited, c) extensive, and/or d) pervasive. The areas of needed support are assessed and identified, followed by the identification of specific functional objectives, individualized outcomes, and a plan for evaluation (Luckasson et al., 2002). The AAIDD (then AAMR) has also published the *Supports Intensity Scale* (SIS) that provides an instrument to assess the need for and intensity of supports for an individual with an intellectual disability (Thompson et al., 2004).

IDENTIFICATION OF ACCOMMODATIONS BY FUNCTIONAL AREA AND BY SYSTEMS

Supports or accommodations can be many different things. When the need for accommodations arises, it is important that they are person-centered, among other factors. Table 6.1 provides a comprehensive list of accommodations by functional area (e.g., vision, hearing), and Table 6.2 provides a list of considerations for accommodations by systems level (e.g., school, work). See pages 104–107 for photographs of examples of devices and equipment used in some of these accommodations.

Although the literature may include a comprehensive discussion of available and recommended accommodations by functional area, there is still distance to cover to make sure that all individuals are accommodated. In a national survey

Table 6.1. Educational and health-related accommodations by functional area

Functional area	Possible accommodations*
Intellectual disabilities	Alternative evaluation options
	Alternative testing arrangements
	Assessment and documentation of health problems as part of individualized health plan/individualized education plan
	Audiotaping or videotaping class sessions
	Books on audiotapes
	Breaking tasks down to simpler and/or smaller steps
	Captioned films
	Computer assisted instruction for self-care, home management, health promotion, and community living skills
	Computer with course software or book
	Computer with enlarged font capacity
	Computer with speech output
	Concrete course instructions including assignments and tests
	Extending the time for tests and assignments
	Hyperlinks
	Instructional demonstrations according to learning style
	Notetaker
	Reducing distractions in class and testing situations
	Repeating instructions and information
	Software to check grammar and spelling
	Talking calculators and other adapted equipment
	Word prediction software
	Use of a facilitator to facilitate understanding/participation in group meetings
Health conditions	Adapted utensils for eating, writing, and physical activity as needed
	Adapted equipment as needed to function in setting
	Allow rest periods for students who get fatigued easily
	Allow use of attendants in the classroom
	Assessment and documentation of health problems as part of individualized health plan
	Assignments in electronic format
	Audiotaping or videotaping class sessions
	Copy of class notes
	Distance education
	Education on health problem management
	E-mail for communication
	Extending the time for tests and assignments
	Flexible attendance requirements for medical-related appointments and/or hospitalization
	Notetaker
	Providing access to health care during before and after-school programs and during field trips
	Providing for counseling as needed
	Scheduling times for delivering medications
	Scheduling times for procedures and/or therapies
	Scheduling core courses for times when the student is least fatigued

(continued)

Table 6.1. *(continued)*

Hearing impairments	Assessment and documentation of health problems as part of individualized health plan
	Audio loops for amplification
	Cochlear implants
	E-mail for communication and discussion groups
	Frequency-modulated systems
	Hearing aid
	Infrared systems
	Interpreter (person who signs)
	Notetaker
	Open or closed-captioned films or videos
	Real-time captioning
	Speaking clearly and at a comfortable, but not fast, rate
	Speaking to the individual's face and not obscuring your mouth
	Telecommunication Device for the Deaf (TDD)
	Visual aids
	Visual warning system for emergencies
	Written assignments, instructions, and/or demonstration summaries
Mental health conditions	Assessment and documentation of mental health problems as part of individualized health plan
	Audiotaping or videotaping class sessions
	Copy of class notes
	Crisis prevention and intervention
	Distance education
	Flexible attendance requirements for medical-related appointments and/or hospitalization
	Provide for needed short- and long-term counseling/therapy
	Extending time on tests and assignments
	Notetaker
	Reducing distractions in class and testing situations or providing alternative settings for testing
Mobility limitations	Accessible classrooms, laboratories, buildings, playgrounds, and gymnasiums and athletic fields
	Accessible locations for fieldtrips and observation experiences
	Adapted utensils for eating, writing, and physical activity as needed
	Adapted equipment for self-care needs (e.g., raised toilet seats)
	Adjustable and movable tables
	Allowing use of attendants in classroom and other learning environments
	Architectural adaptations
	Assessment and documentation of health problems as part of individualized health plan
	Assignments in electronic format
	Computer with input devices for speech and/or alternative keyboards
	Group assignments

Table 6.1. *(continued)*

	Infrared sensors with pneumatic switches
	Mobility devices, such as crutches, braces, and wheelchairs
	Notetaker
	Providing equipment and other needed materials within reach
	Robotic arms
	Switches for a variety of objects
	Touch-sensitive screen
	Voice recognition systems
Speech impairments	Assessment and documentation of health problems as part of individualized health plan
	Augmentative and alternative communication
	Light systems
	Picture book with touch or point system
	Speech output devices
	Switch-operated systems
Vision impairments (including low vision through blindness)	Adapted equipment, such as talking calculators
	Assessment and documentation of health problems as part of individualized health plan
	Assignments in electronic format
	Audiotaped class sessions
	Audiotaped assignment instructions
	Audiotaped texts
	Braille assignments, texts, and lecture notes
	Braille printer
	Braille screen on computer
	Braille signs on equipment and around the environment
	Computer with adapted keyboard
	Computer with enlarged font capacity
	Computer with optical character recognition
	Computer with speech output
	Descriptive video services
	Enlarged print on signage, equipment, and handouts
	Magnified lenses
	Microscope connected to television for larger view
	Prescription glasses
	Raised-line figures
	Screen readers for "text to speech"
	Seeing Eye dog
	Placement at the front of the class
	Special alarms for alerting to emergencies
	Tactile models
	Verbal descriptions of demonstrations and visual aids
	Well-lighted room
	White cane

Adapted from DO-IT, University of Washington, 2005; Hasselbring & Glaser, 2000; Learning Disabilities Association of America, 2005; Thurlow, 2002; U.S. Government Accountability Office, 2005; Wehmeyer et al., 2002; Willliams, 2001.

*Although not all of these accommodations would be deemed "reasonable" for procurement from the setting, there are special programs that the individual and his or her family can be referred to for acquisition of these items.

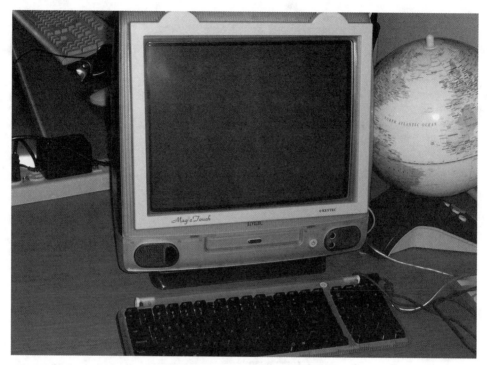

Computers are often used for accommodations. This example shows a touch screen.

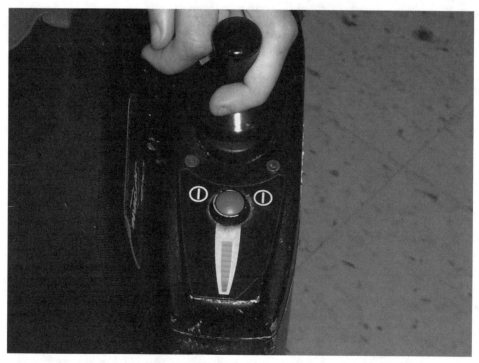

A device to allow an individual to move a wheelchair in desired directions.

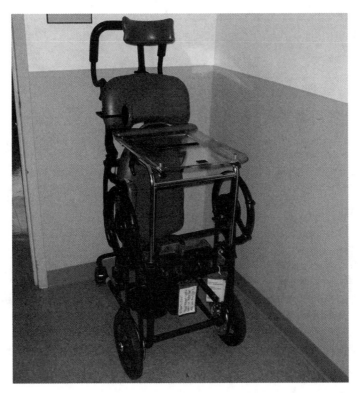

An accommodation to allow the child to stand and be supported.

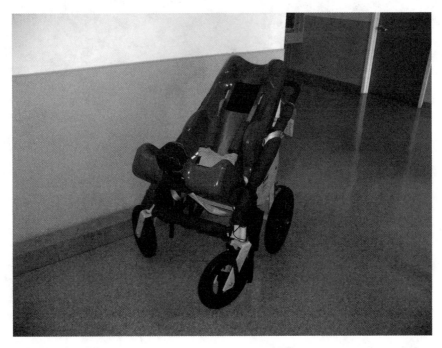

A chair accommodation.

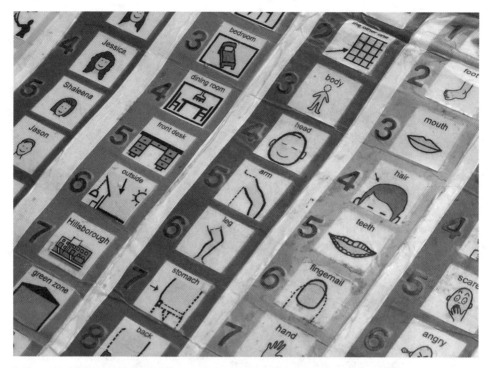

An example of a communication board.

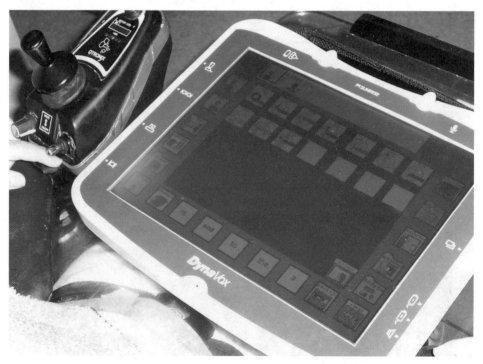

Another example of a communication board.

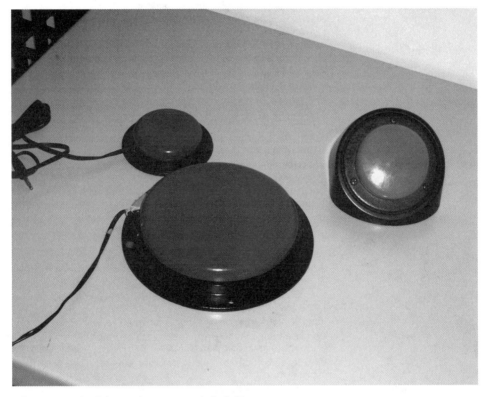

Different types of switches used to operate a desired object.

Table 6.2. Considerations for accommodations by systems

Level of system	Considerations for accommodations
Individual	Developing self-care, home management, and community living skills
	Individualized care
	Identification of a medical home
	Identification of plans for health care transition
	Identification of primary language and translation of materials as needed
	Identification of emergency medical care and resuscitation plan
	Use of a team approach when able
	Able to identify need for medical services
	Able to identify ways to obtain needed equipment and/or supplies
	Access to Disabled Student Services or Office of Disabilities in secondary or postsecondary settings
	Access to Department of Rehabilitation for assistance in obtaining work and job skills
	Participation in health promotion
Family	Understanding of rights and services under applicable federal laws (e.g., Individuals with Disabilities Education Act [IDEA], Section 504 of the Rehabilitation Act, and Americans with Disabilities Act [ADA])
	Understanding of and participates in learning self-advocacy skills
	Understanding of different routes available for health insurance and what plan allows
	Understanding of rights and services under applicable federal laws (e.g., IDEA, Section 504 of the Rehabilitation Act, ADA)
	Helping youth to be independent, including self-care, health promotion, home management, and community living skills
	Identification of primary language and translation of materials as needed
	Identification of the medical home for youth
	Understanding of different routes available for health insurance and what plan allows
	Working with youth to develop transition plan for health care
Secondary school	Presence of school nurse and role on IEP team: • Assesses immunization status • Provides assessment of and information about self-care, home management, health promotion, and community living skills and issues • Provides vision and hearing assessment • Provides nutrition teaching and counseling • Provides skin assessments • Provides education and information on related health topics, (e.g., exercise, safety, sexuality) • Provides referral for dental care and mental health needs as appropriate • Organizes health care procedures, therapies, and medications as detailed in the individualized health plan

Table 6.2. *(continued)*

	• Works with health care team to identify health problems, including secondary conditions, and provides intervention, follow up, and referral as needed
	• Provides referral to community agencies, including summer camps
	• Discusses future planning
	Process for requesting accommodations
	Presence of coordinator for disability services
	Process for individualized health plan to include identification of need, assessment, management, evaluation, information, and needed referrals
	Plan for school absences
	Plan for medical emergencies and resuscitation
	Plan for crisis prevention and intervention
	Plan for development of webpage with frequently asked questions related to accommodations and identification of individuals to contact for further information
	Plan for development of or change in policies and/or procedures
	Plan for development of curriculum that allows for reduced course load and small class sizes (as available)
	Translation of needed materials into student and/or family's primary language
	Adequacy of emergency and safety plan
	Adequacy of plan for transportation and safety on school bus
	Accessibility of building and grounds; need for adaptation
	Availability of tutors
	Understanding of rights and services under applicable federal laws, (e.g., IDEA, Section 504 of the Rehabilitation Act, ADA)
Postsecondary school	Organization of health personnel and role in process for obtaining and following through on accommodations
	Presence of Disability Office or Disabled Student Services
	Identification of Unit Coordinators of Disability Services
	Process for requesting accommodations
	Plan for development of or change in policies and/or procedures
	Plan for school absences
	Plan for medical emergencies and resuscitation
	Plan for crisis prevention and intervention
	Adequacy of emergency and safety plan
	Adequacy of plan for transportation on school bus
	Accessibility of building and grounds; need for adaptation
	Plan for curriculum that allows for part-time study
	Plan for development of web page with frequently asked questions related to accommodations and identification of individuals to contact for further information
	Translation of needed materials into student and/or family's primary language
	Understanding of rights and services under applicable federal laws, (e.g., IDEA, Section 504 of the Rehabilitation Act, and ADA)

(continued)

Table 6.2. (*continued*)

Work setting	Accessibility of building and grounds; need for adaptation
	Organization of health personnel and role in process for obtaining and following through on accommodations
	Presence of Disability Office
	Identification of Unit Coordinators of Disability Services
	Process for requesting accommodations
	Plan for development of or change in policies and/or procedures
	Plan for development of webpage with frequently asked questions related to accommodations and identification of individuals to contact for further information
	Translation of needed materials into employee and/or family's primary language
	Plan for medical emergencies and resuscitation
	Plan for crisis prevention and intervention
	Plan for work absences
	Adequacy of emergency and safety plan
	Understanding of rights and services under applicable federal laws (e.g., Section 504 of the Rehabilitation Act, ADA)

Adapted from Betz & Redcay, 2002; Caldwell et al., 1997; Hart, Zimbrich, & Whelley, 2002; Johnson & Dorval, 2005; National Center on Secondary Education and Transition, 2005; Schultz & Liptak, 1998; Weist, Lowie, Flaherty, & Pruitt, 2001.

of 1,000 school administrators across the country, the National Center for Education Statistics (2000) found that 34% of schools did not have an adequate number of computers for all students with identified disabilities, 35% of schools did not have Internet access, 38% of schools did not have adequate numbers of computers with alternative input/output devices, 39% of schools did not have adequate support and evaluation services to meet technological needs of students with disabilities, and 47% of schools were unable to provide adequate training to teachers on how to use telecommunication devices. A more recent survey has not been done to see if these percentages have decreased.

In all cases, the principles of universal design are tantamount. These principles include the need for accommodations to be appropriate, equitable, flexible, simple, useable, and individualized so that barriers can be removed and success can be achieved (Weymeyer, Sands, Knowlton, & Kozleski, 2002). Universal design must be considered 1) in the presentation of material, such as class material from a teacher to a student or the employer to the employee; 2) in the manner of engagement of the student or employee with the material, such as how the individual takes notes or completes an assignment; and 3) in the way that a student or employee reports back to the teacher or employer through such means as tests or reports. An example of universal design is the use of public transportation. Instructions must be available in picture and written form to accommodate levels of literacy for acquisition of a ticket, and counters in which the ticket is inserted must be at a height appropriate for someone walking or in a wheelchair.

Successfully identifying and putting accommodations in place for an individual in either the school or work setting can be a complicated process that involves many people. It is also important to consider a plan for transitioning an accommodation plan across systems, especially in the case of health-related needs (Reiss & Gibson, 2002).

THE ACCOMMODATION PROCESS FOR SCHOOL AND WORK

Individual primary and secondary schools set the process for the initiation and development of the IEP described in IDEA, which would involve the development of an individualized accommodation plan when needed, as detailed in Section 504. This plan must be individualized to the student and include what the accommodations will be; who will be responsible for training and/or supplying the accommodations; what responsibilities the youth and their parents or guardians have; other needed services or accommodations; and a statement that the parents or guardians have read the plan, are aware of their rights according to the law, and agree to implement the plan (Heiler, 2004; National Association of School Nurses, 2001). Section 504 provides for the denial of requested accommodations based on undue costs or hardships for the schools (Schulzinger, 1999). For more information on the 504 process, refer to Chapter 11.

In the postsecondary school settings (e.g., colleges, universities), policies are in place based on the ADA of 1990 and Section 504 to accommodate students with disabilities. These policies typically can be found on the school's web page, often under headings such as Disability Support Services, Disabled Student Services, or Disability Resource Center. The steps for acquiring and maintaining accommodations are similar to those subsequently outlined for work settings. These policies often include a grievance procedure.

In the arena of work, the Office of Disability Employment Policy of the U.S. Department of Labor supports the Job Accommodation Network (JAN), which provides a comprehensive resource for individuals and agencies concerning job accommodations. JAN has specific web sites for both initiating a job accommodation request (Saab & Batiste, 2005) and the job accommodation process (Saab & Gamble, 2005). The processes described in these web sites are very similar. Luckasson and colleagues' (2002) individualized supports plan is also similar to this process.

JAN's process for requesting an accommodation is based on the ADA of 1990 and involves the following five steps:

1. Request for accommodation

2. Disability determination

3. Acceptance or denial of request and plan if accepted

4. Reassignment

5. Maintenance and evaluation of accommodation effectiveness (Saab & Batiste, 2005)

Request for Accommodation

The request for an accommodation can take place at any time from the time of initial application for employment through any point in time during employment. An employer does not have to make any accommodations if he or she is not informed of the need by an employee. Many employers, especially in large companies, have a formal accommodation process and officer who maintains the process (Saab & Batiste, 2005). An employee seeking an accommodation would need to check on the process in their place of employment. Examples of forms that may be used in the accommodation process can be found at: http://www.eeoc.gov/policy/docs/accommodation_procedures_eeoc.html.

Disability Determination

The next step involves the determination that a disability exists. Specifically, a determination must be made of the symptoms and/or functional limitations that are present for the employee and creating barriers to successful performance, and whether this situation is short- or long-term (Saab & Gamble, 2005). Employers may request medical documentation that a disability exists and that an accommodation is needed. Employers that do not have existing accommodation policies in place may need to develop such a process at this point, and one such policy would be specifically for requesting documentation of an existing disability. This medical information is confidential and needs to be kept separate from an individual's personnel file. Other employees that may be notified of the accommodations are supervisors, health personnel, government officials examining compliance with ADA, state worker's compensation offices, and/or the employer's insurance company (Saab & Batiste, 2005).

Acceptance or Denial of Request and Plan if Accepted

In Step 3, employers must determine if accommodations can be made in the employee's current position. Employers must decide if they can provide each accommodation requested, how they can obtain the accommodations, and if the accommodations would place undue hardship on them. Employers must assess whether modifications are needed for the job, current policies (including the need for a grievance policy), and/or the facility, such as the construction of a ramp or if additional equipment or services are needed. These and other decisions will form the basis of an acceptance or denial of the request (Saab & Batiste, 2005; Saab & Gamble, 2005).

Reassignment

Step 4 will only apply to those situations in which reassignment is an option. Such decisions are complicated by the availability of other jobs in which the person with a disability could participate, whether the available job is equivalent to the old job, and what should take place if the available position is higher or lower than the current position. ADA states that the employer does not have to provide a promotion to make the necessary accommodations (Saab & Batiste, 2005).

Maintenance and Evaluation of Accommodation Effectiveness

The final step in requesting an accommodation involves the maintenance of the accommodation. The employer must determine who is responsible for maintaining and monitoring the effectiveness of the accommodation and identify in what manner and how often communication will take place between this individual and the employee to assess the effectiveness of the accommodation. Most likely, this will be someone from the Department of Human Resources or their designee. In addition, provisions for length of time to provide needed accommodations must be considered in addition to any training required for the employee and the employer concerning new equipment or services. Finally, a process for documentation of this total process including periodic evaluation must be put in place and maintained (Saab & Batiste, 2005; Saab & Gamble, 2005).

The accommodation process is a complicated process that involves a number of people and often the consultation from a number of outside experts. At the center must be the individual with the disability.

SUMMARY

Many individuals with disabilities need assistance through accommodations to be successful in either the school or work setting. Formalized plans for requesting, acquiring, and maintaining these supports are in place in many places and when not, examples of such processes are available for adaptation. Federal laws are further in place to assist in making sure that such accommodations are available. National organizations, such as the AAIDD, provide models and assessment tools for use in making sure that supports or accommodations are properly identified, assessed, planned for, and evaluated (Luckasson et al., 2002). Yet, improvements are still needed across the nation in each setting. Technologies and services continue to improve, and with such improvement, so too will the lives of individuals with disabilities who need them improve. The references listed at the end of this chapter and the resources that appear at the end of this book can provide the reader with places to start to learn more about accommodations, appropriate accommodations, and processes to acquire needed accommodations.

My Story   Mary Ann Scoloveno

Several years ago, I was working as a pediatric nurse practitioner at an urban community clinic in New Jersey. One of my clients was an 8-year old boy who had been diagnosed with severe pervasive developmental disorder (PDD). The family had recently moved from another state in the hopes of finding a place that could help their child. The child was scheduled to attend school in a large urban school district. The school district had made it a policy to try and keep their special needs children within the district because they felt that they could educate them. Further, they believed that there were substantial financial constraints in sending these children out of the school district. It was their practice to place any child with a special health care need into one classroom with a teacher who was not proficient in autism spectrum disorders in general or PDD specifically. After learning of the diagnosis, the school's child study team wanted to adhere to this policy. I went to consult with them on PDD in general and as an advocate for the child and his family. I informed them that this child needed schooling year-long and that the appropriate student–teacher ratio, behavioral therapy needs, and a plan for inclusion did not seem to be available at that school. They said that they did not have a summer program and would not support paying for this child to attend school somewhere else for these needed services.

The parents were divorcing at this time with financial problems and the mother was at a loss of what to do. I informed her of a number of special schools in the state whose mission was to serve children with special needs and that a few specialized in autism spectrum disorders. She consequently visited each and determined that one of these schools could really help her child, but she did not have the money.

I suggested that she go back to the child's school and tell them about this special school with the appropriate services and ask again for them to cover the expenses for attending this school under IDEA. The school again refused.

When the mother told me of this disappointment, I informed her of the Office of Consumer Advocacy and said that she should tell the school that she would contact this office if they would not support her child attending the special school for children with autism spectrum disorders. They again refused and she went to see someone at the Office of Consumer Advocacy. The Office of Consumer Advocacy consequently ruled that the child's school did not have the faculty and curriculum to support the child's educational needs and said that the school would have to pay for the child to attend the special school.

This child did so and improved greatly and was able to return to his original school in a regular classroom within 3 years. The school district has since reassessed their special needs programs and made provisions for individualized care and education of children with similar problems. It is important that a pediatric nurse is able to assist families to place their child in an optimal educational setting where they can achieve to their highest potential. Child and youth advocacy is the hallmark of pediatric practice in schools and in the community.

REFERENCES

American Academy of Pediatrics Committee on Children with Disabilities. (2000). The role of the pediatrician in transitioning children and adolescents with developmental disabilities and chronic illnesses from school to work or college. *Pediatrics, 106,* 854–856.

Americans with Disabilities Act of 1990, PL 101-336, 42 U.S.C. §§ 12101 *et seq.*

Assistive Technology Act Amendments of 2004, PL 108-364, 29 U.S.C. §§ 3001 *et seq.*

Betz, C.L. (2001). Use of 504 plans for children and youth with disabilities: Nursing application. *Pediatric Nursing, 27*(4), 347–352.

Betz, C.L., & Redcay, G. (2002). Lessons learned from providing transition services to adolescents with special health care needs. *Issues in Comprehensive Pediatric Nursing, 25,* 129–149.

Caldwell, T.H., Sirvis, B.P., Still, J., Still, M., Schwab, N., Jones, J., et al. (1997). Students who require medical technology in school. In S. Porter, M. Haynie, T. Bierle, T.H. Caldwell, & J.S. Palfrey (Eds.), *Children and youth assisted by medical technology in educational settings: Guidelines for care* (2nd ed., pp. 3–18). Baltimore: Paul H. Brookes Publishing Co.

Disabilities, Opportunities, Internetworking, and Technology (DO-IT), University of Washington. (2005). *The faculty room.* Retrieved August 28, 2005, from http://www. washington.edu/doit/Faculty/Strategies/Disability/

Hart, D., Zimbrich, K., & Whelley, T. (2002). Challenges in coordinating and managing services and supports in secondary and postsecondary options. *Issue Brief of the National Center on Secondary Education and Transition, 1*(6). Retrieved March 15, 2005, from http://www.ncset.org/publications/printresource.asp?id=719

Hasselbring, T.S., & Glaser, C.H.W. (2000). Use of computer technology to help students with special needs. *The Future of Children, 10*(2), 102–122.

Heiler, K.W. (2004). Integrating health care and educational programs. In F.P. Orelove, D. Sobsey, & R.K. Silberman (Eds.), *Educating children with multiple disabilities: A collaborative approach* (4th ed., pp. 379-424). Baltimore: Paul H. Brookes Publishing Co.

Individuals with Disabilities Education Improvement Act of 2004, PL 108-446, 20 U.S.C. §§ 1400 *et seq.*

Johnson, C.P., & Dorval, J. (2005). *Transitions into adolescence.* Retrieved March 4, 2005, from http://www.sbaa.org/atf/cf/(99DD789C-904D-467E-A2E4-DF1D36E381CD)/adolescence. pdf

Learning Disabilities Association of America. (2005). *Transitioning from college to work.* Retrieved August 8, 2005, from http://www.ldanatl.org/aboutld/professionals/transitioning.asp

Luckasson, R., Borthwick-Duffy, S., Buntinx, W.H.E., Coulter, D.L., Craig, E.M., Reeve, A., et. al. (2002). *Mental retardation: Definition, classification, and systems of supports* (10th ed.). Washington, DC: American Association on Mental Retardation.

Luckasson, R., Coulter, D.L., Polloway, E.A., Reiss, S., Schalock, R.L., Snell, M.E., et al. (1992). *Mental retardation: Definition, classification, and systems of supports* (9th ed.). Washington, DC: American Association on Mental Retardation.

National Association of School Nurses. (2001). *Section 504 of the Rehabilitation Act of 1973.* Castle Rock, CO: Author.

National Center for Education Statistics. (2000). *What are the barriers to the use of advanced telecommunications for students with disabilities in public schools?* (NCES 2000-042) Washington, DC: U.S. Department of Education, Office of Educational Research and Improvement.

National Center on Secondary Education and Transition. (2005). *National standards for secondary education and transition for all youth.* Minneapolis, MN: Author.

National Council on Disability. (2005). *Information technology and Americans with Disabilities: An overview of innovation, laws, progress and challenges.* Washington, DC: Author.

Rehabilitation Act of 1973, PL 93-112, 29 U.S.C. §§ 701 *et seq.*

Reiss, J., & Gibson, R. (2002). Health care transition: Destinations unknown. *Pediatrics, 110,* 1307–1314.

Saab, T.D., & Batiste, L.C. (2005). *Reasonable accommodation and the ADA process.* Retrieved August 8, 2005, from http://www.jan.wvu.edu/media/raproc.html

Saab, T.D., & Gamble, M.J. (2005). *The job accommodation process.* Retrieved August 8, 2005, from http://www.jan.wvu.edu/media/JobAccommodationProcess.html

Schultz, A.W., & Liptak, G.S. (1998). Helping adolescents who have disabilities negotiate transitions to adulthood. *Issues in Comprehensive Pediatric Nursing, 21,* 187–201.

Schulzinger, R. (1999). *Understanding the 504 statute: The role of state Title V programs and health care providers.* Gainesville, FL: Institute for Child Health Policy.

Silverstein, R. (2005). *A user's guide to the 2004 IDEA reauthorization (P.L. 108-446 and the conference report).* Washington, DC: The Center for the Study and Advancement of Disability Policy.

Thompson, J.R., Bryant, B.R., Campbell, E.M., Craig, E.M., Hughes, C., Rothholz, D.A., et al. (2004). *Supports intensity scale: User's manual.* Washington, DC: American Association on Mental Retardation.

Thurlow, M. (2002). Accommodations for students with disabilities in high school. *Issue brief of the National Center on Secondary Education and Transition, 1*(1). Retrieved March 15, 2005, from http://www.ncset.org/publications/printresource.asp?id=247

U.S. Government Accountability Office. (2005). *No Child Left Behind Act: Most students with disabilities participated in statewide assessments, but inclusion options could be improved.* Washington, DC: Author.

Weist, M.D., Lowie, J.A., Flaherty, L.T., & Pruitt, D. (2001). Collaboration among the education, mental health, and public health systems to promote youth mental health. *Psychiatric Services, 52,* 1348–1351.

Weymeyer, M.L., Sands, D.J., Knowlton, H.E., & Kozleski, E.B. (2002). *Teaching students with mental retardation: Providing access to the general curriculum.* Baltimore: Paul H. Brookes Publishing Co.

Williams, J. (2001). *Resources you can use: Adaptations and accommodations for students with disabilities.* Washington, DC: National Dissemination Center for Children with Disabilities.

Health Care Transition Plans

CHAPTER 7

Methods of Assessing Transition Health Care Needs

SUSAN W. LEDLIE

Within the health care community there is an awareness of the need to accommodate the health care and transitional care needs of the growing number of youth with special health care needs and disabilities who are surviving into adulthood (McDonagh, 2005). This is evidenced by a growing body of literature on transition needs and national consensus statements (Betz, 2004). The Centers for Disease Control and Prevention, the National Institute on Disability and Rehabilitation and the U.S. Department of Health and Human Services' *Healthy People 2010*, and the joint consensus statement by the American Academy of Pediatrics (AAP), the American Academy of Family Physicians (AAFP), and the American College of Physicians-American Society of Internal Medicine (ACP-ASIM) (2002) highlight the importance of transitioning youth with special health care needs and disabilities to maximize lifelong functioning and potential through the provision of high-quality, developmentally appropriate health care services that continue uninterrupted from adolescence into adulthood.

Healthy People 2010 established the goal that all youth with special health care needs and disabilities will receive the services needed to make necessary transitions to adulthood, specifically including health care, employment, and independent living. The Maternal and Child Health Bureau (2001) developed a 10-year action plan to facilitate health care transition as an addendum to *Healthy People 2010* and identified six core expectations in achieving community-based systems of services for youth with special health care needs and disabilities. Two of these core expectations are particularly relevant to this chapter and include 1) families of youth with special health care needs and disabilities will participate in decision making at all levels and will be satisfied with the services they receive, and 2) all youth with special health care needs and disabilities will receive the services necessary to make appropriate transitions to all aspects of adult life, including adult health care, work, and independence.

The joint consensus statement on transitioning youth with special health care needs and disabilities into adult health care settings developed by the AAP, the AAFP, and the ACP-ASIM (2002) stated that all youth with special health care needs and disabilities should have a written health care transition plan by the age of 14 years. The goals of transitioning health care include 1) maximizing lifelong functioning and potential through the provision of high-quality, developmentally appropriate, and uninterrupted health care services that continue from adolescence into adulthood and 2) ensuring that all providers who care for youth with special health care needs and disabilities have the knowledge and skills to facilitate the transition from a child-focused to an adult-oriented system of care to ensure uninterrupted, high-quality care.

There is unanimous agreement in the literature that the health care transition from pediatric to adult medical care for youth with special health care needs and disabilities, rather than being a one-time event, is a process that begins at diagnosis for both families and providers (Betz, 1998, 2004; Blum et al., 1993; McDonagh, 2005; Olsen & Swigonski, 2004; Reiss, Gibson, & Walker 2005; Scal, Evans, Blozis, Okinow, & Blum, 1999). Because the transition from pediatric to adult health care is affected by so many forces and factors, it proceeds at different rates within the developmental context of youth with special health care needs and disabilities and their families (Reiss et al., 2005). As the key stakeholders, youth must be motivated to become active participants in, be in agreement with, and be prepared for the transition process (Reiss & Gibson, 2002). Results from studies that have been conducted in the adolescent transition projects funded by the Maternal and Child Health Bureau (2001) indicated that many youth with special health care needs and disabilities have minimal or no experience in managing or discussing their own medical conditions. In addition, these youth and their families struggle to locate information about community resources, deal with ineffective systems of communication, and experience poor health care coordination (Betz & Redcay, 2003). Health care providers and other professionals have been encouraged to engage youth with special health care needs and disabilities and their families in discussion and planning well in advance of the transition. These discussions will serve to empower youth and their families with needed information and resources to proactively manage their care and to plan for the future.

The critical first step to ensuring successful transitioning into adult care systems begins with the health care transition assessment process. This process allows providers to enter into a discussion with youth and their families to identify their needs and goals in order to design a developmentally appropriate written transition plan that should be in place when youth are between 14 and 16 years of age (IDEA 2004). Findings from transition studies have shown that youth with special health care needs and disabilities and their caregivers expressed many concerns regarding transition including leaving familiar people whom they trusted, having to meet a new team of health care providers, and experiencing a possible decline in the quality of care that will be provided (Boyle, Farukhi, & Nosky 2001; Hauser & Dorn, 1999; Madge & Byron, 2002; Scal & Ireland, 2005). Parents were concerned about their child's ability to perform their own health-related self-care, as well as their role in the provision of that care (Boyle et al., 2001). On the other hand, youth expressed concern that their parents refused to let them grow up and take control of their own health care management (Hauser & Dorn, 1999; Patterson & Lanier, 1999). Given these findings, it is incumbent upon providers to systematically plan and assist youth with special health care needs and disabilities and their families in making the transition into adulthood and the adult health care, educational, and vocational systems (Telfair, Alleman-Velez, Dickens, & Loosier, 2005).

This chapter will 1) define the health care transition assessment process and its objectives and goals; 2) describe the transition readiness criteria used to identify the needs of youth with special health care needs and disabilities and their families; 3) illustrate how transition readiness criteria are incorporated into the transition readiness assessment; 4) present three case studies and discuss their clinical application to the individualized education program (IEP), 504 plan, and individualized plan for employment (IPE); 5) discuss how to integrate the findings from the health care transition assessment process into educational and vocational settings; and 6) review resources available to guide providers, youth, and their families through the health care transition assessment process.

HEALTH CARE TRANSITION ASSESSMENT PROCESS

The health care transition assessment process is a comprehensive, ongoing process that attends to the medical needs of youth with special health care needs and disabilities as they move from child-focused to adult-focused health care services (Blum et al., 1993). Transition assessment is also an integral part of the special education process for youth as it provides a framework for identifying their strengths, needs, and interests as they progress through educational, vocational, and postschool environments (Neubert, 2003). Data obtained in the transition assessment process informs the transition plan. This information can assist youth, their families, and health care and school personnel in developing objectives and goals, and identifying services that can be incorporated into the health care transition plan, IEP, 504 plan, and IPE (Stilton, Neubert, & Leconte, 1997).

All youth with special health care needs and disabilities and their families face the same, although individualized, transitions in broad areas of functioning (health care, education, community living, employment, and socialization). This creates psychosocial challenges that youth and their families face in coping with the daily demands of living with a life-changing health concern. For example, parents will experience additional caregiver demands for managing daily treatment regimens such as dressing changes, gastrostomy feedings, postural drainage, and administration of daily medications. Family members will experience the anguish of the uncertainty of the disease course. Many youth with special health care needs and disabilities will experience isolation from their peers due to the perceived stigma of physical disabilities associated with the chronic health condition or disability. However, the degree of differentiation in these areas of functioning will be dictated by the nature and nuances of that condition/disability.

The health care transition assessment process represents an individualized, developmental framework for planning for this multifaceted phase of life that is so important to youth with special health care needs and disabilities. The objectives of the health care transition assessment process are to 1) determine the needs for interventions in transition plans in the health care setting and 2) integrate the findings into school and work settings for the purposes of developing an IEP, 504 plan, and/or an IPE. (For additional information on IEPs, 504 plans, and IPEs, refer to Chapters 6, 10, and 11.) The goals of the health care transition assessment process are to develop a written plan that 1) addresses major concerns, needs, preferences, abilities, and/or desires identified by youth with special health care needs and disabilities and their caregivers; 2) contains relevant data in areas of health care, self-care, community living, education, employment,

careers, sexuality, socialization, lifestyle, personal awareness, and financial resources; 3) fosters independence and communication skills to enable youth to
communicate with education and service providers regarding their health concerns; 4) identifies needed services, supports, accommodations, and linkages; 5)
improves knowledge of youth with special health care needs and disabilities
about managing their health concerns and lifestyle; and 6) promotes health care
decision making as youth become advocates for their health care. An effective
plan will serve to ensure quality outcomes in transitioning youth from pediatric
to adult health systems, as well as in educational, vocational, and community
arenas (Neubert, 2003).

Communication between educators, health care and related service providers, and youth with special health care needs and disabilities and their families is essential during the health care transition assessment process. Youth and
their families must be encouraged to identify their needs and major concerns as
they are the experts in dealing with challenges of living with a chronic condi-
tion/disability. The youth and family's perspective provides essential information
and insights into creating a transition plan that is developmentally age appropriate and meets their needs. Many federal, state, educational, and professional organizations have developed multimedia materials to guide youth with special
health care needs and disabilities, their families, and professional caregivers,
health care providers, and educators through the health care transition assessment process.

TRANSITION READINESS CRITERIA

Betz's (2004) review and analysis of 43 transition studies published from 1982
through 2003 reported that chronological age was the most cited primary criteria
for transitioning youth with special health care needs and disabilities to adult care
systems. The most frequently cited age range for transitioning was reported to
be between 16 and 22 years (Anderson, Flume, Hardy, & Grey, 2002; Court,
1991, 1993; Gennen, Powers, & Sells, 2003; Pacaud, McConnell, Huot, Aebi, &
Yale, 1996; Steinkamp, Ullrich, Muller, Fabel, & von der Hardt, 2001; Westwood,
Henley, & Willcox, 1999).

The concept of *transition readiness* has also been studied (Capelli, MacDonald,
& McGrath, 1989; Hauser & Dorn, 1999; Rettig & Athreya, 1991). Based on the
responses of youth with special health care needs and disabilities, family caregivers,
and professional providers, additional transition readiness criteria and their
components have been identified for initiating transfer to adult health systems
(Betz & Redcay, 2003; Cappelli et al., 1999; Hauser & Dorn, 1999; McDonagh,
2005; Reiss et al., 2005; Rettig & Athreya, 1991; Scal & Ireland, 2005). These include physical and cognitive maturity, current medical status and stability, self-care
skills, adherence to therapies, family functioning, social support systems, self-advocacy, sexuality, educational and vocational planning, financial assistance, and
health insurance. Assessing the components of each criterion listed in Table 7.1 allows for an evaluation of the skills and knowledge needed by the youth to assume
greater or even sole responsibility for his or her self-care. Developmental readiness
to assume aspects of self-care, which relies on physical and psychological readiness
in addition to age, can also be assessed (Table 7.1). For more information related to
interpreting transition readiness criteria, identifying the skills needed for health

Table 7.1. Components of transition readiness criteria

Transition readiness criteria	Components
Maturational/developmental level	Demonstrates some level of parental/family independence and independent life skills
Cognitive ability	Assesses level of cognitive ability related to medical dependence and reliance on parents and other caregivers
Medical condition	Demonstrates an understanding of chronic condition and related complications, knowledge of medications, and knowledge of past medical history; can report illness/functional status; demonstrates skills in decision making about health care
Medical stability	Chronic condition is stable and well controlled; transitioning to adult systems should not be done during periods of illness exacerbations or medication changes
Self-care skills	Demonstrates good health management skills, including daily self-care, illness/disability related self-care, and independent living skills in home, school, community settings
Adherence	Demonstrates adherence to appointments, medications, treatment regimens, and ongoing preventative health care in home, school, community settings
Family functioning	Goes to appointments with parent or primary caregiver; shared management of chronic condition to achieve effective interdependence; family provides appropriate support; family member needs are addressed
Social support system	Identifies family members, peers, resources for ongoing support and advice
Self-advocacy	Demonstrates a working knowledge of the medical system and skills in negotiating health care and related systems such as social services; understands rights and responsibilities
Sexuality	Knowledge of reproductive and sexual health, genetic considerations, impact of chronic condition on puberty and sexual functioning, vulnerability to sexual abuse or exploitation, access to confidential services and sexual health information in community
Educational and vocational planning	Articulates realistic aspirations and plans for future education, vocation, and career; incorporated into individualized education plan, a 504 plan, or individualized plan for employment

(continued)

Table 7.1. *(continued)*

Health and lifestyle	Knowledge of medical condition/ secondary condition effects with regard to lifestyle choices, social activities, mood changes, accident and injury prevention, levels of care; knowledge of and health implications of risky behaviors (e.g., tobacco, alcohol, drugs); ability to participate in community activities to promote a healthy lifestyle and development of social and recreational skills
Financial	Active insurance coverage, availability of entitlements, financial assistance, and social services as determined by chronic condition

care self-care and long-term disability management, and developing strategies to facilitate acquisition of these skills by youth with special health care needs and disabilities, refer to Chapter 4.

TRANSITION READINESS ASSESSMENT

Comprehensive assessment tools that contain transition readiness criteria can serve as a springboard to begin a discussion with youth with special health care needs and disabilities and their families about their knowledge and expectations of adult care systems. Many of these checklists, surveys, and questionnaires have already been developed for professionals, youth, and their caregivers, with a focus on a particular chronic illness/disability (Capelli et al., 1989; Telfair, Myers, & Drezner, 1994). Figure 7.1 presents an example of a questionnaire that incorporates transition readiness criteria in addressing common areas of assessment and planning that might be used for this purpose. Although general in scope, it allows for individual differences dictated by a particular health condition/disability and provides a transition plan for addressing them.

The health care provider can administer this questionnaire to the youth to determine his or her abilities for health and self-care management at visits scheduled specifically to address the health care transition process. These questions can also be discussed with family caregivers as well in determining health-related considerations affecting the youth's future goals and aspirations. Additional background information, including psychological assessments, IQ and academic achievement scores, identified formal and informal supports and accommodations, and life skills abilities can augment that which is obtained in the health care interview to provide a comprehensive assessment (Neubert, 2003).

Based on this assessment, the needs and goals for transition services and resources can be identified. Individualized interventions can be developed, tailored to fit a specific chronic condition/disability, and incorporated into the written transition plan. For example, the renegotiation of health-related self-care, such as medication administration, that takes place in a family with an adolescent who has neurodevelopmental disabilities and cognitive impairment is going to be very different from that of a family with an adolescent who is HIV positive, asymptomatic, and has age-appropriate development. An adolescent with an intellectual disability will require additional, highly structured, and graphic instruction that

Activities of Daily Living

What self-care skills, such as hygiene and dressing, does the youth have?

What housekeeping skills does the youth have for meal planning, shopping, cooking, cleaning, and maintaining living space and clothing?

How will the youth deal with emergencies?

Is the youth organized, enabling tasks to be completed?

What resources and supports are available?

How can they be obtained?

Health-Related Care

What does the youth know about his or her chronic condition, medications, side effects?

What skills does the youth have and/or need to learn to monitor changes in physical condition?

Does the youth participate in therapies and treatment regimens?

Does the youth use any assistive technology?

What other aspects of health-related care does youth do for him- or her-self?

What aspects of health-related care do parents or family caregivers provide?

Does the youth keep health care provider appointments?

Does the youth attend medical appointments alone or with a family member/other person?

Does the youth follow prescribed medical regimen and treatments?

Is the youth's chronic condition under control?

Does the youth communicate independently with health care providers?

Is the youth involved in health care decisions?

What support is available to assist the youth with self-care needs (e.g., personal care attendant, home care nursing services, equipment, supplies)?

How can identified supports and resources be obtained?

What is the youth's source of primary care for general health monitoring, immunizations, preventive health counseling, sexuality education and supports, dental care, mental health support?

(continued)

Figure 7.1.   Areas of assessment and planning for transitioning youth with special health care needs and disabilities. Adapted from Blomquist, Brown, Peersen, & Pressler (1993). Transitioning to independence: Challenges for young people with disabilities and their caregivers. *Orthopaedic Nursing, 17*(3), 27–35.

Figure 7.1. *(continued)*

Living Arrangements

Where does the youth live/wish to live?

With whom does the youth currently live?

What are housing options in the community?

Does the youth require adaptive aids (e.g., ramps, railings, kitchen supports) for independent living?

What are the effects of decisions about living arrangements on the family?

What resources and supports are available?

How can they be obtained?

Mobility

What ability does the youth have to access all facilities used for daily living activities, education, employment, recreation?

What access does the youth have to public transportation or other transportation options in the community?

Is the youth able to access and complete driver's education to become a licensed driver?

What vehicle adaptations, if any, are required?

What adaptation resources are available in the community?

How can they be obtained?

Education

Does the youth attend school or receive home instruction?

What accommodations would be needed to attend school?

Will the youth complete high school or equivalency?

What are the barriers to completing secondary education?

What college or technical school opportunities are available?

What kind of career would youth like to pursue?

What skills and educational programs are required for that career?

Does the youth have enough education/training for the job/career desired?

What other educational options are available (e.g., adult education, continuing education)?

How can they be obtained?

What financial aid is available?

Does the youth understand what rights and protections are available through the ADA laws with regard to education, jobs, and accommodations?

Employment

Has the youth had any home or community jobs?

What skills does the youth have?

What does the youth like to do?

What type of environment does the youth want to work in?

What types of training programs is the youth interested in attending?

What places of employment might fit the youth's choices?

What places of employment/training programs are available in the community?

Are there summer jobs, part-time jobs, in-school jobs, volunteer, non-paid training experiences available?

How can they be obtained?

Finances

What are sources of money for this youth?

What skills in budgeting, bill paying, use of ATMs, checking and savings accounts, and credit cards does the youth have?

What can be learned?

What supports are needed? Are they available? How does the youth access them?

What entitlements does the youth receive?

What financial assistance is the youth eligible for?

How are they obtained?

What are the trade-offs between earnings from work and income from these sources?

Does the youth have active insurance coverage?

(continued)

Figure 7.1. *(continued)*

Socialization

Does the youth have friends?

Is the youth dating?

Is the youth sexually active?

Does the youth identify peers, family members, others who provide advice/ support?

Does the youth identify any role models?

Does the youth attend any counseling activities?

Does the youth attend any illness-related peer support groups?

What counseling opportunities are available?

How would they be obtained?

Lifestyle

What does the youth like to do for fun and for physical and mental fitness?

What skills does the youth have?

Is the youth aware of the way in which his or her medical condition affects activities/lifestyle choices?

What community resources are available for sports, shopping, movies, visiting?

How can they be accessed?

Personal Awareness

How aware is the youth of how he or she interacts with or has an effect on others because of physical, communication, or emotional expression attributes?

How does the youth express anger?

How does the youth mediate conflict?

How does the youth solve problems or make decisions?

Does the youth have a sense of humor?

Does the youth have skills in personal advocacy?

What resources are available to build personal awareness skills?

corresponds with his or her level of cognitive functioning. In contrast, teaching that is more abstract in terms of presentation of content can be used for adolescents whose cognitive competencies correlate to their developmental norms.

The written transition plan should include what services need to be provided, who will provide them, when they will be provided, and how they will be financed. A well planned and successful transition to adult care systems, whether it be medical, educational, or vocational, is critical to ensuring the long-term health, quality of life, and productivity of youth with special health care needs and disabilities. Ultimately, how useful "the fit" of the assessment and subsequent written transition plan is will be determined by the youth and their families (see Chapter 8). Their feedback will inform what interventions were effective in making the transition a successful one and what could be improved. For additional information on evaluation measures to determine the effectiveness of health care transition planning outcomes, refer to Chapter 9.

CLINICAL APPLICATION OF THE HEALTH CARE TRANSITION ASSESSMENT

The following three case studies illustrate the identification of health needs and their incorporation into a written transition plan. A description of how this information can be integrated into an IEP, 504 plan, and an IPE as a mechanism for reinforcing skills learned in the health care setting is presented, as well as examples of interagency collaboration to facilitate coordination of services.

Application to Practice 1: Rosaria's Transition Assessment and IEP

Rosaria has been a patient at a major children's hospital in the region since she was hospitalized in the neonatal intensive care unit as a premature infant with multiple problems. Rosario's diagnoses included tetralogy of Fallot and short bowel syndrome. She has been seen by a team of specialists at the children's hospital who has managed her care. Over the years, the members of the specialized medical team—who included her physicians, nurses, social worker, psychologist, and occupational and physical therapists—worked with her and her family to ensure that they could manage the daily treatment needs required by her conditions.

Now that Rosaria is in high school, team members have begun planning for her transition to adult health services. The team initiated the transition planning process by conducting a thorough assessment using a tool that they adapted from another pediatric hospital. Based on the assessment, the team, in conjunction with Rosaria and her family, developed a transition health care plan that included Rosaria's needs to learn to assume more responsibility for her daily self-care needs, to obtain information on health insurance options, to find adult specialists who are knowledgeable about her childhood acquired conditions, and to inform her teachers and case managers about her continued needs for accommodations in work and community living settings.

Rosaria's specialized, interdisciplinary team determined that the school nurse needed to be contacted about the team's transition planning to discuss what, if any, collaboration was possible between the school and the team. The team's pediatric nursing care coordinator informed the school nurse about the health care transition planning that they had conducted. In response, the school nurse suggested that a member of the specialized health care team participate in Rosario's upcoming transition IEP. The pediatric nursing coordinator responded to the suggestion and participated with the other members of the transition IEP team. Comprehensively, the team members addressed Rosaria's needs for successfully transitioning to adulthood, which included identifying her health-related needs. Rosaria's transition plan for health-related needs included strategies to coordinate activities with her specialized health care team. This invitation to participate in Rosaria's transition IEP resulted not only in having a member of the specialized health care team involved in her transition planning but also in the development of an interagency partnership involving many more specialized teams from this pediatric facility and the school district.

Application to Practice 2: Rob's Transition Assessment and 504 Plan

Rob is 16 years old and has had insulin-dependent diabetes for 10 years. His health care provider initiated the health care transition assessment process by reviewing with Rob what his goals were related to applying for college and gaining employment. Rob indicated that he wanted to attend an out-of-state college and live in a dormitory. His career goal was to become a high school math teacher.

Using a questionnaire similar to the one outlined in Figure 7.1, Rob's nurse practitioner determined what Rob was capable of doing independently and the areas that required additional learning of health care skills to manage his diabetes. The assessment revealed that Rob was knowledgeable in several areas of his health care: he understood his disease process and diet, the symptoms of having and treating a low-blood sugar reaction, the actions of his insulins, and monitoring his diabetes supplies. However, the assessment also revealed that Rob was deficient in some areas of managing his diabetes independently on a long-term basis. For example, he had not assumed responsibility for making his own medical appointments, knowing from where and how to obtain his diabetes supplies, and submitting information to insurance companies. Additionally, Rob had not explored the availability of health care providers in the college student health service or in the town where the college was located. Rob and his health care provider also reviewed the accommodations that would be necessary in the dormitory living arrangements to accommodate his diabetes. Such accommodations included having a refrigerator available in his room to store his insulin, as well as a mechanism for disposing of his lancets and insulin syringes.

Based on this assessment, a plan was devised for Rob to assume greater independency and self-sufficiency in managing his diabetes. The findings were communicated to Rob's parents and his school service coordinator and were integrated into his 504 plan to assist with his transition planning to college life. Having identified that he had an expanded knowledge of his diabetes-related self-care needs, as well as those areas in which he needed to acquire additional health self-care skills, he was able to take a more active role with the school transition team in planning for his college life.

Application to Practice 3: Jared's IPE

Jared has cerebral palsy and attends a 4-year college in the city where he lives. He had participated in the job training program jointly offered by the state Vocation Rehabilitation Department and local school district. Through this program, Jared has been working several hours a week in a local high tech business that develops computer microchips. Jared's interest was piqued in computer technology when he first visited the high tech business two years ago during a career awareness experience at school.

Following high school graduation, Jared continued as a state vocation rehabilitation beneficiary and he worked with his rehabilitation counselor in developing an IPE. His IPE contained his goals for employment, which included his enrollment in the college's

Department of Computer Sciences, computer work station accommodations, and modifications for the computer he uses at school. Jared contacted the social work coordinator of his specialized health care team to request that she participate in a conference call with him and his rehabilitation counselor to provide consultation regarding the type of accommodations needed for his computer and work station. Jared and his rehabilitation counselor plan on reevaluating his IPE after he has completed his first semester of work.

As these three case studies illustrate, multidisciplinary and interagency collaboration is essential to facilitate a team effort that integrates service approaches to ensure successful transitions for youth with special health care needs and disabilities in all areas. However, the overall question remains: How is the information from the health care transition assessment process communicated to and coordinated with other agencies and related systems of care to ensure a successful transition? Historically, the sharing of health-related information between community health care providers and educational/vocational settings has been due to the persistence of individual efforts of parents, professionals, and youth themselves (Betz, 1998; Reiss & Gibson, 2002). Study findings continue to report on the obstacles that exist in integrating information from the health care transition assessment process into educational and vocational settings (Betz, 2004; Reiss & Gibson, 2002). The health care provider may have limited knowledge of community agencies for initiating referrals (Betz, 2004; Olsen & Swigonski, 2004). In addition, the youth's school or vocational program may not request health care provider input (Betz & Redcay, 2005). Educational, vocational, and health care systems are complicated with bureaucratic structures that are extremely difficult to navigate. These organizational characteristics preclude a route that facilitates easy access to and sharing of information (Reiss & Gibson, 2002). Yet, for transition planning to be successful for youth with special health care needs and disabilities, there needs to be collaboration between health care providers and community-based services (Betz, 2004).

INTERAGENCY INTEGRATION
OF THE HEALTH CARE TRANSITION ASSESSMENT

The process by which the health care needs and interventions are integrated into the IEP, 504 plan, and IPE will vary depending on the policies and practices of local communities and states. Ideally, health-related transition needs and a plan of care addressing health and health-related interventions are done in conjunction with the IEP, 504 plan, and IPE team members. The discrepancy between the ideal, as specified by IDEA legislation and/or by evidence-based professional best practices, and actual implementation at the local level is due to a number of factors. These include the lack of collaboration by interagency partners, lack of resources available to fund adequate levels of needed staff, lack of understanding of the transition best practices by local professionals and service providers (Betz, 1999; Flume, Anderson, Hardy, & Grey, 2001; Neubert, 2003; Telfair et al., 2005), and the limitations associated with a system of dissemination of the evidence-based transition best practices to consumers, professionals, and community-based providers in local communities (Reiss & Gibson, 2002). Interagency cross training and discipline-specific education for professionals and service providers who provide transition services to youth with special health care needs and disabilities and their families will assist them in working more effectively with each other.

TRANSITION-RELATED RESOURCES

Many tools have been created and are being integrated into clinical practice to assist professionals, youth with special health care needs and disabilities, and their families in preparing for the transition to adult care systems. A number of interactive resources that can be used in clinical and educational settings are listed below. For additional information on web site resources on transition assessment, refer to Appendix A.

Transition Questionnaires/ Surveys/Checklists/Information Sheets

These resources are available for youth and their families who are beginning the process of transitioning from pediatric to adult health care systems. The resources are helpful in identifying key issues for discussion and allow for identification of needs (e.g., school, medical, financial, legal, vocational) by youth with special health care needs and disabilities and their families. A compendium of resources are available at http://internet.dscc.uic.edu/dsccroot/parents/transition. asp. Similarly, Washington State's Adolescent Health Transition Project offers a comprehensive, informational notebook titled *Working Together for Successful Transition Notebook*. It can be downloaded from http://depts.washington.edu/healthtr/ notebook/content_documents.html.

Life Maps

Life maps identify the end goals of the transition plan. This graphic approach can be used by youth with special health care needs and disabilities and their caregivers to identify what they have considered or planned for life as an adult. Life maps are developmentally appropriate, designed for specific age groups, and allow youth and their families to document completed and anticipated transition activities. These life maps are available from the Healthy and Ready To Work-Kentucky (HRTW-KY) KY Teach project under the "Becoming Independent" link at: http://chfs.ky.gov/ccshcn/ccshcntransition.htm.

Transition Timelines

Transition timelines provide a lifespan framework with a futuristic orientation via a spreadsheet of benchmarks which serve to highlight activities according to age groups that identify parent and child interactions that encourage independence in arranging and managing their own health care and other areas of daily life. The *Transition Timeline for Children and Adolescents with Special Health Care Needs* is available from Washington State's Adolescent Health Transition Project at http://depts.washington.edu/healthtr/Timelines/timeline.htm.

Health Care Skills Checklists

Health care skills checklists are used to assist youth with special health care needs and disabilities as they move toward adulthood in assuming responsibility for their own care. These checklists allow for ongoing measurement of the independent skills that have been achieved. Health care skills checklists identify youths' mastery of skills, as well as skills that still need to be practiced. The *What is Transition?* health care skills checklist is available at http://depts.washington.edu/transmet.

School-to-Work Checklists

School-to-work checklists assist youth with special health care needs and disabilities in planning for their future after high school. Checklists are designed to provide them with key components of planning for independent living, employment, and postsecondary education. The *School to Work Checklist* and the *Employment Information Sheet* are available at http://internet.dscc.uic.edu/dsccroot/parents/transition.asp.

Youth Planners

Youth planners are tools that assist youth with special health care needs and disabilities learn about their health condition and participate in their health care management. Information is compiled in a written database record, which includes health information, changing care requirements, immunizations, medications, contacts, insurance information, emergency planning, school information, and an appointment calendar. On-Trac Youth Transition Services at British Columbia's Children's Hospital provides a planner titled *Your Plan-It*, an excellent resource to assist youth in transition. Copies are available from On-Trac: A Transition Service for Youth, Families, and Health Care Providers, Children's & Women's Health Centre of British Columbia, 4500 Oak St., Room B426, Vancouver, BC V6H 3N1. The cost is $20.00 each plus $5.00 shipping/postage/handling. For more information, contact Dr. Roey Malleson (rmalleson@cw.bc.ca), the director of the Youth Health Program.

Youth Workbooks

Youth workbooks provide opportunities for youth with special health care needs and disabilities to participate in skill development exercises. This is another tool by which youth are supported and encouraged to participate in their health care and transition planning. Workbooks are versatile instructional resources that can be used in health care and/or education, as well as with individual youth or in group workshops. The University of Florida's Institute for Child Health Policy has published *Health Care Transition Workbooks* for youth ages 12–18+ years. To access the workbooks, visit http://hctransitions.ichp.edu/resources.html.

SUMMARY

This chapter presented information on the health care transition assessment process (HCTAP). Description of the transition readiness criteria used to identify the needs of youth with special health care needs and disabilities and their families and illustration of how transition readiness criteria are incorporated into the transition readiness assessment was provided. Clinical examples to demonstrate the application of the HCTAP in educational and vocational settings were discussed. Internet web site addresses have been provided to assist youth with special health care needs

and disabilities and their families to avail themselves of a variety of health care related transition resources. Assessment of the youth health and health-related transition needs is the essential first step in developing a comprehensive plan of care
that addresses their future goals for adulthood. Working collaboratively with
agency providers and youth with special health care needs and disabilities and their
families to implement the written transition plan is critical to ensuring a successful
transition to adult care.

REFERENCES

American Academy of Pediatrics, American Academy of Family Physicians, American
    College of Physicians-American Society of Internal Medicine. (2002). A consensus
    statement on health care transitions for young adults with special health care needs. *Pe-
    diatrics, 110*, 1304–1306.
Anderson, D., Flume, P., Hardy, K., & Grey, S. (2002). Transition programs in cystic fibro-
    sis centers: Perceptions of patients. *Pediatric Pulmonology, 33*, 327–331.
Betz, C.L. (1998). Facilitating the transition of adolescents with chronic conditions from
    pediatric to adult health care and community settings. *Issues in Comprehensive Pediatric
    Nursing, 21*, 97–115.
Betz, C.L. (1999). Adolescents with chronic conditions: Linkages to adult service systems.
    Pediatric Nursing, 25(5), 473–476.
Betz, C.L. (2004). Transition of adolescents with special health care needs: Review and
    analysis of the literature. *Issues in Comprehensive Pediatric Nursing, 27*, 179–241.
Betz, C.L., & Redcay, G. (2003). Lessons learned from providing transition services to adoles-
    cents with special health care needs. *Issues in Comprehensive Pediatric Nursing, 25*, 129–149.
Betz, C.L., & Redcay, G. (2005). An exploratory study of future plans and extracurricular
    activities of transition-age youth and young adults. *Issues in Comprehensive Nursing,
    28*(33), 33–61.
Blomquist, K.B., Brown, G., Peersen, A., & Presler, B. (1998). Transitioning to indepen-
    dence: Challenges for young people with disabilities and their caregivers. *Orthopaedic
    Nursing, 17* (3), 27–35.
Blum, R.W., Garell, D., Hodgman, C.H., Jorissen, T., Okinow, N., Orr, D., et al. (1993).
    Transition from child-centered to adult health-care systems for adolescents with
    chronic conditions: A position paper of the Society for Adolescent Medicine. *Journal of
    Adolescent Health, 14*, 570–576.
Boyle, M.P., Farukhi, Z., & Nosky, M.L. (2001). Strategies for improving transition to adult
    cystic fibrosis care based on patient and parent views. *Pediatric Pulmonology, 32*, 428–436.
Cappelli, M., MacDonald, N., & McGrath, P. (1989). Assessment for readiness to transfer
    to adult care for adolescents with cystic fibrosis. *Children's Health Care, 18*, 218–224.
Centers for Disease Control and Prevention, National Institute on Disability and Rehabilita-
    tion Research, and U.S. Department of Health and Human Services. (2000). Disability
    and secondary conditions. *Healthy People 2010.* Washington, DC: U.S. Public Health Ser-
    vice, U.S. Department of Health and Human Services. Retrieved March 2, 2006, from
    http://www.cdc.gov/ncbddd/dh/schp.htm
Court, J. (1991). Outpatient based transition services for youth. *Pediatrician, 18*, 150–156.
Court, J. (1993). Issues of transition to adult care. *Journal of Paediatrics & Child Health, 29*,
    S53–S55.
Flume, P., Anderson, D., Hardy, K., & Grey, S. (2001). Transition programs in cystic fibro-
    sis centers: Perceptions of pediatric and adult program directors. *Pediatric Pulmonology,
    31*, 443–450.
Gennen, S.J., Powers, L.E., & Sells, W. (2003). Understanding the role of health care
    providers during the transition to adolescents with disabilities and special health care
    needs. *Journal of Adolescent Health, 32*, 225–233.
Hauser, E., & Dorn, L. (1999). Transitioning adolescents with sickle cell disease to adult
    centered care. *Pediatric Nursing, 25*, 479–488.
Individuals with Disabilities Education Improvement Act of 2004, PL 108-446, 20 U.S.C.
    §§ 1400 *et seq.*

McDonagh, J.E. (2005). Growing up and moving on: Transition from pediatric to adult care. *Pediatric Transplantation, 9,* 364–372.

Madge, S., & Byron, M. (2002). A model for transition from pediatric to adult care in cystic fibrosis. *Journal of Pediatric Nursing, 17,* 283–288.

Maternal and Child Health Bureau. (2001). *Achieving success for all children and youth with special health care needs: A 10-year action plan to accompany Healthy People 2010.* Rockville, MD: Maternal and Child Health Bureau.

Neubert, D.A. (2003). The role of assessment in the transition to adult life process for students with disabilities. *Exceptionality, 11*(2), 63–75.

Olsen, D.G., & Swigonski, N.L. (2004). Transition to adulthood: The important role of the pediatrican. *Pediatrics, 113*(3), e159–e162. Retrieved December 5, 2006, from http://www.pediatrics.org/cgi/content/full/113/3/e159

Pacaud, D., McConnell, B., Huot, C., Aebi, C., & Yale, J. (1996). Transition from pediatric care to adult care for insulin-dependent diabetes patients. *Canadian Journal of Diabetes Care, 20,* 14–20.

Patterson, D., & Lanier, C. (1999). Adolescent health transitions: Focus group study of teens and young adults with special health care needs. *Family and Community Health, 22,* 43–58.

Reiss, J., & Gibson, R. (2002). Health care transitions: Destinations unknown. *Pediatrics, 110,* 1304–1306.

Reiss, J.G., Gibson, R.W., & Walker, L.R. (2005). Health care transition: Youth, family, and provider perspectives. *Pediatrics, 115*(1), 112–120.

Rettig, P., & Athreya, B.H. (1991). Adolescents with chronic disease: Transition to adult health care. *Arthritis Care Research, 4,* 174–180.

Scal, P., & Ireland, M. (2005). Addressing transition to adult health care for adolescents with special health care needs. *Pediatrics, 115*(6), 1607–1612.

Scal, P., Evans, T., Blozis, S., Okinow, N., & Blum, R. (1999). Trends in transition from pediatric to adult health care services for young adults with chronic conditions. *Journal of Adolescent Health, 24,* 259–264.

Stein R., & Jessop, D. (1982). A noncategorical approach to chronic childhood illness. *Public Health Reports, 97,* 354–362.

Steinkamp, G., Ullrich, G., Muller, C., Fabel, H., & von der Hardt, H. (2001). Transition of adult patients with cystic fibrosis. *European Journal of Medical Research, 6,* 85–92.

Stilton, P., Neubert, D.A., & Leconte, P. (1997). Transition assessment: The position of the Division on Career Development and Transition. *Career Development for Exceptional Individuals, 2,* 69–79.

Telfair, J., Alleman-Velez, P.L., Dickens, P., & Loosier, P.S. (2005). Quality health care for adolescents with special health care needs: Issues and clinical implications. *Journal of Pediatric Nursing, 20*(1), 15–24.

Telfair, J., Myers, J., & Drezner, S. (1994). Transfer as a component of the transition of adolescents with sickle cell disease to adult care: Adolescent, adult, and parent perspectives. *Journal of Adolescent Health, 15,* 558–565.

Westwood, A., Henley, L., & Wilcox, P. (1999). Transition from paediatric to adult care for persons with cystic fibrosis: Patient and parent perspectives. *Journal of Paediatrics & Child Health, 35,* 442–445.

CHAPTER 8

Developing Transition Health Care Plans

JOHN G. REISS AND ROBERT W. GIBSON

The move from child-centered to adult-oriented health care is only one of the many transitions that all young people must accomplish on the way to adulthood. Good health supported by access to quality health care plays a fundamental role in supporting a young person's capacity to successfully carry out a broad range of activities and responsibilities that come with adulthood, such as finding a job and living independently. This is especially true for youth and young adults with special health care needs and disabilities.[1]

The move from pediatrics to adult-oriented medicine is not simply leaving one health care provider for another. The literature (Reiss, Gibson, & Walker, 2005; Rosen, 1995) tells us that there are significant cultural and practice differences between pediatric and adult-oriented medicine. The expectations and responsibilities of adult patients and the role of their family members are markedly different from the patient role and expectations of families in pediatrics. The change in status from dependent child to independent adult increases the level of responsibility expected in managing daily special health care and disability needs. In addition, reaching adulthood often precipitates changes in access to health insurance coverage and in the type, amount, and duration of services that health insurance will pay for.

To successfully navigate the move from pediatric to adult-oriented medicine it is necessary to plan ahead. A way to objectify this process is to develop a health care transition plan. A health care transition plan is a way to anticipate the changes in accessing and paying for health care and in interacting with adult-oriented providers. A young person's participation in the development and execution of a health care transition plan provides opportunities for the young person to demonstrate independence and readiness to manage his or her special health care needs or disabilities.

Health Care Transition research cited in this chapter was funded by a grant from National Institute for Disability and Rehabilitation Research (RRTC Grant no. H133B001200) and Institute for Child and Adolescent Research and Education Grant, University of Florida No. 2004-03-R.

Health Care Transition Workbooks were developed in part with support from the State of Florida, Department of Health, Children's Medical Service Contract COQFV-R2.

[1]For the remainder of this chapter, youth with special health care needs and disabilities will be referred to as "youth" and young adults with special health care needs and disabilities will be referred to as "young adults," unless specified otherwise.

This chapter discusses strategies for developing and implementing a health care transition plan based on the basic elements of transition planning that were described in the chapters in Section I. The chapter includes a discussion of promising practices and presents examples of health care transition plan formats as well as examples of health-related objectives that could be included in individualized education programs (IEPs), accommodation plans developed under Section 504 of the Rehabilitation Act of 1973 (PL 93-112) (504 plans), and individualized plans for employment (IPEs).

WHAT IS A HEALTH CARE TRANSITION PLAN AND WHO IS IT FOR?

In addition to young people and their families, there can be many other individuals and services involved in the health care transition process. These include a variety of health care providers and individuals from clinics, hospitals, and/or state agencies. Each party has a unique perspective on the process of transition and the goals that are to be accomplished. Thus, transition plans can be written from a variety of perspectives. Although the object of a plan is the smooth transfer of a young person from pediatric to adult-oriented care, each perspective may emphasize different aspects of transition. This chapter discusses the development of a health care transition plan primarily from the perspective of the young person and his or her family. The intent of this approach is two-fold. First, this puts the young person and his or her family at the center of the planning. Second, this approach creates opportunities for the young person to develop and demonstrate the self-determination, communication, and self-care skills needed to interact effectively with the adult-oriented medical system. In addition, we discuss transition-related responsibilities of the health care team and activities that can be carried out by health care providers in support of youth and their families.

STAGES OF TRANSITION

Health care transition had been discussed in the pediatric literature since the early 1980s (Reiss & Gibson, 2002). Despite its longevity as a topic of interest, empirical research on the actual process of transition and the best practices that support health care transition are limited (Betz, 2004; Forbes et al., 2001). To begin to remedy this situation, we initiated a research study in 2000 that explored the lived experience of health care transition. The stages of health care transition and many of the transition recommendations identified in this chapter are a result of that research (Reiss et al., 2005).

The research showed that for families and young adults who were most successful, transition to adult-oriented health care occurred as a developmental process that progressed through three stages: *envisioning a future, age of responsibility,* and *age of transition.* The first stage focused on establishing a future-oriented perspective. The second stage focused on the young person mastering and independently carrying out age-appropriate activities including health care tasks. These two stages laid the foundation for addressing the broad range of the transition-specific activities that occurred during the final stage. An age range is suggested for each of the stages in the discussion below. However, these age ranges are only suggestions since what is most important to consider when judging a person's transition progress is their developmental status and cognitive ability.

Envisioning a Future

This stage was described by family members as beginning shortly after a special health care need or disability was identified. Often this stage was initiated by a health care provider or a member of another family with a child with a disability. Families recalled instances where, despite being overwhelmed by learning that their child had a special health care need or disability, they were prompted by these individuals to acknowledge that their child would reach adulthood and that it was important to plan for this eventuality. Although the specific details of their child's future were difficult to project, parents likened this idea of "envisioning a future" to a new way of thinking about and relating to their child. This change in thinking led families to act in ways that supported their child's future independence.

Participants in the research study acknowledged that plans for the future were subject to extensive revisions as their child's abilities emerged over time. At this stage, what was most important was to ask questions about the future, rather than create plans. Asking questions about future education, employment, independent community living, and future health care needs prompted families and providers to focus on long-term goals and initiate activities that promoted the child's eventual independence. As one parent stated, "He [the child's pediatrician] looked at the kids developmentally. So when Bobby was 3 or 4 months old he said to me, 'where do you want Bobby to be in 20 years?' And because of that I began to think about where it was that I wanted him to be in 20 years."

In conjunction with envisioning and planning for a future, participants recommended starting the transition process early. Both practitioners and parents talked about the importance of starting early. As another parent expressed, "I think a lot has to do with instilling an attitude of self-confidence with the kids early on and just expecting them to do things for themselves."

None of the families in our study developed formal or written transition plans during this early stage. However, it was clear that many families envisioned that their children would be "fully included" in society as adults, and they worked hard to achieve this overarching goal.

Age of Responsibility

During this stage, typically between the ages of 6 and 12 years, family members laid the foundation for future independence by teaching their child to carryout and be responsible for tasks of daily living and medical self-care. Goals for this stage focused on the child acquiring skills and practicing being responsible for daily life tasks. Examples included talking with health care providers, taking medications independently, ordering medications from a pharmacy, and developing positive medical habits and routines. Several participants felt that it was important to transfer responsibilities for medical self-care to the child prior to the onset of adolescence since this avoided some of the inevitable conflicts and struggles for control that are a natural part of the parent–adolescent relationship. The following observation by a parent demonstrates both starting early and the idea of imparting responsibility to the child: "He [the pediatric specialist] was a very firm believer in the children taking responsibility for their own health care. And so when Bobby was two and half years old he started answering his own questions when we came to clinic. And as a family we started rehearsing those questions and answers on the way to clinic."

Age of Transition

This stage was divided into two periods: adolescence (ages 12 to 17) and young adulthood (ages 18 to 23). The dividing point for these periods was flexible but centered on the legal age of adulthood, which is 18 in the United States. With some allowance for developmental delays and cognitive limitations, these age markers are in agreement with the typical expectations for achieving independence by young adults without special health care needs and disabilities (Anderson & Wolpert, 2004; Arnett, 2000; Christie & Viner, 2005; Tong et al., 1998).

It was during this stage that concrete plans for transition were most likely to be developed. The plans were generally informal and focused primarily on practicing independence, self-advocacy, finding new adult-oriented providers, and maintaining health insurance coverage. The following quote from a nurse describes how young people are directed to be more independent in their health care: "So around 14 is when we usually have the child make the appointment or the adolescent." Or as stated by a family member, "Since he's been 16 or 17 years old he's gone to a lot of his [doctor's] visits by himself."

TRANSITION PLANNING TOOLS

During the interviews, families, youth, and health care providers delineated the stages of health care transition and identified many transition-related goals. However, few referred to planning tools or other resources that could be used to help prepare youth and families for the eventual transition to adult-oriented care. Internet and literature searches for transition planning aids yielded only limited results. A listing of some of these transition planning tools can be found in the appendix of resources at the end of this book.

Our review of these tools indicated that these materials had a number of limitations. Some of the tools or checklists were limited because they were designed to be used with a specific disability group or in a particular treatment setting. Some tools focused on assessing developmental skills but were not linked to subsequent transition-related planning and/or activities. Others focused on transition activities without consideration of the developmental nature of the health care transition process. Many of the tools did not recognize the complex nature of transition. Most importantly, the tools did not provide families and young adults, as the central actors in the process of transition, with the means to tailor the transition plan and process to their specific needs and priorities.

In response to the limitations of the available health care transition-related materials, we set out to develop a tool to help families prepare for transition that 1) was designed for families and young adults and was easy to use, 2) was general enough to be used by individuals with a variety of special health care needs and disabilities, 3) was organized in a developmental progression, 4) incorporated the idea of starting early, 5) focused on health care transition, and 6) made linkages with the many other areas (i.e, work, independent living, higher education, further training) in which the transition to adulthood occurs. The resulting tool consists of a set of three workbooks for families and youth—one for youth ages 12–14, one for youth ages 15–17, and one for youth ages 18 and older. Examples from the workbooks are found throughout the remainder of this chapter.

The workbooks for ages 12–14 and 15–17 years contain two sets of work-sheets, one for the young person and the other for parents or family members. The young person's worksheets are divided into two sections and the parent's are divided into four sections. The first two sections of the youth's and parents' part of the workbooks are similar in content and organization.

The first section, "Thinking About Your Child's Future"/"Thinking About Your Future," contains questions about future schooling, employment, and living arrangements and how future health care will be accessed and paid for. This section is designed to contextualize health care transition within the larger process of developing personal independence. The second section, "Health Care Independence," contains seven subsections that address various aspects of health care transition. (See Table 8.1 for a list of subsection content areas.) The questions in this part of the workbook address the adolescent's performance on a variety of health care transition tasks. Most items have three response options: "the activity is carried out independently," "the activity is done with some help," or "the active requires a lot of help/cannot be done." *Independently* is defined as including the ability to direct others if the adolescent lacks the physical ability to carryout the task. In some instances, "yes" and "no" responses are used.

The third and fourth sections appear only in the workbook for family members. The third section, "Parents' Health Care Transition Activities," contains questions about things that parents can do to support their child's health care transition. Some of the questions have three response options: "I do this often or regularly," "I do this sometimes," and "I do this rarely or never." Other questions have two response options: "I have done this" and "I have not done this."

Table 8.1. Health care independence

Subsection	Content	Sample item
Basic knowledge	Ability to share knowledge about health condition	I can tell someone what my diagnosis, disability, or health condition is.
Health care practices	Ability to carry out health care task	I make good choices about friends, food, exercise, alcohol, and smoking in order to stay healthy.
Medications, medical tests, equipment, and supplies	Ability to carry out medical tasks related to medication, tests, and equipment	I can name my medications (using their proper names) and the amount and times I take them.
Doctors' visits	Ability to carry out behaviors related to health care visits	I answer many of the questions during a health care visit.
Health care transition	Ability to carry out activities that support health care transition	I have talked with my doctor or nurse about going to different doctors when I am an adult.
Transition to adulthood	Ability to carry out general transition activities	I advocate for myself so that I get the accommodations I need and so that my legal rights are not violated.
Health care systems	Ability to share knowledge about health care systems	I can tell someone about the limitations of my health insurance plan and about the problems I need to watch out for when ordering supplies and/or medication and other equipment.

The final step in the workbook for family members is to complete the "Health Care Transition Plan Family Worksheets." To help develop the health care transition plan, the parent and the youth are instructed to first look at their answers to the questions in the first section of their workbooks and talk about the differences and similarities in the answers to the questions about where the youth will live, who he or she will live with, and what kind of job he or she will have.

Parents and adolescents are to discuss answers to the questions in the "Health Care Independence" and the parents are to share their answers to the "Parents' Health Care Transition Activities" section, to talk about the differences and similarities in their perceptions, and work together to identify several activities that either the youth could do more independently or the parents could do to help the youth become more independent.

Finally, with these discussions in mind, the family is to agree on and write down several health care transition-related goals and to describe the activities that the young person and family members will undertake, in order to achieve the identified goals.

The workbook for families and young adults age 18 and older is similar to the other two workbooks, but the "Thinking About Your Future" section has additional questions about independent community living, and the "Health Care Transition Plan Family Worksheets" section is included in the young adult's rather than the parent's part of the workbook.

These workbooks have been designed to raise awareness of health care transition issues; help young people and their families perform self-assessments of their current knowledge, skills, and behaviors; and develop answers to the key questions about what might promote a smooth transition to the adult-oriented health care system. Table 8.2 provides a list of key transition issues that young people and their families will need to address in developing an individualized health care transition plan.

Two health care transition planning areas, paying for health care and ongoing supports for young adults with limited cognitive abilities, present significant challenges that often require additional attention. It is not possible to adequately address either of these areas in the limited space of this chapter. The following discussion serves only as an introduction to these areas. For additional information on these topics, refer to Chapters 3 and 6.

Paying for needed health care services can be challenging because young adults with special health care needs and disabilities are less likely to have health insurance when compared with healthy young adults (Callahan & Cooper, 2004; Collins, Schoen, Tenney, Doty, & Ho, 2004; Fishman, 2001; White, 2002). In addition, the services and supports covered under a public health insurance program for adults are typically not equal to those covered under health insurance programs for children and adolescents.

The lower rate of health insurance coverage for young adults with special needs and disabilities is related to the fact that most individuals with health care insurance in the United States have employment-based health insurance. Employment-based health insurance plans typically have age limits (generally between the ages of 19 and 23 years), after which coverage for dependent children is no longer offered (Collins et al., 2004). The young person then has to secure his or her own insurance through employment or some other means. Employment rates for young adults with special health care needs and disabilities are low. Therefore, they are less likely

Table 8.2. Key transition issues

Key issues	Rationale	Questions
Future goals	This is the context for all transition activities	What are the young person's future goals for education, employment, and living arrangements?
Knowledge and skills	Knowledge or skills needed to live with a chronic illness	What knowledge and skills will the young person need to be independent in addressing their medical needs?
Adult medical services	Medical services necessary to maintain good health and function during adulthood	What kind of primary or specialty health care, diagnostic procedures, and treatment related to aging will the young person need during adulthood?
Adult-oriented providers	Adult service providers	Who will provide the young person's medical services during adulthood?
Health care costs	Health care financing and insurance	How will medical services be paid for? What arrangements are necessary to ensure continued health insurance?
Guardianship	Assistance in health care decision making	Is guardianship a necessity for managing future medical decision making and care?
Transfer target date	Transition outcome	When will health care services be transferred to adult-oriented providers?

than their healthy peers to obtain employment-based insurance (Fishman, 2001; White, 2002). While young adults with special health care needs are more likely than their peers to be insured through state Medicaid programs (McManus, Flint, & Kelly, 1991), Medicaid typically provides a significantly lower rate of payment to providers than does employment-based coverage or Medicare. This may discourage physicians from accepting Medicaid patients (Kaiser Family Foundation, 2002). Youth who are insured through Medicaid because they qualify as disabled under the Supplemental Security Income (SSI) program may lose both SSI and Medicaid at age 18. The SSI disability criteria for children, age birth to 17, are less restrictive than the criteria for adults age 18 and older (Loprest & Wittenberg, 2005; Reiss, Wallace & McPherson, 2002; Sandler et al., 2001).

In addition, there are differences in the scope of health plan coverage for children and adolescents compared with that for adults, especially in public programs. Medicaid, the State Children's Health Insurance Program, and the state Title V Children with Special Health Care Needs Programs offer benefits to children that are not equally available to adults in need. For example, Medicaid's Early and Periodic Screening, Diagnostic, and Treatment (EPSDT) program, which covers recipients younger than 21, requires that specified services be provided to children even if a state's Medicaid program does not cover the service for other beneficiaries (Centers for Medicare and Medicaid Services, 2005). The EPSDT program also requires state programs to provide information to families and help them use available services appropriately.

Unfortunately, the scope of this coverage as written is not matched by the actual delivery of services. The U.S. General Accounting Office (2001) has reported that Medicaid-eligible children often do not receive critical EPSDT services. Notwithstanding this shortfall, many children with special health care needs and disabilities experience a loss of financial access to certain services when they become adults, even if they continue to be covered by Medicaid. This can complicate the transition to adult care and frustrate patients, their families, and providers. For additional information on health insurance options for youth with special health care needs and disabilities, refer to Chapter 3.

The need of young adults with limited cognitive abilities for ongoing supports and accommodations and special legal arrangements also presents significant challenges that need to be specifically addressed in the individual's health care transition plan. Regardless of cognitive level, a young person's chronological age and their increase in physical size will probably require them to access health care from adult-oriented providers and facilities. Most pediatric providers and children's hospitals have policies that mandate patients older than 21 be transferred to the adult health care system. This transfer must be planned for and carried out prior to the time when medical care is needed from the adult system. Because the young adult has a limited capacity to make medical decisions and provide informed consent, family members often stay involved in the care of these individuals, and this ongoing, active involvement must be accommodated in the transition process. Health care transition for this subpopulation may not involve a significant increase in the young adult's level of independence, but it will nonetheless involve changes in medical providers and services. For young adults older than 18 years old who will not be able to direct their medical care, additional legal arrangements, such as guardianship, will need to be established (Millar & Renzaglia, 2002). Guardianship can take many forms but is generally easier to accomplish before the young person turns 18 year old. For additional information on guardianship, refer to the resource section of this chapter and Chapter 2.

IMPLEMENTING HEALTH CARE TRANSITION IN THE EDUCATIONAL SYSTEM

In addition to health care transition plans developed by young people and their families, another valuable resource is the school-based transition plans developed as part of IEPs and 504 plans.

The Individuals with Disabilities Education Improvement Act (IDEA) of 2004 (PL 108-446) defines transition services within an IEP as a coordinated set of activities for a child that focus on improving the academic and functional achievement of the child with a disability to facilitate the child's movement from school to postschool activities, such as work, further education or training, and independent living (U.S. Department of Education, Office of Safe and Drug-Free Schools, 2004). A 504 plan defines ways for making sure a student with disabilities is afforded an equal opportunity to participate in academic, nonacademic, and extracurricular activities. While Section 504 does not specifically address the issue of transition, the purpose of this part of the Rehabilitation Act of 1973 is to promote full participation of individuals with disabilities in all aspects of life, including health care (Council for Exceptional Children, 2003). For more information on 504 plans, refer to Chapters 10 and 11.

The literature clearly indicates that, for youth with special health care needs and disabilities, being able to access and use needed health care is a key functional skill and is an important part of independent living and community participation (McDonagh, 2005; Reiss et al., 2005). Therefore, we believe that it is in keeping with the intent of IDEA and Section 504 that schools provide students with opportunities that are designed to improve their ability to manage their disability and/or health care needs in the school setting, work effectively with health care providers, take a lead role in directing the actions of others, and do the things they want to do more independently. However, despite the shared goals of health and educational transition, health care–related goals and activities are not typically included in the transition component of IEPs or in 504 plans (Heller & Tumlin, 2004; Reiss et al., 2005). For information on integrating health-related needs into IEPs and 504 plans, see Chapter 10.

Results of a survey of school personnel, outside agency representatives, and family members in Florida who served on county-wide committees that support academic transition provide some insight into why health care transition is often not included in IEPs, 504 plans, or other aspects of the academic process (Repetto et al., 2005). Fifty-six percent of the 187 survey respondents reported that they never heard of or knew little about health care transition. Respondents who were more familiar with health care transition indicated that they were interested in helping address the issue of health care transition in school but lacked the experience, knowledge, and tools to do so. Together, these findings suggest that school personnel did not oppose including health care transition–related issues in IEPs and 504 plans in the school setting; that many were not aware that health care transition was a problem, while others needed additional health care transition–related training, resources, and supports.

Many students with complex health care needs also have an individualized health care plan (IHP) that defines the roles and responsibilities of the school nurse and other education staff in delivering appropriate health care to the student while in school. These plans have typically been used to provide health care services to the student and have not focused on increasing skills and independence in the area of personal health (Haas, 1993). However, a recent study suggests that IHPs could be expanded to include actions that classroom teachers and school nurses could take in carrying out a medical treatment program and to include ways that students can be more involved in their own care (Heller & Tumlin, 2004).

Schools may also be reluctant to promote student independence in self-care, because this may mean that the student has more responsibility for administering his or her own medications and keeping these drugs secure and away from other students. Some school systems have not allowed students to be independent in their health self-care because they mistakenly believed that allowing students to carry medications and medical equipment was in conflict with the federal Department of Education's Drug-Free School policies, although the U.S. Department of Education, Office of Safe and Drug-Free Schools has issued guidance clarifying that "a student's prescription drugs, and related equipment, are not illegal drugs and are not prohibited by the [Safe and Drug-Free Schools and Communities Act]" (2004). An excellent example of this can be seen in the current debate about allowing students to keep asthma inhalers on their person rather than requiring that they be held in a secure location by school personnel. Policies vary by state and school district; however, the trend is now for schools to allow students greater independence in managing their own inhalers and other medications (Jones & Wheeler, 2004; Juvenile Diabetes Research Foundation International, 2006; National Asthma Education and Prevention Program-School Subcommittee, 2003).

Because health care transition is a new issue for schools, there are few examples that can be used to guide school staff as they work to incorporate health

Table 8.3. Sample adaptation of individualized education plan goals to support health care transition

Goal	Standard activity	Transition-related activity
Carry out multiple-step activity	Complete multiple-step academic task	Set up, clean, and put away medical equipment used during school hours
Assertiveness, communication skills	Role play returning unwanted items to a store	Role play speaking with a doctor to discuss a change in treatment or need for additional services
Telephone skills	Find and dial a phone number and request information or services	Using the telephone during an emergency; calling a doctor's office to request or make an appointment
Written communications, organizing information	Keep a class notebook of completed assignments	Keeping a medical journal or assembling a medical notebook containing health and treatment information
Information/knowledge	Academic subject material	Information on healthy lifestyles and health promotion, disability rights

care transition into school activities. For teachers, nurses, and therapists, this involves integrating health care–related issues into the student's overall educational plan and providing the young person with opportunities to generalize relevant life management skills to self-care and other aspects of medical management. (For additional information on self-care/self-management, refer to Chapter 4.) For examples of lesson plans that can be used by educators to support the development of health care transition and self-determination skills, see the *Standing Up for Me* curriculum (Florida Department of Education, 2004). Also see Table 8.3.

While schools do not typically include self-care and other health care transition–related competencies in IEPs and 504 plans, we believe that doing so has several advantages for students and families. The skills used in health care transition, including planning, self-determination, self-responsibility, communications, and using transportation services are similar to the skills that schools are already working on to prepare students for work, independence, future education, and other aspects of community living. There are significant parallels between competencies involved in being independent in medical tasks and competencies that are typically addressed in IEPs and 504 plans.

Schools are practical, comfortable, natural learning environments, where a number of different individuals may be available to support the youth in planning for and practicing independence. In addition, by promoting skill development and independence in managing one's own health care, the school can help to reinforce the idea that the youth is increasingly autonomous, and has a growing responsibility to monitor and manage his or her health in "real world" settings.

IMPLEMENTING TRANSITION PLANS IN THE HEALTH CARE SYSTEM

There are multiple ways in which health care providers can help youth plan for and successfully carry out the transition to adult-oriented health care and other aspects of adulthood, including providing age- and developmentally appropriate health care; facilitating the development of the adolescent's self-care skills; and promoting the adolescent's self-determination, sense of autonomy, and active participation in health care and other life activities.

In order to successfully negotiate the adult health care system, youth need to learn how to communicate effectively with health care providers, make health care decisions, and, ultimately, take responsibility for their own health care. Health care providers can actively support the development of these skills and behaviors by educating both the parents and the child about the condition and treatments, soliciting input from the child regarding his or her understanding of and preferences about the plan of care, and directing some specific clinical questions to the child as soon as he or she is to communicate effectively (using an augmentative communicative device if necessary).

Health care providers can also strive to obtain *assent*—an affirmation that the child understands and is willing to participate in the plan of care (in keeping with his or her level of cognitive development)—well before the child has the legal authority to consent to treatment. Research indicates that children as young as 9 are able to make reasoned decisions about treatment preferences, and that 14-year-olds are as competent as 18- and 21-year-olds to make medical treatment decisions (Bailey, O'Connell, & Pearce, 2003; Roth, Meisel, & Lidz, 1977; Weithorn & Campbell, 1982).

As discussed previously, the process of health care transition should begin at diagnosis and initially involves parents and family members envisioning their child growing up to be an adult. Health care providers can support this process by encouraging parents to take a step back from their child's day-to-day health care problems and to focus periodically on the long term. Health care providers can model this in their interactions with the child and family by being sure to ask children with special health care needs and disabilities some of the same questions they ask their typically developing patients, such as "What chores do you have at home?" "What's your favorite subject in school?" "What do you do with your friends after school?" and "What are you going to do after high school?" Further, providers can promote a broader vision of future possibilities. For example, if a youth is planning to go to a local community college, the provider can ask what stands in the way of their going to a school that is larger or farther away.

When a patient reaches early adolescence (usually around age 12), it is advisable for health care providers to initiate a discussion of the issue of health care transition with the patient and family in a more formal and structured fashion. This discussion might involve informing the youth and his or her family about any upper age limit policies of the individual practitioner and the practice setting (e.g., clinic, children's hospital), setting expectations about patient responsibilities for knowledge of their condition, seeing providers alone for a portion of the health care visit, promoting the learning of self-care skills, and so forth. This is also a good time to revisit the issue of long-term goals. It is at this age that many youth make the transition from elementary to middle school; begin the developmental process of separating from their family; make meaningful friendships with peers; and think more seriously about their goals for further education, work, living independently, and having a family of their own. Independence in health care can be framed within the context of the adolescents' inherent desire to be more autonomous and self-reliant in other aspects of their lives.

As affirmed in *A Consensus Statement on Health Care Transition for Young Adults with Special Health Care Needs*, pediatric providers should prepare and maintain an up-to-date medical summary for use by the patient and family that is portable and accessible (American Academy of Pediatrics [AAP], American Academy of Family Physicians [AAFP], American College of Physicians-American Society of Internal Medicine [ACP-ASIM], 2002). This summary of key health care information is critical for a successful health care transition because it provides a common knowledge base for adult-oriented providers to whom the young adult may transfer and other health care professionals involved in the care and transition of the young adult patient. Giving a portable medical summary to youth and young adults also provides key information to the patient. This medical summary is in keeping with the goal of putting young adults in control of, and being responsible for, their personal health information. For examples of model medical summary forms, see Hait, Arnold, & Fishman, 2006; LoCasale-Crouch & Johnson, 2005; and Rubin, 2003.

Further, a written health care transition plan should be developed when a patient reaches age 14. At a minimum, this plan should include "what services need to be provided, who will provide them, and how they will be financed" (AAP, AAFP, ACP-ASIM, 2002, p. 1305). The introduction and development of a transition plan when the child is in early adolescence can serve to raise the awareness of families and youth about the importance and complexity of health care transition and can provide sufficient time to address important issues such as incorporating health care transition goals and activities into school-based IEP and 504 plans, maintaining health insurance coverage, identifying and transferring to adult-oriented primary and specialty care providers and facilities, and addressing the issue of guardianship for youth with diminished decision-making capacity. As noted by a parent in the transition video titled *College and Beyond*, "Families don't know what they don't know about health care transition" (Reiss, Gibson, & Miller, 2004).

Health care providers also need to work directly with parents and other family members to help them carry through with the often anxiety-provoking process of transitioning out of the role of "doer," turning over lead health care responsibilities to the youth, and gradually assuming the role of "coach" or "guide" (Kieckhefer & Trahms, 2000). While the written health care transition plan can serve as a guide to parents and other family members, providers can further support parents in this process by letting parents know that it is normal for them to be uncomfortable when changing roles. Some parents find it helpful to talk with others who have been through this process and to be reassured that the road to independence may be a rocky one, but that the end results—a young adult who is able to successfully negotiate the adult health care system—is worth the effort. Health care providers can play a facilitative role, by linking parents of youth in the early states of transition with parents of young adults, or with the young adults themselves.

In addition, pediatric providers need to "say good-bye" to young adult patients and/or renegotiate their relationship with the young adult and their family in a psychologically positive manner and make explicit the role they are willing to play in the young person's care in the future (Reiss & Gibson, 2002; Rosen, 2004).

The final pediatric visits can be used to review and validate the gains and accomplishments that the young person and his or her family has made, to affirm and empower the young person to continue to develop the skills needed to take the lead in his or her own health care, to reaffirm the young person's future goals and objectives, and to mutually acknowledge and address the feelings associated with loss and change.

It is important to make it clear to patients that when they leave the pediatric practice, their new adult-oriented physician is responsible for their care. Some pediatric providers would like to be informed about former patient's future medical status and be copied on letters sent by the adult-oriented provider to their former patients regarding health status and plan of treatment. Some pediatric providers are willing to serve as a "sounding board" when their former patients need to make decisions about treatment options, or they may be willing to assist, if things don't work out with the new adult doctor, and to help find other adult-oriented health care providers who might better meet the youth's needs and preferences. It is important to discuss these future contingencies as the young person is in the final stages of transition.

It may also be helpful for the pediatric provider to reframe the end of pediatric care as a major accomplishment, like graduating from high school and college. Doctors and clinics don't usually give their patient-graduates a certificate and a party, but doing so might make saying good-bye a little easier.

In addition, health care providers need to address systems-level issues, which impact the transition of youth with special health care needs and disabilities. This involves developing and implementing policies, procedures, and practices that ensure an efficient transfer of clinical information among pediatric and adult-oriented providers and the continuous provision of high-quality, coordinated care that is responsive to the priorities, values, and preferences of the young person and their family.

Pediatric providers can also support the health care transition process by fostering positive working relationships with a set of primary and specialty care providers who are interested in and willing to provide care to young adults, and can play an active role in linking older patients to their new providers. Researchers have indicated that some youth and their families do not follow through on referrals to new, adult-oriented physicians, while others see the new physician only once, then go without care, because they are not comfortable with or prepared for the manner in which care is provided in the adult system (Flume, Anderson, Hardy, & Gray, 2001; Viner, 2001; Watson, 2005; Webb, 2003). While difficult to arrange, a "transitional visit" has been identified as very helpful for some young adults. During a transitional visit, the young person sees both the pediatric and the new adult provider at the same time. The physicians are able to share information about the patient and the current course of treatment face-to-face, and there is an opportunity to develop a future plan of care that is acceptable to all (Baldassano et al., 2002; Boyle, Farukhi, & Nosky, 2001; Rosen, 2004).

Adult-oriented providers need to acquire the medical knowledge they need to care for young adults with childhood onset chronic conditions (Rosen, 2004). They also need to effectively address the challenges involved in establishing a positive working relationship with patient/families who have had long-standing relationships with pediatric providers and whose experiences are limited to the pediatric health care system. Strategies for "getting off on the right foot" include not initially making significant changes in the medical regimen, ordering a minimal number of initial medical tests and procedures, not making disparaging remarks about pediatric providers, and asking youth what worked and what did not work for them in their pediatric care. The leadership of pediatric and adult health care organizations also has a critical role to play in making transition a priority and in addressing the financial, procedural, and inter-professional issues that can impede the smooth transfer of youth with special health care needs and disabilities to the adult health care system.

SUMMARY

This chapter has discussed the multiple participants and their roles in the health care transition planning process. Every young adult and their family will face unique hurdles in the transition process. For some, transition may be relatively smooth and trouble free. For others, health care transition will be time consuming and present seemingly insurmountable obstacles. Regardless of how health care transition unfolds, asking questions about the future in general and health care specifically lays the foundation for planning and anticipating future health care needs. Transition planning tools and activities have been suggested to help make the process of HCT more manageable and organized. The longest journey always begins with one step—health care transition planning is that step.

My Story   Joy and John Ryan Mudry

An important aspect of health care transition planning and independence is its perception. The following vignette demonstrates that even within one family there are both shared and unique understandings of the transition process. In this vignette John Ryan and his mother share their perspective on health care transition and John Ryan's future.

John Ryan

We're all in a card game called Life. God is the dealer. You keep what is dealt. Some hands are good, some bad. You just keep playing 'til you cash out.

That is a pretty good way to look at it I think. It is really not what you have; it's how you look at it. Take me and my family, for instance. Dad sees mostly negative; Mom sees mostly positive. You're either living in a dark, gothic castle, or you're living in Disney World. Me, I'm a realist. I look at both positive and negative aspects of life and then base my judgments, views, and predictions on what things really are. Yes, I have several chronic illnesses, yes I will have a shorter life, but I can still have fun, go out with friends and all that. I just have to make choices like having a regular soda versus having a dessert. That extra piece of pie or more insulin. In economics that's called an opportunity cost. What you give up for something else. I think I manage my health affairs pretty reasonably, but shush! Don't let my parents know! They still think I can't handle it just because I do things a little late or change the order around a bit.

What can I say? Parents, oh bless them! I reason that they did a pretty decent job of transitioning me from pediatrics to adult medical care. I mean, as long as I'm still conscious I can handle any problem that should arise. I make decisions even when my nurses are not sure. I've been handling all my own insulin and medicines since I was 12. At first Mom did everything, then I started injecting the needle myself, then I would draw up what my mom would tell me to do, and finally I can make all the decisions for myself. In fact, Mom doesn't do anything in that area anymore. I can talk to doctors, explain what is going down and decide what medicines I need and when to take them. I've learned how to read my pulmonary function tests numbers well enough to know whether I'm sick or not. Mom used to check all my meds to see if I was running low, and now I check them and send the order into the pharmacy myself. About the only thing I can't handle yet is the dollar end of it. Those prices are really high and I don't even have a job yet. But I could handle the numbers if need be. I have three bank accounts and I can balance a checkbook. So all in all I reckon I came out all right. Thanks most in part to my parents.

Joy: John Ryan's Mother

I believe that I have been transitioning John Ryan since he was born. Going from a crib to a "big boy" bed, then lately into a queen size. Moving from pre-K into regular school, then middle school, then high school, and now looking into colleges. The medical aspect is just one more transition that must be made.

I first started the transition process by never allowing John to make excuses for his illnesses. He has always been expected to do well in school, to do his chores at home, and take part in physical education classes. We have helped him learn his limitations and when to give in to them. His dad and I determined early on that he would be treated just like any other kid. Today you would never know he had problems to look at him or talk to him.

John has numerous health issues. He has cystic fibrosis, Type I diabetes (not related to the cystic fibrosis), hypothyroidism, short-gut syndrome, asthma, sporadic croup, and nasal polyps. He has had eight surgeries in the last 18 years. Before he went to kindergarten, he could do all his own finger-sticks for blood glucose monitoring, and take all his enzymes at meals. I met with every kindergarten teacher, the resource teachers, the nurse, all office staff, and all of the administrators before he went to school. They worked with me to keep him as independent as possible at school. I stayed in constant touch with a beeper and frequent meetings. Every year in elementary school I would go and talk to his teachers and anyone new that would have contact with him. We were very blessed with a wonderful school and very caring people who helped us make the transition from home to school a smooth one.

John started learning to draw up his own insulin and inject himself when he was around 9. He learned to keep good records and start recording events that affected his health and/or his blood glucose. I went back to work teaching when he was in third grade, and was able to work at the same school where he was until eighth grade, so contact was easily made when a problem came up. However, he did a very good job of talking to the teachers about his health and of keeping up with his work when he had to be out. I'm very proud to say that he has maintained honor roll status through out his entire 12 years in school.

Cystic fibrosis means frequent stays in the hospital. I learned to question everything and ask lots of questions when he was very young. Without even realizing it, John has learned to mimic me and he does the same. We used to stay with him all the time when he was in the hospital, then gradually leave him at night. His last stay he was able to sign himself in, talk to the doctors and nurses, get his percutaneous intravenous catheter line in, and get his room set up before I even got there from work. He checks everyone's badges when they come in, keeps his own records, and handles all of the hospital stay like a pro.

Toward the end of middle school, I started making John responsible for keeping track of his medicines, keeping them well stocked and calling for refills when they would get low. I also had him start calling the nurses at Pulmonary and Endocrine to report any problems or concerns. They would talk to him first, then to me for my input. He has gradually taken over all of the calls to the specialists, and all of the medicine orders. He goes to the pharmacy to pick them up, and writes the check to pay for them. By the time he started high school, he could rattle off the names, doses, and costs of all of his medicines. I wrote a letter to his teachers introducing him during preplanning and he went to them to talk about his health issues and how they could help. He also started talking directly to his doctors during clinic visits at that time. He would look to me for some assistance. Now, just this past December he went to several clinic visits alone. He discussed everything with the doctors and made return appointments.

We still have a long ways to go to move him to total independence. He recently brought home a brochure about a college in Miami. I must confess that I laughed and thought he was kidding. He wasn't, and we had to have big discussion about his readiness to move that far away from the doctors, nurses, hospital, and parents who know him inside out. Transition has been a work in progress from the time he was born. As a parent and full-time caregiver, it has been difficult in some ways, and easy in others. John is a great kid, who, for the most part, handles his illnesses well. My goal throughout his life has been to make him as healthy and happy as possible, so that eventually he could be an independent adult with as great a life as possible.

REFERENCES

American Academy of Pediatrics, American Academy of Family Physicians, & American College of Physicians-American Society of Internal Medicine. (2002). A consensus statement on health care transition for young adults with special health care needs. *Pediatrics, 110,* 1304–1306.

Anderson, B.J., & Wolpert, H.A. (2004). A developmental perspective on the challenges of diabetes education and care during the young adult period. *Patient Education and Counseling, 53,* 347–352.

Arnett, J.J. (2000). Emerging adulthood: A theory of development from the late teens through the twenties. *American Psychologist, 55,* 469–479.

Bailey, S., O'Connell, B., & Pearce, J. (2003). The transition from paediatric to adult health care services for young adults with a disability: An ethical perspective. *Australian Health Review, 26*(1), 64–69.

Baldassano, R., Ferry, G., Griffiths, A., Mack, D., Markowitz, J., & Winter, H. (2002). Transition of the patient with inflammatory bowel disease from pediatric to adult care: Recommendations of the North American Society for Pediatric Gastroenterology, Hepatology and Nutrition. *Journal of Pediatric Gastroenterology & Nutrition, 34,* 245–248.

Betz, C. (2004). Transition of adolescents with special health care needs: Review and analysis of the literature. *Issues in Comprehensive Pediatric Nursing, 27,* 179–241.

Boyle, M.P., Farukhi, Z., Nosky, M.L. (2001). Strategies for improving transition to adult cystic fibrosis care, based on patient and parent views. *Pediatric Pulmonology, 32,* 428–436.

Callahan S.T., & Cooper, W.O. (2004). Gender and uninsurance among young adults in the United States. *Pediatrics, 113,* 291–297.

Centers for Medicare and Medicaid Services. (2005). *Medicaid early and periodic screening and diagnostic treatment benefit: Overview.* Baltimore: Author.

Christie, D., & Viner, R. (2005). ABC of adolescence: Adolescent development. *British Medical Journal, 330,* 301–304.

Collins, S., Schoen, C., Tenney, K., Doty. M., & Ho, A. (2004) *Rite of Passage? Why young adults become uninsured and how new policies can help.* The Common Wealth Fund Issue Brief May 2004. Retrieved December 4, 2006, from http://www.cmwf.org/programs/insurance/collins_riteofpassage_ib_649.pdf

Council for Exceptional Children. (2003). *Section 504 of the rehabilitation act.* Retrieved August 28, 2006, from http://ericec.org/faq/sectn504.html

Fishman E. (2001). Aging out of coverage: Young adults with special health care needs. *Health Affairs, 20,* 254–266.

Florida Department of Education. (2004.) *Standing up for me: Strategies for teaching self-determination skills.* Tallahassee, FL: Bureau of Exceptional Education and Student Services.

Flume, P.A., Anderson, D.L., Hardy, K.K., & Gray, S. (2001). Transition programs in cystic fibrosis centers: Perception of pediatric and adult program directors. *Pediatric Pulmonology, 31,* 443–450.

Forbes, A., While, A., Ullman, R., Lewis, S., Mathes, L., & Griffiths, P. (2001). *A multimethod review to identify components of practice which may promote continuity in the transition from child to adult care for young people with chronic illness or disability.* National Coordination Centre for National Health Service, Service Delivery and Organization R & D.

Haas, M. (1993). Individualized health care plans. In Marykay Haas, (Ed.), *The school nurse's source book of individualized healthcare plans* (pp. 41–54). North Branch, MN: Sunrise River Press.

Hait, E., Arnold, J.H., & Fishman, L.N. (2006). Educate, communicate, anticipate: Practical recommendations for transitioning adolescents with inflammatory bowel disease to adult health care. *Inflammatory Bowel Disease, 12*(1), 70–73.

Heller, K., & Tumlin, J. (2004). Using expanded individualized health care plans to assist teachers of students with complex health care needs. *Journal of School Nursing, 20*(3), 150–160.

Individuals with Disabilities Education Improvement Act of 2004, PL 108-446, 20 U.S.C. §§ 1400 *et seq.*

Jones, S.E., & Wheeler, L. (2004). Asthma inhalers in schools: Rights of students with asthma to free appropriate education. *American Journal of Public Health, 94,* 1102–1108.

Juvenile Diabetes Research Foundation International. (2006). *Diabetes in school.* Retrieved February 13, 2006, from http://www.jdrf.org/index.cfm?page_id=103439.

Kaiser Family Foundation. (2002). *National survey of physicians part IV: Doctor, payers and low income patients.* Publication #3223. Menlo Park, CA.

Kieckhefer, G., & Trahms, C. (2000). Supporting development of children with chronic conditions: From compliance toward shared management. *Pediatric Nursing, 26*(4), 354–381.

LoCasale-Crouch, J., & Johnson, B. (2005). Transition from pediatric to adult medical care. *Advances in Chronic Kidney Disease, 12*(4), 412–417.

Loprest, P., & Wittenburg, D. (2005). *Choices, challenges, and options: Child SSI recipients preparing for the transition to adult life.* Washington, DC: The Urban Institute. Retrieved December 4, 2006, from http://www.urban.org/Template.cfm?NavMenuID=24&template=/TaggedContent/ViewPublication.cfm&PublicationID=9277

McDonagh, J.E. (2005). Growing up and moving on: Transition from pediatric to adult care. *Pediatric Transplantation, 9*(3), 364–372.

McManus, M., Flint, S., & Kelly, R. (1991). Adequacy of physician reimbursement for pediatric care under Medicaid. *Pediatrics, 87*(6), 909–920.

Millar, D.S., and Renzaglia, A. (2002). Factors affecting guardianship practices for young adults with disabilities. *Exceptional Children, 68*(4), 465–484.

National Asthma Education and Prevention Program-School Subcommittee, National School Boards Association, American School Health Association, American Diabetes Association, American Academy of Pediatrics, Food Allergy and Anaphylaxis Network, & Epilepsy Foundation. (2003). Students with chronic illnesses: Guidance for families, schools, and students. *Journal of School Health, 73*(4), 131–132. Retrieved February 13, 2006, from http://www.nhlbi.nih.gov/health/public/lung/asthma/guidfam.pdf

Reiss, J., & Gibson, R. (2002). Health care transition: Destinations unknown. *Pediatrics, 110,* 1307–1314.

Reiss, J., Gibson, R., & Miller, R. (2004). *Health care transitions: College and beyond* [Streaming-video]. Institute for Child Health Policy. Retrieved December 4, 2006, from http://video.ichp.ufl.edu/collegeandbeyond.htm

Reiss, J., Gibson, R., & Walker, L. (2005). Health care transition: Youth family and providers perspectives. *Pediatrics, 115,* 112–120.

Reiss, J., Wallace, H., & McPherson, M. (2002). Supplemental Security Income program for children. In H. Wallace et al. (Eds.), *Health and welfare for families in the 21st century* (2nd ed.) Sudbery, MA: Jones and Bartlett.

Repetto, J., Reiss, J., Lubbers, J., Gibson, R., Gritz, S., & Garvan, C. (2005). Integrating health care transition into existing public school transition strategies. Unpublished final report. University of Florida, College of Education.

Rosen, D. (1995). Between two worlds: Bridging the cultures of child health and adult medicine. *Journal of Adolescent Health, 17,* 10–16.

Rosen, D. (2004). Transition of young people with respiratory diseases to adult health care. *Paediatric Respiratory Reviews, 5,* 124–131.

Roth, L.H., Meisel, A., & Lidz, C.W. (1977). Tests of competency to consent to treatment. *American Journal of Psychiatry, 134*, 279–284.

Rubin, K. (2003). Transitioning the pediatric patient with Turner's syndrome from pediatric to adult care. *Journal of Pediatric Endocrinology & Metabolism, 16*, 651–659.

Sandler, A.D., et al. (2001). The continued importance of Supplemental Security Income (SSI) for children and adolescents with disabilities. *Pediatrics, 107*(4), 790–793.

Tong, E.M., Sparacino, P.S., Messias, D.K., Foote, D., Chesla, C.A., & Gilliss, C.L. (1998). Growing up with congenital heart disease. *Cardiology in the Young, 8*, 303–309.

U.S. Department of Education. (2005). Individuals with disabilities education improvement Act of 2004. Retrieved December 20, 2005, from http://www.ed.gov/policy/speced/guid/idea/idea2004.html

U.S. Department of Education, Office of Safe and Drug-Free Schools. (2004). Guidance for state and local implementation of programs. Retrieved August 25, 2005, from http://www.ed.gov/programs/dvpformula/legislation.html

U.S. General Accounting Office. (2001). Medicaid: Stronger efforts needed to ensure children's access to health screening services. Washington, DC: Author. Retrieved August 18, 2006, from http://frwebgate.access.gpo.gov/cgi-bin/useftp.cgi?IPaddress=162. 140.64.21&filename=d01749.pdf&directory=/diskb/wais/data/gao

Viner, R. (2001). Barriers and good practice in transition from paediatric to adult care. *Journal of the Royal Society of Medicine, 94*, 2–4.

Watson, A.R. (2005). Problems and pitfalls of transition from paediatric to adult renal care. *Pediatric Nephrology, 20*(2), 113–117.

Webb, G. (2003). Challenges in the care of adult patients with congenital heart defects. *Heart, 89*, 465–469.

Weithorn, L.A., & Campbell, S.B. (1982). Competency of children and adolescents to make informed treatment decisions. *Child Development, 53*, 1589–1598.

White, P. (2002). Access to health care: Health insurance considerations for young adults with special health care needs/disabilities. *Pediatrics, 110*, 1328–1335.

CHAPTER 9

Looking for Applause

Determining Transition Health Outcomes

KATHLEEN B. BLOMQUIST, LINDA M. GRAHAM, AND JENNIFER THOMAS

All the world's a stage,
And all the men and women merely players:
They have their exits and their entrances;
And one man in his time plays many parts,
His acts being seven ages.

William Shakespeare, *As You Like It*

Youth in transition are like actors. Actors learn basic acting techniques; practice to develop familiarity, comfort, and skill in executing their roles; and audition at every available opportunity to expand their repertoires and get closer to achieving their personal goals. Similarly, children and youth develop attitudes, behaviors, and skills to successfully take on the roles of adulthood. The outcome of successful transition is the performance of adult roles and responsibilities. This chapter examines the context and measurement of adult roles and responsibilities; the leading men and women; the supporting cast of families; desired outcomes from the national playwrights; and the agents, directors, prompters, and sceneshifters in the lives of young people. The spotlight is on health outcomes, but included are outcomes related to work, education, recreation, and independence that enrich the lives of young people and motivate them to stay healthy so that they can participate in life. The following is an overview of the optimal health-related and postsecondary transition outcomes that youth with special health care needs and disabilities can achieve with the appropriate services and supports (Arnett, 2000; Brown, Moore, & Bzostek, 2004; Clark & Davis,

For the purposes of this chapter, the term *youth with disabilities* represents the range of chronic conditions that youth with special health care needs and disabilities experience.

Writing of this paper was partially funded by MCHB Cooperative Agreement U39MC0004, the HRTW National Center. We greatly appreciate the contributions of the staff of Kentucky Commission for CSHCN and Alabama Children's Rehabilitation Service for their transition expertise. Particular appreciation goes to Theresa Glore for enthusiasm for the theme and writing expertise. Special thanks to Stacy Brock and her family for their stories and to Alabama CRS Youth Advisory Board members Jicoria Robinson, Ashley Farr, and Andy Phelps for their insights on the outcomes youth want.

2000; Holmes & Hazel, 2003; KY TEACH Project, 2002; National 4-H Council, 2004; SEARCH Institute, 2005).

Health condition

- Can describe condition to others and understands body systems involved and how condition affects them

- Can determine when condition is worsening, when secondary disabilities (e.g., decubiti, urinary tract infection, constipation, contractures) are occurring and how to take preventive and corrective actions

- Knows what equipment does and how to fix minor problems

- Knows names of medications, their actions, and side effects, and takes medications independently (or can instruct attendant)

- Can perform self-care and treatments or instruct attendant

- Knows how condition affects sexuality; knows about birth control, safe sex, and reproductive concerns (e.g., genetics, pregnancy); girls can care for menstrual needs

- Knows how tobacco/drugs/alcohol/foods affect body and mind and illness/disability and how they interact with medications; knows how to read labels

- Eats nutritious diet and maintains healthy weight

- Maintains physical fitness with regular exercise

- Has someone to talk with for coping/mental health issues/problem solving

- Perceives life to be satisfying in general; has hope and optimism

Providers

- Knows primary care provider, dentist, and specialists (name, address, phone, how to contact); has had experience talking with these people alone; makes own appointments, asks questions, and follows through with medical recommendations

- Has a plan for getting help in an emergency

- Knows how to contact pharmacies and equipment suppliers and other health-related providers

- Has plans for finding or has found new providers in another location, and adult providers if still seeing pediatricians; knows personality factors and expertise wanted in medical and dental care providers

- Has started process to transfer records to providers in the community of new school/work setting

- Keeps summary medical file

Insurance

- Knows insurance plan's name, address, case manager contact information; responsible for health insurance ID card

- Knows what benefits are covered and not covered and is prepared to make co-payments; knows how to make benefits inquiries; knows codes for counseling

- Knows how to submit bills for payment and follow up disputes

Family and friends

- Socializes with family, friends, neighbors, and others

- Is dating, possibly thinking of marriage; physical and psychological intimacy satisfying to both partners

- Has experience with children in preparation for parenting

Independent living

- Has plans for transportation and knows how to use public and private options

- Has a driver's license or state identification card

- Can budget money; has opened and uses a bank account; pays bills responsibly

- Has found housing with needed accommodations; nutritional, safety, and rest needs are met

- Has cooking, meal planning/nutrition, housekeeping, laundry, and clothing care skills, and has a plan for housekeeping help if needed

- Has a personal attendant or plans to hire one if needed for personal care

Employment and postsecondary education and training

- Can use a computer to search the Internet, word process, and can use various software

- Can advocate for self regarding accommodations needed in school, work, community, or home, and can determine their effectiveness

- Has a resume and model letter requesting recommendations

- Can complete a job application and interview for a job

- Has obtained vocational training in the community through volunteer work, visited employment sites, has participated in "shadowing" employees, and has been employed in part-time and/or summer jobs

- Has developed the interpersonal skills necessary to maintain employment

- Can identify people and agencies to assist in job searches

- Identifies activities of interest and can find community education courses

- Identifies personal learning styles, career interests, and opportunities

- Knows how to register to take college entrance exams (e.g., ACT/SAT)

- Knows how to apply to postsecondary institutions and for financial aid, scholarships, loans, work-study, and contact disability support and counseling services

Recreation and leisure

- Has plans for having fun in health-promoting ways
- Has developed a variety of specific recreation and leisure skills
- Has spectator or audience member skills
- Identifies affordable recreation and leisure activities
- Can arrange social activities
- Has identified social supports through family, peer group, mentors, and community resources

Other general skills

- Knows strengths and limitations; accepts responsibility for own actions
- Knows laws, policies, rights, and responsibilities for adults with disabilities; has participated in transition planning meetings; identified and contacted community agencies; knows rights regarding physical accessibility
- Is aware of community resources and options
- Identifies acceptable dress behavior for a variety of situations
- Has shopping skills
- Can order and dine in restaurants, pay for service, and tip
- Has personal safety skills (e.g., navigating streets, reading maps, using phone and cell phone, wearing seatbelts, gun safety)
- Has developed communication skills and can interact with peers, authority figures, and community members
- Accepts legal responsibilities at age 18; has registered to vote and for military selective service (if appropriate); signs legal documents
- Participates as a responsible citizen in the community; stays out of the criminal justice system
- Has explored guardianship issues (if appropriate)

STATUS OF YOUTH AND ADULTS WITH DISABILITIES

Information on the status of youth and adults with disabilities comes from surveys of adults with and without disabilities, special education students, and graduates of pediatric systems of care.

The National Organization on Disability/ Harris Survey of Americans with Disabilities

These telephone and on-line surveys of adults ages 18 to 64 years with and without disabilities have provided data at varying intervals since 1986. The findings of the 2004 National Organization on Disability (NOD)/Harris Survey (NOD, 2004) indicate what outcomes are of concern to people with disabilities, policy makers, and the public. For each finding, changes over the years and information about the 18-to-29-year-old subgroup, if available, are noted.

- Employment: Only 35% of people with disabilities reported being employed full or part time, compared with 78% of individuals without disabilities. Employment of individuals with disabilities has been slowly increasing from a low of 29% in 1998. Two thirds of those unemployed would prefer to work. For the 18-to-29 age group, 57% were working compared with 72% of their typically developing peers—a promising trend.

- Income: Three times as many people with disabilities lived in poverty with annual household incomes less than $15,000 compared with the general public (26% vs. 9%). The gap between 18- to 29-year-olds with and without disabilities is only 9 percentage points. The percent of people with disabilities living in poverty has been slowly decreasing.

- Education: People with disabilities were twice as likely to drop out of high school compared with students without disabilities (21% vs. 10%). Approximately 8 out of 10 students with disabilities graduated from high school in 2004 compared with 6 out of 10 in 1986.

- Transportation: People with disabilities were twice as likely to have inadequate transportation compared with individuals without disabilities (31% vs. 13%).

- Social/community activities: People with disabilities were less likely to socialize, eat out, or attend religious services than their typically developing peers (85% vs. 70%). These statistics have not changed over the past decade. More positively, 18- to 29-year-old people with disabilities were almost as likely as their typically developing peers to socialize with close friends, relatives, or neighbors (about 90% for both groups).

- Life satisfaction: Thirty-four percent of people with disabilities said they were very satisfied with life compared with 61% of individuals without disabilities; there has been little change in this statistic in the past decade. The gap was smaller for 18- to 29-year-olds, with 44% of younger people with disabilities saying they are very satisfied with life compared with 57% of those without disabilities.

- Job discrimination: Twenty-two percent of employed people with disabilities reported encountering job discrimination—this percentage has dropped from 36% in 2000.

- Health care: Eighteen percent of people with disabilities said they did not get needed health care on at least one occasion in the past year compared with 7% of people without disabilities.

- Health insurance: People with and without disabilities were equally likely to have health insurance (about 90% for both groups). However, people with disabilities were more likely to have special needs that were not covered by their health insurance as compared with people without disabilities (28% vs. 7%).

- Concern about health: People with disabilities were much more worried about their future health and well-being than individuals without disabilities. Fifty percent worried about not being able to care for themselves or being a burden to their families compared with 25% of other Americans.

- Assistive technology: One third of individuals with disabilities said that they would lose their independence without this technology.

The severity of disability makes a significant difference in all of the life areas, and people with severe disabilities as reported in this survey experienced much greater disadvantages.

National Longitudinal Transition Studies

The National Longitudinal Transition Studies (NLTS) documented the experiences of two national samples of secondary special education students over several years as they moved from secondary school into adult roles (Wagner, Newman, Cameto, & Levine, 2005). The first study was conducted in 1987, and the second study (NLTS-2) was conducted in 2003. The findings of the NLTS-2 revealed that students with disabilities have made significant progress in their transition to adulthood during the past 25 years with lower dropout rates, an increase in post-secondary enrollment, and a higher rate of gainful employment after leaving high school. Comparison of the findings from the NLTS and the NLTS-2 revealed that the incidence of students with disabilities completing high school rather than dropping out increased by 17 percentage points to 70%. The postsecondary education participation of students with disabilities more than doubled to 32% during this relatively short period of time. And, the employment prospects improved as the percent of students with disabilities out of school for up to two years who had paying jobs increased from 55% to 70%.

The demographic profile of the NLTS-2 revealed that 75% of youth with disabilities were males, 33% were poor, 33% lived in single-parent families, 21% (vs. 10% of all U.S. families) lived with family members with less than a high school education, and 35% of heads of households were unemployed. Outcomes for youth in various disability groups differed greatly. Those with emotional and behavioral difficulties or multiple disabilities had the poorest outcomes, while those with learning disabilities and hearing impairments demonstrated the best outcomes in terms of health conditions affecting their daily activities, missing school, inadequate health insurance, unmet needs for health care services, difficulty obtaining referrals, and not having a personal doctor or nurse (Bethell, Read, & Blumberg, 2005; Wagner, Cameto, & Guzman, 2003).

Surveys of Graduates of a State Children with Special Health Care Needs Agency and Pediatric Hospital in Kentucky

As part of the evaluation of the Kentucky Healthy & Ready to Work Project, graduates of the Commission for Children with Special Health Care Needs and Shriners Hospital for Children were surveyed. Respondents were 18 to 23 years of age, 61% were female, and 69% reported being independent in activities of daily living. Survey findings included:

- Eighty percent of young adults with disabilities had a family doctor or clinic but used the emergency room at almost double the rates of their typically developing peers (40% vs. 25%).

- Forty-one percent of young adults with disabilities said their health was excellent or very good compared with 63% of their typically developing peers.

- Thirty percent of young adults with disabilities smoked compared with 39% their typically developing peers.

- Eighteen percent of individuals with disabilities had children, and 47% of those individuals were unwed mothers.

- Twenty-nine percent of individuals with disabilities lacked health insurance compared with 36% of their typically developing peers.

- Twenty percent of young adults with disabilities had dropped out of high school compared with 15% of their typically developing peers.

- Forty-four percent of young adults with disabilities were working compared with 88% of their typically developing peers.

- Eighty-two percent of young adults with disabilities had never been married compared with 77% of their typically developing peers.

- Fifty-seven percent of young adults with disabilities lived with their parents compared with 56% of men and 43% of women in the general population.

Of great concern is that 26% of young adults with disabilities were not working, were not in school, or were not home with children, although 47% of these idle young adults reported they were independent in function, 48% used computers, and 41% drove (Blomquist, 2006).

These surveys indicated that although young adults with disabilities were doing better than older people with disabilities in terms of education and work, they were still significantly below the levels of their typically developing peers. They had concerns about their health and insurance coverage for their special needs, they were much more likely to live in poverty and lacked access to transportation and opportunities for community socialization, and their life satisfaction and perception of health were much lower than their typically developing peers.

THE LEADING MEN AND WOMEN: WHAT DO YOUTH WITH DISABILITIES WANT?

What researchers decide are appropriate outcomes for youth with disabilities may not be what youth want. Youth with and without disabilities express many of the same dreams. Stacy Brock, a young adult from Alabama, says

> For my future, I want to have a loving and productive relationship with first a boyfriend and then my husband. I feel that this will be a key element of my success as an adult. If I'm not happy at home, I can't be happy at work, and if I'm not happy at work, I can't do my job well. I also feel that the happiness of my children will depend greatly on my happiness with my husband. I also feel that maintaining strong relationships with friends and family is crucial to my happiness and success as an adult. Even though many non-disabled people place the same importance on having a family and friends, many of them seem surprised that I need these things.
>
> Until some people get to know me they often think I have the intellect, emotions, and desire for intimacy of a toddler. The idea that I would pursue a career in the field of theater and film is also perceived as totally ludicrous. People are to-

tally baffled by the fact that I bond more quickly and easily with my peers that are not disabled than those who are. For example, my Mom sent me to a camp for youth with disabilities thinking I would get in touch with my disabled side. I only formed a friendship with one of the other campers, but many of the staff members who worked that summer are part of my extended family now.

Perhaps my optimistic and carefree perspective on life comes from the fact that I feel that my disability has enhanced my quality of life by allowing me to meet people I would not otherwise have met and challenging me to make who I am clear. When I talk to other people with disabilities some of them seem to feel deprived and isolated from the rest of the world. I hardly ever feel deprived or isolated because of my disability. If I ever do feel this way, I blame it on my family's lower-than-average income or the rural area that I live in.

Maybe I am in denial, but I think I'm better off. Even though my disability is severe physically (quadriplegic cerebral palsy) I am healthy, which allows me to fill my time like any other 21-year-old woman, as long as I have dependable attendant care. My favorite hobbies are being in beauty pageants, watching movies, reading, listening to music, and taking 2 to 4 college courses every semester, with a little flirting in between. My wish for the future is to have a successful career and a happy family.

When asked what they want, youth with special needs seldom put health as a top priority. However, they know if they do not stay healthy, they cannot do what they want to do. Using input from youth discussion groups and a review of the literature, the Alabama Youth Advisory Council for the state's Title V Children with Special Health Care Needs program generated a list of outcomes youth want for their lives. Based on the findings, a framework depicting the range of youth desires was generated. This framework is depicted below.

To have opportunities, such as:

- Being heard and listened to

- Speaking for themselves

- Trying new things: school, work, recreation

- Experiencing success in a challenging school environment

- Knowing how to make things happen in their lives

- Knowing what steps to follow and what an experience might be like

- Striving for a goal that will result in their achieving it instead of being hindered

- Asking for accommodations to make education, work, and community living fair and accessible, not based on giving greater advantage (see Chapter 6)

To be included and accepted by:

- Having choices and supports needed

- Being able to get around in an accessible community

- Having a sense of self-worth and belonging

- Contributing through paid work or volunteer activities

- Giving back through service to others

- Having roles in families
- Being active citizens in the community
- Having rights and privileges that other citizens want and deserve to have
- Having friends who respect them and are trustworthy
- Having positive social interactions in which young people are valued and supported by friends and family

To be independent by:

- Taking the lead in making decisions about their lives
- Developing an "I want to do it myself" attitude
- Learning responsibility
- Having self-determination regarding choices, opportunities, and activities
- Having family members who expect them to be successful adults
- Learning how to set goals and "stick up" for themselves

To be educated about:

- Functioning of their bodies and disabilities or special health care needs
- Staying healthy
- Recognizing and knowing how to cope with signs of change
- Making decisions about health including treatments, providers, therapies, and insurance

To experience health and wellness by:

- Having physical and emotional states of well-being
- Staying as active as possible, including participating in physical activity and exercise
- Developing coping strategies
- Controlling pain
- Accepting themselves as they are and moving forward with their lives
- Having respectful, concerned, and informed health providers who treat the whole person
- Getting a good doctor who treats adults
- Anticipating what could happen if condition gets worse
- Having a plan for what to do in an emergency
- Knowing how to get health insurance
- Exchanging ideas and feelings on living with the special needs with others with similar conditions

- Having a sense of purpose and hope for the future (Alabama Children's Rehabilitation Service Youth Advisory Council, personal communication, August, 2005; Konopka Institute, 2005; Peterson, 2004; National Collaborative on Workforce and Disability for Youth, 2005; PACER Center, 1997; Powers, Turner, & National Youth Leadership Network, 1997; Putnam et al., 2003)

As these responses indicate, youth want opportunities to have a voice that is heard by those around them, to set and strive to achieve goals, to practice new roles, to stay healthy, and to hear applause for their performance to know that they are valued.

THE SUPPORTING CAST: WHAT DO FAMILIES WANT?

As these responses indicate youth grow up in families who have expectations for their children and themselves for the future. Families set the stage and affect the scripts for individual members. Comedy, tragedy, and fantasy interact to create the character in each member. Stacy Brock who related her dreams for the future receives support from her parents and grandparents to achieve her dreams. Her grandparents, Faye and L.D. Burt, say:

> To Our Rosebud: We watched as Stacy grew from a 2½ pound preemie into a beautiful young lady. We were there as she conquered challenge after challenge, which took a lot of patience, grit, and determination. Our wish for Stacy is that she will find her soul mate and keep chasing her dreams, never losing her sense of humor, trust in God, or her love for life. You have now spread your petals and become a rose in full bloom. But to us, you will always be our rosebud. Love, Nanny and Papaw.

Stacy's parents, Denise and Mack Brock, say:

> As parents, we wish for Stacy to be happy in life, no matter what her endeavor. We hope this will come through a good education and the right opportunities in her chosen field of theater and film. Stacy is working on a degree in this area now and hopes to one day attend the New York Film Academy. When she was in high school, she was told this was an unrealistic goal for her to pursue, and teachers were surprised that her parents were supportive of this goal. We told them we had always told Stacy she could do anything she worked hard enough for and she believed us. Now it is time for us to provide the resources for her to follow her dreams.
>
> We want Stacy to be successful in her career. She is physically dependent on others for attendant care and she will need to be able to pay for it as we age and are not able to provide it for her. We hope she will always have dependable people in her life, because she has the determination to succeed if she has the support for her physical needs. Having attendant care from someone with whom she has a professional rather than family relationship seems to foster her feelings of independence and decision making. This is the situation that allows her to attend college now, without having to have her mother or father drive her and stay with her throughout the day. As family members we tend to second guess or assume what her decisions might be.
>
> We feel it would be most rewarding for Stacy to have a family of her own. Even though she is healthy, Stacy will need help to care for her children because of her limited functional movement due to cerebral palsy. We hope there will be support services available if she needs them and that she will find a supportive husband who will be a partner in her life.

Private insurance has played a big role in Stacy's good health, and we hope this remains an option for Stacy in her adult life. It allows her to have the individualized care program to maintain a high quality of life. Stacy's disability requires specialized equipment and services that Medicaid does not pay for. For instance, she needs standing equipment on her wheelchair. This helps her maintain strong bones allowing her to help with transferring and also keeps her digestive system working well. In the long run this decreases the down time she might experience from illness and decreases her medical expenses. At this point in Stacy's life, our focus is to allow her the freedom to make decisions for her future while being as supportive and nonjudgmental as we can force ourselves to be.

Families want their teens and young adults to have friends and fun, to have a full range of educational and employment opportunities, and to have living options with supports needed. They want their children to stay healthy, manage health insurance, and to be safe and free from fear and harm. Families want their children's conditions to have minimal impact on family members' physical and mental health, quality of life, prosperity, and involvement in community. They want to be able to navigate the system and obtain assistance when needed and to have community supports in place for the youth so that family members can work in the community for pay if they so desire. They want to be involved in care/service planning that is strength-based and consistent with cultural values and expectations. They want to be knowledgeable about adolescent and adult growth and development, age appropriate developmental tasks, medical condition/disability, health care, and social service systems. Young people and their families must both adjust to youths' growing need for independence while remaining emotionally related. Parents are still very much a part of their children's lives—but in different ways. Young adults still rely on parental input, support, and resources, but not in the same way as when they were younger. Families want support in "letting go" so that they can support developing independence in their children with confidence in the community support system (Newman, 2005; Olsen & Swigonski, 2004).

THE NATIONAL PLAYWRIGHTS: DESIRED HEALTH OUTCOMES FROM NATIONAL POLICIES

Several initiatives of the federal government describe health outcomes desired for youth and youth with special health care needs and disabilities. These initiatives provide direction for educators and health care and social service providers in developing health and health-related transition objectives for individualized education programs and 504 plans, health care transition planning services and programs, health education programs for youth and their families, and continuing education programs for professionals and providers who work with youth with special health care needs and disabilities.

New Freedom Initiative

President Bush's *New Freedom Initiative* (NFI), announced in February 2001, is part of a nationwide effort to remove barriers to community living for people with disabilities. More than 54 million Americans live with disabilities, representing about 20% of the population. A report to the Interagency Committee on Disability Research (2003) found that 67 separate laws define disability for federal purposes alone (Interagency Committee on Disability Research, 2003). Some programs use definitions that encompass person, physical surroundings, and social environment. Others define disability on the basis of specific activities of daily living, work, and other functions essential to full participation in community-based living, sometimes for a specific length of time. In addition, there are more than 25 million family caregivers and millions more who provide aid and assistance to people with disabilities. The NFI is a comprehensive plan that represents an important step in working to ensure that all Americans with disabilities have the opportunity to learn and develop skills, engage in productive work, make choices about their daily lives, and participate fully in community life. NFI goals are to:

- Increase access to assistive and universally designed technologies
- Expand educational opportunities
- Promote homeownership
- Integrate Americans with disabilities into the workforce
- Expand transportation options
- Promote full access to community life

Integrated into the NFI are the Maternal and Child Health Bureau's (MCHB's) six national performance measures for children with special health care needs. The six performance measures include early and continuous screening, youth and family involvement, medical home, health insurance, coordinated services, and transition. These six interrelated measures were designed to increase the probability that youth with special health care needs transition more successfully to adult health care, work, and independent living. Performance measure six addresses transition to adulthood, which is the outcome of a successful service system that has provided ongoing health and related services and supports for children with special health care needs. To support this measure, MCHB has funded the *Healthy & Ready to Work* initiative of state projects and a national resource center.

Surgeon General's Call to Action to Improve the Health and Wellness of Persons with Disabilities

As part of the NFI, the *Surgeon General's Call to Action to Improve the Health and Wellness of Persons with Disabilities* (2005) recognized that with good health, individuals with disabilities have the freedom to work, learn, and engage actively in their families and communities. As identified in the *Call to Action,* challenges to health and wellness come from insufficient knowledge due to inadequate access to information and opportunities for appropriate health care and wellness promotion. Other challenges are the product of provider and community attitudes and behaviors and service systems that do not make use of innovative and creative approaches to enhancing the health and wellness of individuals with disabilities.

The *Call to Action* identified barriers to overcome and provided a number of recommendations to improve health at the federal, state, tribal, and community levels in 1) policy and programs, 2) infrastructure and education, and 3) the hearts, minds, and actions of individuals with disabilities and their families, health care providers, and the public. The goals of this *Call to Action* include:

- People nationwide will understand that individuals with disabilities can lead long, healthy, productive lives

- Health care providers will have the knowledge and tools to screen, diagnose, and treat individuals with disabilities with dignity

- Individuals with disabilities will promote their own good health by developing and maintaining healthy lifestyles

- Accessible health care and support services will promote independence for individuals with disabilities

Initiatives such as the ones described emphasize the importance of health to enable people with disabilities to participate fully in mainstream society.

AGENTS, SCENESHIFTERS, DOORKEEPERS, BACKSTAGE PROMPTERS, MEDIA CRITICS, AND THE AUDIENCE: OTHERS IMPORTANT IN THE LIVES OF TRANSITIONING YOUNG PEOPLE

A variety of people come in and out of the lives of children, youth, and young adults with special health care needs and disabilities as they develop the knowledge, skills, behaviors, and attitudes important for roles in adulthood. Included in this group are primary care and specialty physicians and other pediatric and adult health care providers, mental health professionals, social and legal service providers, teachers and counselors and others in the school systems, workforce development personnel and employers, and members of the communities. Each of these groups and individuals within every group have expectations based on cultural scripts and their own attitudes, knowledge, and hopes for the young people with whom they work, and for themselves. They can become the advocates and mentors who are essential to helping the young people advance in their adult roles, or they can be the critics who impede or even halt the transition.

Physicians

Physicians are major scriptwriters and agents for young people with disabilities. Pediatricians and pediatric specialists offer their best estimates as to the future prospects for children with disabilities, instilling a sense of hope or lack thereof. The ability of physicians to provide anticipatory guidance for the future is very important for families and youth to develop the competencies necessary to grow and develop and reach their highest potential. Various health care guidelines exist to assist physicians and other health care providers to focus young people on learning the knowledge, behaviors, and attitudes important for success in adulthood. HEADS (Goldenring & Cohen; 1988; Goldenring & Rosen, 2004), the American Academy of Pediatrics's Bright Futures (2002), the American Medical Association's Guidelines for Adolescent Preventive Services (2005), and the U.S. Preventive Services Task Force Guidelines for Clinical Preventive Services (2005) are examples of anticipatory screening tools and recommendations for health care guidance. (For more information on transition assessment, refer to Chapters 1 and 7.)

Responsibility for oneself is an adult expectation. Major responsibilities for youth with special health care needs and disabilities to learn regarding their health needs are health promotion, management of their chronic conditions, and use of the health care system, including insurance. The extent to which youth with special health care needs and disabilities can assume responsibilities for their health care needs can be used as indicators of outcomes and content for teaching youth to become more responsible for their health and health care. There are a variety of ways to track outcomes related to health and health behaviors. The CHOICES Transition Guidelines developed by the Kentucky HRTW project funded by the federal Maternal and Child Health Bureau and Shriners Hospitals for Children is an example of health care outcomes for youth with special health care needs and disabilities. The CHOICES Transition Guidelines provide outcome criteria and possible interventions for health care providers working with children and youth with special health care needs and disabilities. The CHOICES Transition Guidelines are composed of seven categories that include health promotion and disease prevention, health problem management, development and self-care, self-perception, coping and stress, family and community support, and school and work. An example of CHOICES Transition Guidelines for health problem management outcomes and interventions for youth 11 to 21 years old is listed in Table 9.1.

Health Insurance and Other Benefits Providers

Young adults ages 19 to 29 years old are the largest segment of the population without health insurance in the United States. Young adults often lose coverage under their parents' policies at age 19 or when they graduate from college. Nearly 40% of college graduates and half of high school graduates not going on to college endure a time without health insurance in the first year after graduation (Collins, Schoen, Kriss, Doty, & Mahato, 2004). The transitional nature of young adults' lives following their 19th birthdays makes it difficult for them to secure a stable and consistent source of health insurance coverage. Having health insurance is an important outcome and affects other health outcomes for young adults.

Health insurance and benefits providers want young people to make use of the benefits allowable under their health insurance plans. Young people who have health insurance benefits need to learn to use health care resources and services appropriately as well as identify problems and get treatment early. Other skills young people need to acquire are knowing how to document their condition and treatment and knowing how and when to use the appeal process. It is important for young people to know their legal rights and responsibilities associated with insurance coverage, so they can promptly report changes in income, residency, and so forth that are critical factors in Medicaid eligibility. (For more information about health insurance, refer to Chapter 3.)

Table 9.1. Example of CHOICES transition guidelines with outcomes and interventions for ages 11 to 21: Health problem management

Outcomes	Interventions
Young person interacts directly with physicians, nurses, therapists	Direct questions to young person rather than parents
	Provide privacy and time without parents
	Assess current level of understanding
Young person demonstrates competence in health problem management skills such as:	Assess competence with appropriate healthcare skills checklist and/or observation
treatments	Teach young person about health problem(s) and how to manage care
medications	
therapy	Provide with culturally appropriate information including Internet sites relating to disability
exercise	
orthopedic appliance	Encourage independence in health case management to the greatest extent possible
latex allergy	
bowel program	Complete appropriate health problem management plan/worksheets and include in transition workbook
bladder program	
prevention of skin breakdown	
Young person demonstrates health practices that will prevent secondary disabilities such as:	Assess risk status for secondary disabilities
obesity or under nutrition	Teach young person about risk of secondary disabilities associated with health condition and cues to early identification
contractures	Teach to monitor for secondary disabilities
skin problems	Individualize prevention and monitoring activities and include in a transition workbook
constipation	
urinary tract infections	

Developed by CHOICES Transition Project, funded by federal Maternal and Child Health Bureau and Shriners Hospitals for Children, Betty Presler, and Kathy Blomquist, 2001. CHOICES Transition Guidelines for ages 11–21 are available at http://www.hrtw.org and http://chfs.ky.gov/ccshcn. Adapted with permission.

Educators

Teachers and others in the schools have great influence on attitudes, expectations, and experiences of youth. Examples of education outcomes desired by educators, families, and youth include progressing through school with inclusion and special services using IDEA and 504 provisions (see Chapters 10 and 11); having the ability to not only participate in testing for math and English but also meet the state standards as required by the federal *No Child Left Behind* legislation and state programs; and developing reading, computer, and math skills needed for future employment and full community participation. Educational performance is greatly influenced by a youth's health status. Academic achievement is influenced by health-related concerns, as evidenced by the need to have consistent attendance with health care planned outside of school hours and not losing school days because of health conditions, disease exacerbations, or health care needs. Learning to independently seek assistance for special health care needs/health problems from teachers and school nurses is important to prevent problems from getting worse. Other educational outcomes to assess are youths' involvement in peer activities/relationships at and outside of school and their participation in art, music, sports, service, and clubs. Other outcomes include growing independence from parents, self-control, and personal responsibility for planning and enacting life plans, completing high school with job skills, and planning for and completing college/technical school.

Employers

Good workers support employers' goals of making profit, growing, and developing markets for their goods and services. Employers want workers who come to work regularly, are willing to learn, and work in team settings. They want workers who manage their health and health care outside of work time so attendance is consistent. They want employees who have the ability to ask for and use reasonable accommodations. Employers are often willing to develop natural supports within the work setting or develop customized jobs that offer youth opportunities to use their talents within the constraints of their conditions. Employers want workers who have had volunteer and service learning experiences, part-time jobs, and mentorship experiences, so they can see positive work patterns. Therefore, it is important that youth with disabilities have opportunities to practice skills and have experiences that are transferable to the workplace. Youth need families, educators, and communities that expect them to work (Bullis & Chaney, 1999; Gramlich, Crane, Peterson, & Stenhjem, 2003; Stapleton & Burkhauser, 2003). (For additional information on employment issues, refer to Chapter 12.)

Communities

Community members want and need their youth to be productive members of society. Communities are different in terms of their support for people with disabilities. Communities that are supportive of youth with disabilities value their creativity, talents, and contributions. Community support is evidenced by accessibility and having information and communication networks so people know how to access services, programs, and policies that facilitate transition processes. As mentioned in Chapter 1, the ideal comprehensive transition service system is one that has a single point of access to transition services that are coordinated, responsive, and culturally competent to eliminate duplication.

SUMMARY

Although the outcomes in terms of health, education, work, and community integration for youth with disabilities are improving, they still are behind their peers. Youth with disabilities want the same experiences and high expectations that all youth want. They want to be listened to, encouraged, and applauded when they do well. They want to stay healthy but also take risks just like everyone else and be challenged. The federal government will continue to promote coordinated transition services through the NFI and other programs mentioned in this chapter. It is the people surrounding the youth, namely, their families, health care providers, teachers, potential employers, and people in the community who help youth with disabilities become all they can be.

My Story
Jennifer Thomas

Although I advocate for care being given to the whole person, at times I fail to see the big picture when it comes to my own health. Having a disability, radial club hands, also known as phocomelia, affects every area of my life, and the fact that I need support is always present. As a result, I have managed to somehow separate my disability and the experiences that come with it from my health in general. As I reflect on my 22 years, I realize that it all goes together, and the expectations of those who have taken part in my drama played a major role in the development of my script for life.

My production team consists of a few different playwrights, all possessing their own ideals and desires for my life. The lead playwright is my mother. She encouraged my independence as much as possible, teaching me basic skills that I would need throughout life. I was not excluded from household chores, whether it meant pulling the covers up on my bed the best I could using my feet or wiping the table after eating. My mother also taught me to speak for myself. If I wanted to eat at McDonald's, I had to place my own order. At the grocery store, it was my job to find items on the list, and my mother would place them in the cart. When it was time to transport the bags of groceries to the car, I carried the lighter bags. At the laundromat, I alerted my mother or my siblings when clothes were done. Whether I liked it or not, my mother expected my best and made sure that I had a role in our household.

My siblings were playwrights with desires of their own, my younger sister being the most outspoken. We got along great sometimes and fought sometimes and both of us wanted to take center stage. My sister greatly influenced the script because she was given a huge responsibility—me. Because I was unable to dress myself, I had to call on my sister when it was time to get ready for bed. When I needed to go to the bathroom, I had to call on her. We were always together because I needed her so much, leaving us both feeling like we needed our own lives. She got tired of my having to rely on her so much; so did I! She constantly expressed her wish for me to be able to do things for myself while I wished that I were more adequate as a big sister. In no way did I want to be a burden to her or to anyone else, so I learned to mask my self-pity and insecurities. I was determined to become a big sister who my siblings could be proud of. It took some time, but my sister's words motivated me to find my inner strength and step into my role.

My grandmothers were also involved in the writing of the script. Just as they did with their other grandchildren, they both desired that I do well, that I prosper. My maternal grandmother observed how I functioned using my feet and encouraged my mother to allow me to explore the house barefooted. She showed me that it was okay that I played, ate, and so forth, differently, and she made sure that my siblings and cousins understood this. However, she was protective and sometimes had others help her with things instead of me, in fear that I would get hurt. My paternal grandmother, a preschool teacher, taught me how to be assertive. "Look people in the eye and don't whisper when you are talking to them!" she would say. When I visited her, we would spend hours in her garden. She would do her best to answer my questions about everything and regularly praised my accomplishments. Her main contributions to my life were her high expectations for me; no matter what, she has always expected me to try.

After the script was written, technical assistance was needed so that the saga of Jennifer could go forth. Included under technical personnel were my community primary physician and specialty service providers. My primary physician's task was to help me stay well, providing an overall assessment, information, and preventive services. I hated being immunized, but nothing was worse than having to undress and be eyeballed and poked at. Eventually, I began seeing the female partner in the practice and my mother sat in the waiting room at my request. The doctor expected my questions and seemed to look forward to them. I wanted to be a walking book of knowledge concerning my body. This was of more importance to me when terrible cramps began around age 14. All of my friends had begun menstruating, but I had not. After multiple tests, the pediatric gynecologist discovered that I was missing an ovary and my uterus failed to develop completely. The specialist let me know about everything he found and gave his recommendations. I learned more about my body. I was not planning to have children the next day, but the news did impact my future decisions. In my freshman year of college I confronted a new issue called migraines. An MRI was negative, I was placed on medication and learned how to cope with my migraines.

In 2004, I began occupational therapy (OT). I had OT in the past, but it was definitely time for me to rehearse that scene again. A major breakthrough occurred. I learned how to dress myself completely! I was now an adult and wanted to be as independent as possible in as many areas as possible. There were some tools that I had had for years that needed some adjustments made to them so that I could use them with ease. I was placed on an exercise plan to help strengthen my muscles. The process itself was mostly trial-and-error. There were some days in which major successes occurred, and there were other days when I just wanted to give up. I haven't learned how to comb my hair, ride a bike, swim (learning to swim wasn't in my treatment plan for OT), or do a host of other things YET, but I will. Dressing myself and going to the bathroom on my own seemed so far away at one time, but it happened. My therapist and I both wanted it, and together we willed it to happen.

So what's a drama without props? My community, the set designers in my life, made sure that I had plenty of these, adding clarity and beauty to my life. I gained many of the props for my life as I attended church. This was like a second home for me all of my life. I obtained my first taste of leadership here as I participated in the youth choir, youth ministry, and several other activities. I was never excluded from anything and was always expected to succeed. I was given support, as well as responsibilities.

Ever since the seventh grade, I have been involved in a community service organization of some form or another. Being included in something greater than myself always made me feel human, like a citizen doing her part. I became a delegate for the Alabama Governor's Youth Leadership Forum (YLF) for High School Students with Disabilities. This was my first time being away from home by myself and realizing that living on my own was far more possible than I had ever imagined. Attending YLF led me to the CRS Youth Advisory Committee (YAC) and, eventually, to KASA (Kids as Self-Advocates). Both of these groups encouraged me to voice my opinions as a youth with a disability. YAC provided me with options, skills for assertiveness, and training. KASA has helped me to identify more with the disability community, teaching me about its history and culture.

Employment opportunities have also provided props to support my life. In the past, I worked as a counselor with Goodtimes, an after-school program offered through the YMCA. In this first job I learned very quickly how to function in a team with my coworkers to get things done. My supervisor made it evident that she valued me by making sure that I had the accommodations I needed. I was able to complete work-study as a receptionist during my freshman year of college. Currently, I work as the State Youth Consultant for Children's Rehabilitation Service. It's funny how the roads we take often lead us to where we began. I am the first and only Youth Consultant for the Title V Program in the state of Alabama (and the United States). Each job that I have had has added to who I am today. I have gained a strong work ethic, leadership skills, and knowledge about life. Most importantly, I have gained validation. Now I know my worth, and I don't have to feel like a burden because I am helping to take care of me and others.

There were other set designers that I can't leave out—my friends. These people accept me for who I am and whatever comes along with me. They act as counselors, chauffeurs, loan officers, comedians, and medical advisors. They taught me how to skate, and they listen when I talk about disability culture. They attend my poetry readings, even when poetry isn't their favorite thing, and they motivate me to kick my bad habits.

Before a drama can be performed successfully, many roles have to be fulfilled. Responsibilities have to be taken care of, and trustworthy people are needed to help plot the course. Much of the casting in my life took place before I was able to make decisions for myself, but gradually, the responsibility is being turned over to me. Support is great to have, and I appreciate having it. There were times where I wasn't well, and there were times when I simply needed help. Though people came to the rescue, I needed to learn about myself for myself. I am not saying that I want my life to be a monologue. What I am saying is that when the curtains rise, I want to be the director. I believe that ultimately youth should have a major role in directing their own performance, their drama called life.

REFERENCES

American Medical Association. *Guidelines for Adolescent Preventive Services*. Retrieved November, 10, 2005, from http://www.ama-assn.org/ama/pub/category/1980.html

Arnett, J.J. (2000). Emerging adulthood: A theory of development from the late teens through the twenties. *American Psychologist, 55*(5), 469–480.

Bethell, C.D., Read, D. & Blumberg, S.J. (2005). Mental health in the United States: Health care and well being of children with chronic emotional, behavioral, or developmental problems — United States, 2001. *Morbidity and Mortality Weekly Report, 54*(39), 985–989. Retrieved October, 3, 2005, from http://www.cdc.gov/mmwr/preview/mmwrhtml/mm5439a3.htm

Blomquist, K.B. (2006). Health, education, work, and independence of young adults with disabilities. *Orthopaedic Nursing, 25*(3), 168–187.

Brown, B.V., Moore, K.A., & Bzostek, S. (2004, August). A portrait of well-being in early adulthood. *CrossCurrents, 2*, 1–8. Retrieved August 6, 2005, from www.hewlett.org/archives/publications/portraitofwellbeing.htm

Bullis, M., & Chaney, D. (1999). Vocational and transition interventions for adolescents and young adults with emotional or behavioral disorders. *Focus on Exceptional Children, 31*(7), 1–24.

Clark, H.B., & Davis, M.A. (2000). *Transition to adulthood: A resource for assisting young people with emotional or behavioral difficulties*. Baltimore: Paul H. Brookes Publishing Co.

Collins, S.R., Schoen, C., Kriss, J.L., Doty, M.M., & Mahato, B. (2006). Rite of passage? *Why young adults become uninsured and how new policies can help*. New York: The Commonwealth Fund. Retrieved November, 2006, from http://www.cmwf.org/publications/publications_show.htm?doc_id=374136

Goldenring, J.M., & Cohen, E. (1988). Getting into adolescent heads. *Contemporary Pediatrics, 5*, 75–90.

Goldenring, J.M., & Rosen, D. (2004). Getting into adolescent heads: An essential update. *Contemporary Pediatrics, 21*, 64–90.

Gramlich, M., Crane, K., Peterson, K., & Stenhjem, P. (2003). Work-based learning and future employment for youth: A guide for parents and guardians. *Information Brief, 2*(2). Retrieved October 3, 2005, from http://www.ncset.org/publications/viewdesc.asp?id=1222

Holmes, A.B., & Hazel, K. (2003). *Young adults in South Carolina: A comprehensive report on the lives of South Carolinians ages 18 to 29*. Retrieved June, 2005, from http://www.scyoungadults.org/yac-mainpage.html

Interagency Committee on Disability Research. (2003). *Federal Statutory Definitions of Disability*. Retrieved October, 2005, from http://www.icdr.us/documents/definitions.htm

KY TEACH Project. (2002). *Competencies for young people transitioning to postsecondary school and/or work, compiled by K. Blomquist, A. Peersen, B. Presler, and others*. Retrieved August, 2005, from http://chfs.ky.gov/ccshcn/ccshcntransition.htm

Konopka Institute at the University of Minnesota. (2005). *Konopka Institute for Best Practices in Adolescent Health*. Retrieved August, 2005, from http://www.allaboutkids.umn.edu/konopka/

National Collaborative on Workforce and Disability for Youth, NCWD_YOUTH (2005). Retrieved June, 2005, from www.ncwd-youth.info

National Longitudinal Transition Studies (1987 and 2003). Retrieved June, 2005, from http://www.nlts2.org

National Organization on Disability. (2004). *NOD/ Harris Survey of Americans with Disabilities.* Retrieved November, 2005, from http://www.nod.org

New Freedom Initiative. Retrieved August, 2005, from www.hhs.gov/newfreedom

Newman, L. (2005). Family expectations and involvement of youth with disabilities. *NLTS2 Data Brief, 4*(2), 1–7. Retrieved November 10, 2005, from http://www.ncset.org/publications/viewdesc.asp?id=2473

Olsen, D.G., & Swigonski, N.L. (2004). Transition to adulthood: The important role of the pediatrician. *Pediatrics, 113,* 159–162.

PACER Center. (1997). *Teens speak out: A survey of teens with chronic illness and disabilities in transition.* Retrieved December 6, 2006, from http://www.pacer.org/publictaions/transition.htm

Peterson, K. (2004). Supporting dynamic development of youth with disabilities during transition: A guide for families. *NCSET Information Brief, 3,* 2. Retrieved June, 2005, from http://www.ncset.org/publications/viewdesc.asp?id=1432

Powers, L., Turner, A., & National Youth Leadership Network (2003). *Building a successful adult life: Findings from youth-directed research.* Working paper, National Youth Leadership Network.

Presler, B., & Blomquist, K. (2001). *CHOICES Transition Guidelines.* Retrieved November, 2005, from http://chfs.ky.gov/ccshcn/ccshcntransition.htm

Putnam, M., Geenen, S., Powers, L.E., Saxton, M., Finney, S., & Dautel, P. (2003). Health and wellness: People with disabilities discuss barriers and facilitators to well being. *Journal of Rehabilitation, 69*(1), 37–45.

Stapleton, D.C., & Burkhauser, R.V. (2003). *The decline in employment of people with disabilities: A policy puzzle.* Kalamazoo, MI: W. E. Upjohn Institute for Employment Research.

Surgeon General's call to action to improve the health and wellness of people with disabilities (2005). Retrieved August 22, 2005, from http://www.surgeongeneral.gov/library/disabilities

U.S. Preventive Services Task Force. (2005). *U.S. Preventive Services Task Force guidelines for clinical preventive services.* Retrieved August 22, 2005, from http://www.ahrq.gov/clinic/pocketgd.pdf

Wagner, M., Cameto, R., & Guzman, A.M. (2003). Who are secondary students in special education today? *NLTS2 Data Brief, 2,* 1. Retrieved June 10, 2005, from http://www.ncset.org/publications/viewdesc.asp?id=1008

Wagner, M., Newman, L., Cameto, R., & Levine, P. (2005). *Changes over time in the early postschool outcomes of youth with disabilities: A report of findings from the National Longitudinal Transition Study and the National Longitudinal Transition Study-2.* Menlo Park, CA: SRI International. Retrieved November 15, 2005, from http://www.nlts2.org/reports/str6_report.html

Interagency Services

Integrating Health-Related Needs into Individualized Education Programs and 504 Plans

CECILY L. BETZ AND WENDY M. NEHRING

Living with a special health care need and/or disability requires continuous management throughout the day, including time spent at school. However, even excellent ongoing care with careful attention to the details of treatment needs does not provide absolute assurance that complications and disease exacerbations will not occur. Living with special health care needs and disabilities results in serious disruptions in schooling, which leads to higher levels of school absences, higher levels of family stress, and negative psychosocial consequences (e.g., lower levels of self-esteem, higher incidence of mental health problems, disruptions in social relationships).

Ultimately, having a special health care need and/or disability means learning to live with the uncertainty of a condition—the ups and downs and in-betweens. Youth with special health care needs and disabilities, even those who have achieved a high level of independence, need assistance and support managing the requirements of their treatment regimen at home and at school.

School nurses serve as the liaisons between educators, health care professionals, parents, and other members of the individualized education program (IEP) team to ensure continuity between service systems for the student with special health care needs and disabilities. The school nurse serves as the facilitator to implement the care plan originally developed in the health care setting to ensure that the student's long-term management needs are met. For example, a student with Type I diabetes would need ongoing assistance and monitoring in the school setting to assure that the student does not have hypoglycemic or hyperglycemic episodes while attending school. Not only would the nurse be involved with monitoring of the student's diabetes, but he or she would also support and supervise the youth's self-management of his or her diabetes and ensure necessary supplies, equipment, and accommodations were available as needed to assure that academic performance is not adversely affected.

This chapter presents information on the process of integrating health-related needs into IEPs and 504 plans. The chapter begins with an overview of the prevalence of children and youth with special health care needs and disabilities in the schools, focusing on the impact of health upon learning and care needs of youth with special health care needs and disabilities. The chapter then provides an overview of the federal legislation and initiatives related to the health and learning of students with special health care needs and disabilities. Integral to this discussion will be a presentation of the role of school nurses and their importance as liaisons between the service systems of health and education as well as a member of the IEP/504 plan teams. This discussion will include an examination of the professional standards and guidelines that direct school nursing practice. The chapter concludes with information about integrating health-related concerns into IEPs and 504 plans, including the relationship of the individualized health plan (IHP) and emergency action plan (EAP) to both. A case study is then presented as an application example.

PREVALENCE OF CHILDREN AND YOUTH WITH SPECIAL HEALTH CARE NEEDS AND DISABILITIES IN THE SCHOOLS

The United States government conducts regular surveys to ascertain the numbers of children and youth with special health care needs and disabilities. These surveys provide statistics, for example, on the numbers of children and youth with certain conditions, type of limitations, type of school environment attended, and number of school days missed based on illness or injury. These figures provide an understanding of the number of children and youth with special health care needs and disabilities in the school system that impact the delivery of education in the classroom as well as the delivery of health care by the school nurse.

Prevalence of Special Health Care Needs

According to the results of a National Survey of Children with Special Health Care Needs (NSCSHCN) in 2001, 48,690 (12.8%) of children and youth between birth and 17 years of age were reported to have a special health care need (van Dyck et al.). Specifically, there were 13,915 children and youth (28.7%) with a behavioral, developmental, or emotional condition. The majority of these children and youth were between the ages of 6 to 11 years (19,214, 14.6%) and 12 to 17 years (20,752, 15.8%), most likely due to diagnosis during these years of learning and other health-related conditions. The figures for children birth to 5 years were 8,694 (7.8%). More boys (29,021, 60%) were reported to have special health care needs than girls (19,636, 40%) (Child and Adolescent Health Measurement Initiative, 2005).

According to the U.S. Census Bureau (2002) in their profile of the population in 2000, 6% of children between the ages of 6 and 14 years had learning, mental, or physical delays. An additional 5% of children in this age group had a learning disability, 2% had a motor or speech impairment, 2% had an emotional or social delay, and less than 1% were diagnosed with mental retardation or a hearing or vision impairment.

Bloom and Dey (2006), in their analysis of the results of the National Health Interview Survey in 2004, found the following:

- 9 million children and youth younger than 18 years of age (12%) were diagnosed with asthma. Boys were more often diagnosed with asthma than girls (15% vs. 9%).

- Approximately 5 million children and youth between the ages of 3 and 17 years (8%) were diagnosed with a learning disability. Again, boys were more frequently diagnosed than girls (10% vs. 6%).

- Attention deficit hyperactivity disorder (ADHD) was found in 4.5 million children and youth between the ages of 3 and 17 years (7%) with the condition more often diagnosed in boys (10%) than girls (4%).

- Children from low-income families were more likely to be diagnosed with a learning disability (12%) than a child not living in poverty (8%).

In this survey, parents were asked to rate their child as being in excellent, very good, fair, or poor health. Those parents who ranked their children as having fair or poor health also indicated that their children had a learning disability five times more often than parents who said that their children were in excellent or good health (30% vs. 6%). Similarly, parents who said that their child had fair or poor health were twice as likely to say that their child also had ADHD (16% vs. 7%). These figures are interesting since these two conditions do not generally affect health.

Conditions that affect a child's or youth's mental health are often not included in general discussions about special health care needs; however, Hootman, Houck, and King (2003) found that one in five children have mental health conditions that interfere with their learning and affect their development. Witt, Kasper, and Riley (2003) found that children with special health care needs and poor psychosocial adjustment often did not receive needed mental health services. Specifically, younger children and African American children were less likely to have obtained these services.

When examining the prevalence of children and youth, birth to 17 years, with special health care needs in various racial/ethnic categories, there are more Caucasians diagnosed with a special health care need (35,950, 74.1%), followed by African Americans (5,036, 10.4%), Hispanics (4,302, 8.9%), other (1,658, 3.4%), and multiracial (1,581, 3.2%). In each category, there are more boys than girls, as shown in Table 10.1 (Child and Adolescent Health Measurement Initiative, 2005).

Prevalence of Limitations of Daily Activities

Children and youth can have a variety of short- and long-term conditions that create limitations in their daily activities that may affect their academic progress and/or

Table 10.1. Percentages of children and youth with special health care needs ages birth to 17 years by gender and race/ethnicity in 2001

Race/ethnicity	Male	Female
Hispanic	61.3%	48.8%
White	51.5%	48.5%
Black	50.4%	49.6%
Multiracial	49.4%	50.6%
Other	50.2%	49.8%

Adapted from Centers for Disease Control and Prevention, National Center for Health Statistics (2001).

experiences in moving around school during the day. In 2001, the Federal Inter-agency Forum on Child and Family Statistics (2003) reported that approximately 8% of children and youth between the ages of 5 to 17 years experienced limitations in their activities of daily living. They also found that children living in poverty experienced more limitations in their activities of daily living than did children not living in poverty (12% vs. 8%).

In the same year, there were 48,690 children and youth between the ages of birth and 17 years with special health care needs with conditions that affected their activities of daily living, according to the NSCSHCN (Child and Adolescent Health Measurement Initiative, 2005). Of that number, 18,179 (36.7%) had conditions that required taking prescription medications; 11,862 (23.7%) had conditions that required prescription medications plus the regular use of medical, mental health, and/or other services; 10,430 (21.4%) had functional limitations; and 8,219 (18.2%) had conditions that required the regular use of medical, mental health, and/or other services.

Missed Days in School

Children and youth with special health care needs often need to miss school based on their health, levels of limitation, health care visits, hospitalizations, and/or appointments for health-related therapies or services. Specifically, the Centers for Disease Control and Prevention (2004) found that children with asthma miss 14 million school days annually. In 2001, according to the results of the NSCSHCN, 32,923 days of school were missed by children and youth with special health care needs. The majority of these children and youth missed 3 days or less (17,251, 50.7%), followed by 4 to 6 days (6,668, 20.3%), 11 days or more (4,793, 15.8%), and 7 to 10 days (4,111, 13.2%). Table 10.2 illustrates missed days of school as categorized by the health needs and/or limitations of children and youth with special health care needs, and Table 10.3 details the categories of missed school days by race/ethnicity (U.S. Department of Health &

Table 10.2. Days of missed school in past 12 months due to illness or injury by health needs/limitations of special health care needs in 2001

Health needs/limitations of special health care needs	0–3 days missed	4–6 days missed	7–10 days missed	11+ days missed	Total
Functional limitations	2,655 (36.8%)	1,318 (19.8%)	1,021 (15.5%)	1,894 (27.9%)	6,888 (100.0%)
Managed by prescription medications	7,498 (57.5%)	2,693 (21.9%)	1,374 (11.6%)	964 (9.0%)	12,529 (100.0%)
Above routine need/use of services	2,899 (54.7%)	1,026 (18.6%)	611 (11.4%)	649 (15.3%)	5,185 (100.0%)
Prescription medications and service use	4,199 (49.6%)	1,631 (19.4%)	1,105 (14.8%)	1,286 (16.2%)	8,221 (100.0%)

Adapted from Centers for Disease Control and Prevention, National Center for Health Statistics (2001).

Table 10.3. Days of missed school in past 12 months due to illness or injury by race/ethnicity in 2001

Race/ethnicity	0–3 days missed	4–6 days missed	7–10 days missed	11+ days missed	Total
Hispanic	1,399 (50.2%)	531 (21.2%)	342 (11.7%)	445 (16.9%)	2,717 (100.0%)
White	13,031 (50.0%)	5,184 (20.6%)	3,161 (13.7%)	3,539 (15.7%)	24,915 (100.0%)
Black	1,723 (54.9%)	552 (18.8%)	329 (11.5%)	451 (14.8%)	3,055 (100.0%)
Multiracial	498 (46.9%)	183 (16.9%)	137 (17.3%)	150 (18.8%)	968 (100.0%)
Other	530 (54.4%)	195 (18.8%)	131 (11.0%)	190 (15.8%)	1,046 (100.0%)

Adapted from Centers for Disease Control and Prevention, National Center for Health Statistics (2001).

Human Services, Health Resources and Services Administration, Maternal & Child Health Bureau, 2004).

Prevalence of Children and Youth in Special Education

The number of children requiring special education in this country continues to grow. In 2002, approximately 5.9 million children, ages 6 to 21 years, required special education, and the most growth was found in children diagnosed with autism (U.S. Department of Education, Office of Special Education Programs, 2003a). In 2004, this number had increased to a little more than 6.1 million children served under IDEA, Part B. More than half were White (58.7%), followed by Black (20.5%), Hispanic (17.2%), Asian/Pacific Islander (2.1%), and American Indian/Alaska Native (1.5%). Table 10.4 provides the numbers and percentages of 3 to 21 year olds served under IDEA, Part B in 2004 by diagnosis. The greatest numbers of students were diagnosed as having a learning disability (41.8%) or speech/language impairment (21.8%). The fewest number of students were diagnosed with visual impairments (0.4%), traumatic brain injury (0.4%), and deaf/blindness (0.1%) (U.S. Department of Education, Office of Special Education Programs, 2003b). The ratio of boys to girls in special education is about 2 to 1. Children in poor families are more likely to be placed in special education, but poor Hispanic children are less likely to be placed in special education than poor White children. Also, children living in the Northeast and in the Midwest are more often placed in special education than are children living in the South or in the West (Centers for Disease Control and Prevention, National Center for Health Statistics, 2006).

The classroom setting is also important in describing the environment in which students learn and where they may receive any health treatments or therapies. Table 10.5 specifies the different school environments experienced by children 6 to 21 years served under IDEA, Part B in 2004 by their diagnosis. Most children spend their time during the school day in the regular classroom, but depending on their diagnosis—such as mental retardation, emotional disorders, multiple disabilities, or autism—more time may be spent in a specialized classroom (U. S. Department of Education, Office of Special Education Programs, 2003b).

Table 10.4. 2004 numbers and percentages of students, ages 3–21 years, served under IDEA, Part B, by age groups

Diagnosis	3–5 year olds	6–12 year olds	13–17 year olds	18–21 year olds	Total
Learning disability	13,736	1,244,112	1,448,309	147,273	2,853,430
	(0.5%)	(43.6%)	(50.7%)	(5.2%)	(41.8%)
Speech/language	333,290	1,043,331	102,453	5,476	1,484,550
	(22.5%)	(70.3%)	(6.9%)	(0.3%)	(21.8%)
Mental retardation	22,636	232,049	264,232	71,499	590,416
	(3.8%)	(39.3%)	(44.8%)	(12.1%)	(8.6%)
Emotional disorder	5,853	185,220	269,600	29,668	490,341
	(1.2%)	(37.8%)	(55.0%)	(6.0%)	(7.2%)
Multiple disabilities	8,434	62,583	52,843	17,938	141,798
	(5.9%)	(44.1%)	(37.3%)	(12.7%)	(2.1%)
Hearing	7,824	38,640	29,224	4,762	80,450
	(9.7%)	(48.0%)	(36.3%)	(6.0%)	(1.1%)
Orthopedic	8,599	37,010	23,666	4,776	74,051
	(11.6%)	(50.0%)	(32.0%)	(6.4%)	(1.1%)
Other health	12,838	267,577	225,916	18,376	524,707
	(2.4%)	(51.0%)	(43.1%)	(3.5%)	(7.7%)
Visual	3,322	13,971	10,246	1,913	29,452
	(11.3%)	(47.4%)	(34.8%)	(6.5%)	(0.4%)
Autism	25,929	111,568	45,280	9,576	192,353
	(13.5%)	(58.0%)	(23.5%)	(5.0%)	(2.8%)
Deaf/Blind	259	794	700	231	1,984
	(13.1%)	(40.0%)	(35.3%)	(11.6%)	(0.1%)
Traumatic brain injury	1,054	10,041	10,917	2,290	24,302
	(4.3%)	(41.3%)	(44.9%)	(9.4%)	(0.4%)
Developmental delay	258,175	74,377	0	0	332,552
	(77.6%)	(22.4%)	(0.0%)	(0.0%)	(4.9%)
All	701,949	3,321,273	2,483,386	313,778	6,820,386
	(10.3%)	(48.7%)	(36.4%)	(4.6%)	(100.0%)

The developmental delay category only includes children ages 3–9 years.
Adapted from U.S. Department of Education, Office of Special Programs (2004).

FEDERAL LEGISLATION RELATED TO THE HEALTH AND LEARNING OF STUDENTS WITH SPECIAL HEALTH CARE NEEDS AND DISABILITIES

There are a number of federal statutes and initiatives that influence the provision of health and educational services to students with special health care needs and disabilities in school settings. These statutes include the Individuals with Disabilities Education Act (IDEA), the No Child Left Behind Act of 2001, Section 504 of the Rehabilitation Act of 1973, the Family Education Rights and Privacy Act (FERPA) of 1974, and the Health Insurance Portability and Accountability Act (HIPAA) of 1996. Federal initiatives include the *New Freedom Initiative* and *Healthy People 2010*. The legislative provisions of these statutes are known primarily in terms of their application for educators; their implications for school nurses and health care professionals are less well known. A brief overview of each of these statutes and initiatives will be presented in terms of their implications for students with special health care needs and disabilities and the health care professionals who respond to their needs.

Table 10.5. 2004 numbers and percentages of students, ages 6–21 years, served under IDEA, Part B, in different school environments

Diagnosis	Outside the classroom			Public separate facility	Private separate facility	Public residential facility	Private residential facility	Home or hospital environment	Total
	<21%	21%–60%	>60%						
LD	1,464,407 (51.5%)	1,006,343 (35.4%)	339,455 (12.0%)	9,447 (0.3%)	10,496 (0.4%)	2,721 (0.1%)	1,838 (0.1%)	4,978 (0.2%)	2,839,685 (46.4%)
SP/Lang	1,018,046 (88.3%)	75,641 (6.6%)	53,852 (4.7%)	1,457 (0.1%)	2,521 (0.2%)	491 (0.04%)	240 (0.01%)	650 (0.05%)	1,152,898 (18.8%)
MR	78,199 (13.8%)	166,636 (29.3%)	286,528 (50.5%)	25,085 (4.4%)	5,831 (1.0%)	1,494 (0.3%)	1,600 (0.3%)	2,445 (0.4%)	567,818 (9.3%)
ED	156,965 (32.4%)	106,414 (22.0%)	137,734 (28.4%)	34,696 (7.2%)	27,829 (5.7%)	5,689 (1.1%)	9,473 (2.0%)	5,727 (1.2%)	484,527 (7.9%)
Multiple disabilities	17,369 (13.1%)	22,400 (16.8%)	60,096 (45.1%)	16,808 (12.6%)	10,636 (8.0%)	1,206 (0.9%)	1,774 (1.3%)	2,949 (2.2%)	133,238 (2.2%)
Hearing	34,185 (47.1%)	13,556 (18.7%)	15,192 (20.9%)	3,113 (4.3%)	1,939 (2.7%)	4,247 (5.8%)	293 (0.4%)	127 (0.1%)	72,652 (1.2%)
Orthopedic	31,751 (48.5%)	12,724 (19.4%)	16,796 (25.6%)	2,584 (4.0%)	530 (0.8%)	73 (0.1%)	87 (0.1%)	954 (1.5%)	65,499 (1.1%)
Other health impairments	275,851 (53.9%)	149,584 (29.2%)	69,454 (13.6%)	4,104 (0.8%)	4,162 (0.8%)	635 (0.1%)	909 (0.2%)	7,254 (1.4%)	511,953 (8.4%)
Visual	14,801 (56.8%)	4,179 (16.0%)	3,833 (14.7%)	934 (3.6%)	536 (2.0%)	1,449 (5.6%)	213 (0.8%)	136 (0.5%)	26,081 (0.4%)
Autism	48,568 (29.1%)	29,565 (17.7%)	69,717 (41.8%)	9,098 (5.5%)	7,778 (4.7%)	165 (0.1%)	1,146 (0.7%)	608 (0.4%)	166,645 (2.7%)
Deaf/Blind	331 (18.8%)	267 (15.1%)	623 (35.3%)	166 (9.4%)	118 (6.7%)	129 (7.3%)	49 (2.8%)	81 (4.6%)	1,764 (0.1%)
TBI	8,739 (37.6%)	6,605 (28.4%)	6,030 (25.9%)	615 (2.7%)	721 (3.1%)	53 (0.2%)	130 (0.6%)	360 (1.5%)	23,253 (0.3%)
DD	42,246 (56.8%)	18,778 (25.2%)	12,433 (16.7%)	519 (0.7%)	160 (0.2%)	62 (0.1%)	27 (0.1%)	150 (0.2%)	74,375 (1.2%)
All	3,191,458 (52.2%)	1,612,692 (26.3%)	1,071,743 (17.5%)	108,626 (1.8%)	73,257 (1.2%)	18,414 (0.3%)	17,779 (0.3%)	26,419 (0.4%)	6,120,388 (100.0%)

The developmental delay category only includes children ages 3–9 years.

Diagnosis labels: LD, learning disability; SP/Lang, speech/language; MR, mental retardation; ED, emotional disturbance; TBI, traumatic brain injury; DD, developmental delay.

Adapted from U.S. Department of Education, Office of Special Programs (2004).

Individuals with Disabilities Education Act

IDEA refers collectively to educational personnel who provide health and health-related services as *related services personnel*. School nurses, occupational and physical therapists, speech and language therapists, physicians, dieticians, and school psychologists all are considered related services personnel according to IDEA. The most recent authorization of IDEA (Individuals with Disabilities Education Improvement Act, 2004) specifies that transition planning begins formally at age 16; however, it does not preclude transition planning beginning earlier depending on the needs of the student. Related services personnel are designated as responsible for addressing the health and health-related needs of students with disabilities (terminology used in IDEA to refer to students whose condition meets the categorical criteria for special education services) that interfere with their academic performance and are enrolled in special education programs. As such, related services personnel are expected to participate on the youth's IEP team to provide input on health and health-related concerns that can not only negatively impact the transition to adulthood but adulthood itself (Betz, 2001, 2003; Individuals with Disabilities Education Improvement Act, 2004; Schulzinger, 1999). An example of this application is presented later in this chapter.

No Child Left Behind Act of 2001

The No Child Left Behind Act of 2001 is designed to reform elementary and secondary education as a means of enhancing the achievement outcomes of disadvantaged students. This goal is achieved by improving the quality of instruction provided by 1) creating standardized achievement tests to measure student progress in learning to read and perform math, 2) altering the mechanism for appropriation of federal funds at the state level based on local needs, 3) providing options for disadvantaged families to have expanded school choice and supplemental instructional programs, and 4) offering financial incentives and additional training to improve the quality of teachers (U.S. Department of Education, 2005a, 2005b, 2005c).

Initially, significant concerns were raised by educators about the appropriateness of the No Child Left Behind Act requirements for students with disabilities, including students who are enrolled in special education programs. In response to those criticisms, adaptations have been made to accommodate the needs of students with disabilities including those with significant cognitive limitations. Provisions were made to accommodate the needs of students with disabilities who were unable to perform at expected levels of achievement according to grade level. *Modified achievement standards* are designed for those students with disabilities who are either general or special education students who cannot achieve grade-level expectations within the academic year and as determined by the IEP team. It is estimated that 1% of students in the general population and 10% of students with disabilities enrolled in special education are entitled to alternative methods of assessment (No Child Left Behind Act of 2001; U.S. Department of Education, 2004a). Students with disabilities who can perform at grade level at a slower pace and with the assistance of accommodations can be assessed using alternative methods of assessment that are aligned with statewide assessment methods. Two percent of students are entitled to this form of assessment. The impact of this act has yet to be determined, as the program is in the early stages of implementation (No Child Left Behind Act of 2001; U.S. Department of Education, 2004a).

Section 504 of the Rehabilitation Act of 1973

Section 504 of the Rehabilitation Act of 1973 (Betz, 2001; Schulzinger, 1999) provides protections to individuals with disabilities by prohibiting discrimination against them in publicly funded programs. For students with disabilities, Section 504 ensures that they have equal access to education. Students who qualify for Section 504 protections are eligible to obtain the accommodations needed to enable them to participate fully in school activities and academic programs. For additional information on Section 504, refer to Chapter 11 and Moses, Gilchrest, & Schwab (2005).

Family Education Rights and Privacy Act of 1974

FERPA provides families rights regarding their children's educational records (20 U.S.C. § 1232g; 34 C.F.R. Pt. 99). FERPA confers to families the rights to have full access to their children's academic records. Additionally, parents are given the sole authority to provide consent for the release of their children's educational records. FERPA regulations have implications for educational and related service personnel as it pertains to sharing of information between service systems. That is, consents must be obtained from parents or the youth (if youth has the legal authority) for any educational records to be released to providers outside of the educational system.

Health Insurance Portability and Accountability Act of 1996

HIPAA ensures the confidentiality of consumer health records. The intent of HIPAA was to protect the private health information of consumers from being disseminated indiscriminately to people or agencies whose interest in acquiring the data was not for clinical purposes. HIPAA regulations do not pertain to elementary and secondary schools, however, as FERPA regulations are in effect. HIPAA regulations do permit health care professionals to share information with school nurses for treatment purposes. Information shared is restricted to that which is medically necessary for treatment purposes (U.S. Department of Health and Human Services, Office on Civil Rights, 2006).

New Freedom Initiative

The President's *New Freedom Initiative* (NFI), issued in 2001, proposed a comprehensive plan to promote the full inclusion of individuals with disabilities in society (U.S. Department of Health and Human Services, 2003). NFI is based on the collective input of agencies within the federal government, including the U.S. Department of Health and Human Services, to address the goals of societal inclusion, such as living independently in the community of choice, having access to training and education needed to acquire the knowledge and skills needed for gainful employment, having a network of friends, and obtaining employment with health insurance coverage. This initiative was created in response to the Supreme Court *Olmstead* decision in 1999, which supported the rights of individuals with disabilities to live inclusively in the community rather than in institutional settings (The Center for an Accessible Society, 1999).

As part of the NFI, in *Delivering on the Promise*, the Maternal Child Health Bureau of the Health Resources and Services Administration "will take the lead in developing and implementing a plan to achieve appropriate community-based service systems for children and youth with special health care needs and their families" to eliminate barriers to full community participation (U.S. Department of Health and Human Services, 2002, p. 43). One of the major barriers identified was related to the successful transition of youth with special health care needs from pediatric and child services to adult health care and other adult community services. This initiative is of particular interest to school nurses as it addresses the health related component of transition planning for youth with special health care needs and disabilities. Comprehensive health care transition planning involves the coordination of health-related transition concerns with school nurses and pediatric and adult health care professionals in community-based and health care organizations (U.S. Department of Health and Human Services, 2002).

Healthy People 2010

Objective 16-23 of *Healthy People 2010* specifies that "comprehensive community-based systems of care will be developed and implemented for children with special health care needs and their families within the State Title V Children with Special Health Care Needs (CSHCN) Program" (U.S. Department of Health and Human Services, 2000). This lifespan approach for comprehensive health services for children and youth with special health care needs is integrated into the State Title V CSHCN Program available for income-eligible families in every state and territory in the United States. The range of services offered through the State Title V CSHCN Programs extends from early intervention and preventive services for infants and toddlers to transition services for youth who exit the program when their eligibility for services terminates. Title V CSHCN Programs work closely with schools to ensure children and youth enrolled in this program receive ongoing chronic care services in school-based clinics and programs.

THE ROLE OF SCHOOL NURSES

There are approximately 60,000 nurses who provide services to students in school settings (National Association of School Nurses [NASN], 2002a). The U.S. Department of Health and Human Services (2000) in *Healthy People 2010* recommended that there are 750 students to every school nurse in the general school population. In addition, there should be 225 students to every school nurse in the mainstreamed population and 125 students to every school nurse in the developmental disabilities and/or severely chronically ill population.

It is essential that a school nurse, preferably one that is certified, is present to care for the health needs of children in the school setting, as school children are *entitled* to health services in school (American Nurses Association [ANA], 2005b; Costante, 2001). NASN (2002b) stresses that

> The registered professional nurse is the health care provider who has the knowledge, education, experience and authority to manage and provide the full range of health services in the education system. The ultimate goal of school nursing practice is to support students' optimal state of health to promote student's capacity for successful learning. (p. 1)

Research has demonstrated that children with special health care needs and disabilities have had fewer missed school days due to the presence of a full-time school nurse in the school setting (Telljohann, Dake, & Price, 2004; Vought-O'-Sullivan, Meehan, Havice, & Pruitt, 2006). Costante (2001) further emphasized that the school nurse must be able to elucidate the need for qualified health services provided by a school nurse to an educational audience.

School nurses provide a wide array of health services to students on school campuses. These services include but are not limited to health screenings (including vision and hearing testing), health assessments and health histories, health care procedures, administration of medications, case management, counseling and advocacy, direct care for acute and chronic conditions, equipment troubleshooting, provision of immunizations, health education and consultation, and provision of first aid and care for minor illnesses. In addition, the school nurse works with the child's interdisciplinary health team in the community and/or hospital to assure continuity of care in the school setting (American Academy of Pediatrics [AAP], Committee on School Health, 2001; ANA, 2005b; NASN, 2005b). It is important to note that medication errors are significantly lower when a school nurse administers the medication as opposed to any other school personnel (McCarthy, Kelly, & Reed, 2000).

The dimensions of care provided to students with special health care needs and disabilities by school nurses include 1) ensuring their safety, 2) preventing and/or reducing situations requiring emergency responses, 3) managing emergencies when they occur, 4) collaborating in managing long-term special health care needs, and 5) instituting accommodations and services to reduce the effects of the special health care needs on academic performance (NASN, 2005b). School nurses caring for children and youth with special health care needs and disabilities should use the following texts to guide their practice: *School Nursing: Scope and Standards of Practice* (ANA and National Association of School Nurses, 2005) and *Intellectual and Developmental Disabilities Nursing: Scope and Standards of Practice* (ANA and the American Association on Mental Retardation, 2004). The NASN has also issued a number of issue briefs and position statements related to the care of children and youth with special health care needs and disabilities in the schools, and these are listed at the end of this chapter under Recommended Readings.

The importance of ongoing care provided to children and youth with special health care needs and disabilities by school nurses has been affirmed by the U.S. Supreme Court. In *Cedar Rapids Community School District v. Garrett F.,* the Supreme Court issued a precedent-setting ruling that school districts were required to provide school nursing services to students who had specialized health needs. The Court recognized that school-based nursing services were pivotal to enabling the full participation of the student with special health needs in school. The importance of school nurse services for students with special health care needs and disabilities has been echoed by advocacy groups, federal agencies, and professional associations such as the Centers for Disease Control and Prevention; the Asthma & Allergy Network, Mothers of Asthmatics; and the American Academy of Pediatrics (NASN, 2003). For additional reading on significant court cases and their findings related to the health-care services for children and youth with special health care needs and disabilities specifically related to medication administration, emergency care, do-not-resuscitate orders, and so forth, see Thomas and Hawke (1999).

School nurses face numerous challenges in providing health services in educational settings. Since the 1980s, the role responsibilities of school nurses have extended beyond conducting health screenings, immunizations supervision, and health education, to case managing the ongoing health needs of students with complex special health care needs and the provision of services that are both time-intensive and complicated—in some instances requiring a high level of clinical skills and knowledge. Such direct services include ostomy care, ventilator care, and trachesotomy care (ANA, 2005b).

Coupled with the increased level of acuity of students' special health care needs and disabilities requiring the provision of direct treatment services are the more complex psychosocial needs of students. Students come from diverse ethnic and cultural families whose primary language is not always English, and many students are disadvantaged with few resources available for enrichment opportunities and recreational pursuits. Efforts to reach out to low-income families may be difficult due to linguistic and cultural differences.

School nurses face other psychosocial challenges when dealing with families that are not only clinically problematic but also legalistic and ethical in nature. Nuclear families are now one of many family configurations that school nurses deal with on a daily basis. Children today live in families who are blended, separated, divorced, and same-sex. For school nurses, knowing who to contact in cases of an emergency, with whom to share confidential student health information, and from whom consent is obtained are complicated given these contemporary family units.

On many elementary and secondary campuses comprehensive primary health care services are provided to ensure that disadvantaged students who do not have health insurance receive well child and preventive care. School-based clinics are typically staffed by pediatric nurse practitioners and enable improved access to health services for students with inadequate or no health insurance. In some schools, comprehensive interdisciplinary services are offered to students with multiple health and psychosocial needs by a team of health care professionals composed of members such as a pediatrician/adolescent medical specialist, psychologist, social worker, dietician, and drug counselor (AAP, Committee on School Health, 2001).

Delegation of Nursing Tasks

An important issue facing the practice of school nursing is the delegation of nursing tasks by school nurses who are registered nurses to unlicensed assistive personnel (UAP) for the purpose of providing care to students with special health care needs and disabilities. Although registered nurses can delegate care to an UAP, the registered nurse continues to be accountable for the care provided (ANA, 1994; NASN, 2005a). This service arrangement was created to address the increased demands for nursing services due to the increasing numbers of students with special health care needs and disabilities while attempting to contain costs of care. For example, the school nurse-to-student ratio has risen to as high as 1 to 5,000, whereas the recommended ratio is 1 to 750.

Although delegation has been acknowledged as a service delivery model by professional associations and enacted by state nurse practice regulations, a number of concerns exist regarding implementation. These concerns include consideration of the following factors: 1) the safety of the student receiving care provided by the UAP, 2) the regulations governing delegation activities in state nurse practice acts, and 3) the scope and acuity of health needs of students with special health care needs and disabilities (ANA, 2005a). The decision to delegate nursing care provided to students with special health care needs and disabilities has to be individualized and based on the assessment of the student's needs. According to the NASN's Guiding Principles to Determine When Delegation is Appropriate, there are five criteria that can be used to evaluate the appropriateness of delegation of nursing care to UAP, as listed below.

1. **The Right Task**—Is the task within the nurse's scope of practice? Is the task reasonably routine with a predictable outcome? Is it based on medical orders? Is it one that is repeated frequently? Is it performed according to an established sequence of steps, without modification? Is the task one that does not involve assessment, interpretation, or decision-making?

2. **The Right Person**—Who is immediately available to the student, willing, and competent to do the task at the required time?

3. **The Right Direction**—How much training will be required by the UAP to perform the task in a safe and appropriate way? What are the learning needs of the UAP? How many tasks will the UAP need to learn?

4. **The Right Supervision**—How much initial and ongoing supervision will be needed by the school nurse for the performance of this task? What type of supervision will be needed?

5. **The Right Circumstance**—Is the child particularly vulnerable due to age, developmental level, cognitive abilities, gender, or specific health issues? Is the environment safe for UAP to perform the delegated task as planned? (NASN, 2005)

Given the current circumstances school nurses face in their roles as providers of health and health-related services to students with special health care needs and disabilities, they encounter numerous demands in their positions to ensure that the health needs of all students, including students with special health care needs and disabilities, are met.

The Role of the School Nurse on an IEP and 504 Plan Team

The school nurse's role on an IEP or 504 team is essentially the same for transition-aged youth, although the nursing functions will differ. As the team member with expertise on the health-related needs of the students, the school nurse shares assessment data gathered from and about the student and serves as a consultant to other team members on devising interventions to address the student's health-related needs that interfere or could potentially impede the student's academic performance, as an informational resource on health topics, and as an advocate to ensure that the health-related needs of the student are sufficiently addressed in either the IEP or 504 Plan (Zimmerman, 2006).

Individualized health plans (IHPs) are plans of care developed by school nurses for students who have special health care needs that require nursing actions (NASN, 2002b). Unlike IEPs, the IHP is composed by the nurse and is focused on the health-related needs of the student. The IHP focuses on ensuring the student's health needs are being met as well as the accommodations needed to mitigate the untoward effects of the student's special health care needs on academic performance. For example, the student with Type I diabetes may need to have access to water when thirsty. The student may need to have a bottle of water at his or her desk thereby eliminating the need to leave the classroom to obtain water from a drinking fountain.

The nurse's responsibility includes ongoing monitoring of the student's condition to ensure or prevent untoward change in the student's condition and determining the need for accommodations for the student should some manifestation of a condition interfere with his or her ability to learn. For example, a student with hemophilia may need to have scheduled rest period(s) during the school day that could be taken in the school nurse's office. Other nursing actions related to managing the student's condition at school include monitoring the administration of medications, performing urinary catheterization, and administering inhalation treatments for the student with cystic fibrosis

IHPs can be developed for both students who are enrolled in special education and in general education who have special health care needs. Special education students will have IEPs that specify the goals and objectives of their educational programs that are meant to guide the selection of learning and daily life skills experiences needed to achieve developmental competencies typical for their age group. For many students enrolled in special education programs, their level of achievement will not be equivalent to their typically developing peers and they will lag far behind what is considered to be typical for their age. Whatever the student's level of expected achievement is as specified in the IEP, the goals of the school nurse remain basically the same. The school's nurse primary goal is to minimize the untoward impact of the student's disability/special health care needs upon his or her academic performance. To achieve this, the school nurse will work with the IEP team to ensure that the health-related needs of the student are integrated as IEP objectives (Zimmerman, 2006).

How might the school nurse's IHP be integrated into the student's IEP? The primary foci of school nursing actions in an IHP are to 1) identify the accommodations needed to perform academically, whether it be in the classroom, on school campus, and/or in work/community-based settings; 2) monitor continuously the student's physical status and stamina in the school setting; 3) serve as an advocate and troubleshooter in circumstances wherein the student's full rights and protections are not fully acknowledged or realized; 4) serve as a liaison between the educators at the school and professionals in the health care setting; and 5) identify the nursing services required to manage the student's daily health-related treatment needs (Betz, 2001; NASN, 2005b; Zimmerman, 2006). An example of an IHP is displayed in Figure 10.1.

The process for transferring relevant components of the student's IHP into the IEP/504 plan begins with the recognition and support for the school nurse's

Student health problem: Student lacks self-sufficiency with management of diabetes.

Student will demonstrate knowledge and skill in managing diabetes as evidenced by

   a. Administration of insulin injections

   b. Monitoring serum glucose

   c. Ability to identify signs and symptoms of hypoglycemia/ hyperglycemia

   c. Identifies actions to prevent/treat hypoglycemia/hyperglycemia

   d. Demonstrates ability to manage nutritional intake according to dietary guidelines

   e. Demonstrates ability to balance daily exercise with insulin and dietary requirements

Interventions

1. Assess student's ability to

   a. Administer insulin injections

   b. Perform serum glucose monitoring

   c. Recognize signs and symptoms of hypoglycemia/hyperglycemia

   d. Perform preventive health care including skin care

   e. Engage in daily exercise

   f. Engage in behaviors to prevent infections

   g. Engage in self-care management

2. Instruct and reinforce instruction on diabetes self-care management as identified in #1.

3. Coordinate diabetes self-care management with parents/primary caregivers and diabetes special health care team.

4. Refer to mentorship program with adult role models with diabetes for ongoing support and instruction.

5. Keep student's parent(s), teachers, members of special health care team apprised of developments.

Student outcome

1. Student demonstrates proficiency in managing daily treatment regimen.

Figure 10.1. Individualized health plan.

participation on the IEP team. Curiously, nurses are not always invited to join the student's IEP/504 plan team. Unless it is the policy of the school to include the school nurse as a team member as indicated by the student's needs for school nursing services, it is the school nurse's responsibility to contact the IEP/504 team. School nurses whose caseload includes students who have an IEP/504 plan or who require some type of nursing service for special health care needs management can take the initiative to inform the IEP transition/504 plan coordinator of their desire to be involved with IEP transition/504 planning. An example of an IEP with health-related objectives is listed in Figure 10.2.

In school districts wherein the school nurse's involvement in IEP transition/504 planning is not customary, it may be necessary for the school nurse to provide an explanation of the rationale for participating on the IEP/504 plan team. In these circumstances, the role and value of school nurse participation in IEP/504 planning may not be well understood.

Emergency Action Plan

Emergency action plans (EAPs) are developed by the school nurse for educational personnel who may come into contact with students who have special health care needs to avert or manage medical crises that may occur while in school. The EAP specifies a plan for dealing with a health care emergency prior to the arrival of emergency medical services personnel. Although the school nurse is likely to be the first responder in managing the medical emergency, such as initiating CPR, treating shock, or stabilizing an injury, EAPs are developed for all educational personnel. Educational personnel may include cafeteria workers, bus drivers, school teachers, and school counselors. For additional information on this type of plan, see Heller & Turnlin (2004) and Zimmerman (2006).

The majority of school emergencies are due to respiratory distress associated with asthma and shock due to massive blood loss. Nearly half of health emergencies among children and youth with special health care needs and disabilities, however, are not associated with their special health care needs (Hazinski et al., 2004). An example of an EAP is presented in Figure 10.3.

It should be noted that part of an EAP may be for do-not-resuscitate (DNR) orders. In a national survey of 81 school districts, Kimberly, Forte, Carroll, and Feudtner (2005) found that 80% did not have any policies, protocols, or regulations in place for how to deal with DNR orders. Of interest is that 76% stated that they would not honor these orders if present or did not know if they could. Of the school districts that did have a policy, protocol, or regulation in place that would allow them to honor the DNR order (*n*=16), 10 prohibited their school personnel from carrying out these orders. Of further note, 13 of the school districts that would honor the DNR order are in states that do not have any laws in place that would protect personnel from a law suit or criminal liability if they withheld CPR.

Components of the nursing process used in IHP and EAP are presented in Table 10.6. A comparison of IEP, IHP, EAP, and 504 plans highlighting purpose, focus of the plan, legal authority, responsible professionals, and professional involved in the plan development is presented in Table 10.7.

The following case study illustrates the experience of a youth with special health care needs and a disability and the family in the school setting. The role of the school nurse is important for a successful experience both academically and socially.

Nursing diagnosis: Infection, at risk for during times of infectious outbreaks at school.

Student will be protected from getting ill due to infectious contacts from students/school personnel.

1. Student will be seated at the front of the classroom to minimize close contact with students who are ill or potentially contagious.

2. Student will be encouraged to wash hands frequently during the day, especially after meals, recreational breaks, and hygiene breaks.

3. Student may be required to wear a mask to prevent contact with students who have colds or infections.

4. Student may be home-schooled during periods of hospitalization and infection outbreaks at school.

5. Student will report to school nurse for temperature taking as necessary.

6. Teacher will make advanced arrangements for work assignments when absent from class.

7. Teacher will contact parent(s) directly to schedule home schooling arrangements.

Student outcome

1. Student will be free of infections.

2. Student's school absences will be fewer than those of the previous year.

Figure 10.2. Individualized education program with health-related objectives. Adapted from Betz, 2001; Betz & Sowden, in press; North American Nursing Diagnosis Association, 2004; Zimmerman, 2006.

Emergency action plan

Student's name: _____

School: _____

School nurse: _____

Contact information (e-mail/phone/fax): _____

Parent/primary caregiver: _____

Emergency contact (name): _____

Home address: _____

Work address: _____

Work phone number: _____

Home phone number: _____

Cell phone number: _____

E-mail address: _____

Health care provider(s) (name): _____

Work address: _____

Work phone number: _____

Cell phone number: _____

E-mail address: _____

Hypoglycemia (low blood sugar)

The following signs and symptoms indicate the student has low blood sugar:

   a. Skin appears flushed

   b. Acts agitated, irritable

   c. Confused, has problems with concentration

   d. Sweating profusely

   e. Wants to eat, states is hungry

   f. Aggressiveness

   g. Vertigo (dizziness)

   h. Lethargic (tired)

   i. Weak

   j. Pale skin color

   k. Abrupt mood change

   l. Seizure activity

Figure 10.3. Emergency action plan. Adapted from Betz, 2001; Betz & Sowden, in press; North American Nursing Diagnosis Association, 2004; Zimmerman, 2006.

Treatment of low blood sugar includes

   a. Give piece of candy or glass of juice (milk, orange juice)

   b. Contact school nurse

   c. If has seizure, protect from injury (lie on floor, remove objects student may hit)

Hyperglycemia (high blood sugar) (serum glucose higher than 300 mg/dl)

The following signs and symptoms indicate the student has high blood sugar:

1. Thirsty

2. Increase in urination

3. Gets up at night to use bathroom

4. Enuresis-incontinent when asleep

5. Has difficulty concentrating

6. Blurred vision

7. Energy level is decreased

8. Changes in personality and/or behavior noted

9. Has fever or feels "sick"

Treatment of high blood sugar includes:

1. Administer rapid acting insulin

2. Can use restroom freely without having to raise hand to ask teacher/obtain classroom pass to use restroom.

3. Check urine for ketones (student/school nurse)

4. Monitor for diabetic ketoacidosis (Kussmaul respirations, elevated serum glucose, fruity odor with breath, dehydration)

J.T. was diagnosed with Down syndrome at birth. His infancy and childhood years were uneventful in terms of his health status until his diagnosis of acute lymphocytic leukemia (ALL) at 15 years of age. Prior to his diagnosis, J.T. had visited the school nurse's office several times with complaints of feeling tired and "sick" and having aching joints. At that time, the nurse took his vital signs (pulse and respiratory rate, blood pressure, and temperature). His vital signs were within normal range except that he had a temperature of 101°F, so his mother was called and she picked him up from school. At that time, the school nurse advised Mrs. T. that it was likely that J.T. had the flu, which many of the students were suffering from at the time. She recommended that Mrs. T. treat J.T. symptomatically and if his symptoms did not resolve in the next few days, then the school nurse recommended that J.T. be taken to his pediatrician.

Table 10.6. Components of the nursing process used in individualized health plan (IHP) and emergency action plan (EAP)

Nursing assessment	Assessment of the student's health related needs that negatively impact academic performance. Data are gathered from numerous sources that include student's medical records, consultation with members of youth's specialized health care team, teachers, interviews with youth and parents, identification of medications taken and procedures needed. Information gathered is done in compliance with Health Insurance Portability and Accountability Act and Family Education Rights and Privacy Act.
Nursing diagnosis	Nursing diagnoses are formulated based on the identification of the youth's health problems. The terminology of nursing diagnoses is based upon classifications developed by nurses to identify client problems that can be treated by nurses independently. Examples of nursing diagnoses frequently encountered in school settings are Ineffective Coping, Knowledge Deficient, Ineffective Breathing Pattern, and Pain.
Nursing interventions	The independent actions undertaken by nurses to ameliorate health problems of the client. Examples of independent nursing functions include ongoing monitoring of a student's respiratory function who is ventilator dependent, hearing and vision screening, reinforcing the use of proper techniques for continuous intermittent catheterization, and educating school personnel on recognizing the symptoms of hypoglycemia in a student with Type I diabetes.
Nursing evaluation	Criteria are developed to assess the effectiveness of the nursing interventions. Nurses will identify the expected outcomes and timelines of changes expected due to the nursing actions. Examples of student outcomes are fewer absences and the ability to perform intermittent catheterization independently using proper technique, and improvement in school performance.

Source: North American Nursing Diagnosis Association (2004); Zimmerman (2006).

J.T.'s symptoms did not resolve and only worsened. The pediatrician referred J.T. to the hematology specialty team at the local children's hospital as he realized after examining the laboratory test results that J.T. needed additional diagnostic evaluation. J.T. was hospitalized wherein the diagnosis of ALL was made and his chemotherapy treatment was initiated.

The advanced practice nurse (APN) in the hematology specialty team contacted the school nurse while concurrently the social worker contacted the school teacher (after signed permission from Mrs. T.) to discuss the process of school reintegration. Both the APN and the school nurse reviewed what health-related accommodations were needed for J.T.

The APN reviewed the projected chemotherapy regimen J.T. would be on for the next two to three years if he continued to be in remission. The school nurse was advised about the current medications J.T. was receiving, including the monitoring for side effects of the chemotherapeutic agents that J.T. would receive if he continued to be in remission. Some of the side effects that J.T. might experience would not only include physical symptoms of discomfort (e.g., nausea, vomiting) and observable changes (e.g., alopecia [hair loss], skin color changes, skin rashes, red and infectious eyes) but also side effects that could impact his academic performance resulting in learning

Table 10.7. Comparison of individualized education program (IEP), individualized health plan (IHP), emergency action plan (EAP), and 504 plans for transition-age youth

	IEP	IHP	EAP	504 plan
Purpose	Specifies student's interagency and interdisciplinary transition IEP	Specifies nursing action plan for student's school performance/transition planning	Specifies school personnel emergency response to student's medical emergency	Specifies the accommodations the student requires to learn
Focus of plan	Educational focus	Health focused	Emergency plan for student with chronic illness who has a medical emergency	Educational focused
Legal authority	Specified by federal law (IDEA)	None	None	Specified by federal law (Rehabilitation Act of 1973)
Professional responsibility for plan	Transition IEP special educator	School nurse	School nurse	504 Coordinator
Service recipient	Student focused	Student focused	Educational personnel	Student focused
Professionals involved in plan development and implementation	Interdisciplinary members (special and general education teachers, parent, youth, and interagency representatives invited by parent/youth). Nurse is not mandated as member of transition IEP; considered a "related service" personnel	School nurse	School nurse	504 Coordinator and other members involved depending on needs of students (general and special education teachers, school counselor, and school nurse is not required)
Eligibility criteria	Category of students with disabilities specified in IDEA	Students who have special health care needs that require ongoing management of their condition	Students who have special health care needs that require ongoing management of their condition	Students with disabilities; students with a record of having a disability and student is regarded as having a disability
Assessment process	Formalized assessment process conducted by professionals to determine student's interests, preferences, and needs as specified in IDEA	Nursing assessment based on identification of student's needs and strengths related to cognitive, developmental, and health domains	Nursing assessment	Assessment process not specified and may include nonstructured educational assessments, classroom observations

(continued)

197

Table 10.7.   (continued)

Service plan	Goals and objectives of service plan based on individualized interests, preferences, and needs	Nursing interventions based on identification of student needs (nursing diagnoses) enabling student to manage special health needs independently and perform academically	Nursing interventions based on nursing diagnoses	Specifies accommodations, services, and aides needed to facilitate access and participation in educational program
Evaluation/review of plan	Reviewed annually; re-evaluation every 3 years or sooner if requested by parent or youth	Reviewed annually	Updated annually	Reviewed annually
Plan approval	Approved by parent/youth (mandatory)	Approved by parent/youth (not mandatory)	Approved by parent/youth (not mandatory)	Approved by parent/youth (not mandatory)
Plan distribution	Interdisciplinary team, youth, parents	Teachers, educational personnel	Distributed to school personnel who have contact with student: teacher, bus driver, cafeteria worker, teaching assistant	Teachers, 504 Plan team members, youth, parents
Linkages between plans	IHP/EAP can be integrated into IEP	EAP can be integrated into IHP; IHP/EAP can be integrated into IEP	EAP can be integrated into IHP; IHP/EAP can be integrated into IEP	IHP/EAP can be integrated into 504 Plan

The term *youth* refers to youth who have attained age of majority. Adapted from Betz, 2001; Betz & Sowden, in press; Zimmerman, 2006.

disabilities. The APN indicated that she would send an instructional sheet listing J.T.'s medications together with possible side effects that could be used for later reference. Both the school nurse and the APN identified the parameters for notifying each other should J.T. exhibit chemotherapy side effects.

They also discussed the care of the infusion port that J.T. would have while receiving chemotherapy. It was apparent that J.T.'s physical education program would be altered to avoid contact sports to prevent damaging it. The nurses reviewed infection control procedures, including avoidance of classmates during times of flu/infection outbreaks, and J.T.'s hygiene practices while at school, including the possibility of J.T. wearing a mask during periods of schoolwide illness outbreaks.

Both nurses also discussed J.T.'s school absences that would be necessary for chemotherapy treatments and diagnostic and laboratory testing and any academic arrangements that could be made in advance. Also, the possible scenarios related to the occurrence of complications such as seizures, bleeding and infections, and unforeseen hospitalizations were reviewed, including the accommodations that would be needed to ensure that J.T's schooling would continue and his IEP objectives would be achieved. Additionally, the school nurse queried the APN as to the application of accommodations in job-training settings, as J.T. had a job training placement in a local nursery (Betz, 2003; Betz & Sowden, in press).

Although the APN was unable to attend J.T's IEP transition planning meeting, the school nurse ensured that his health-related needs were integrated as IEP objectives to minimize their negative impact on his academic and functional performance. The school nurse's IHP included the information from J.T's IEP but was more expansive, as it included information on nursing actions that were required for ongoing management such as administration of medications and monitoring of his infusion site. In addition, an EAP was developed and distributed to the classroom teachers, physical education teacher, bus driver, and cafeteria workers in the event of a health-related emergency such as a seizure or bleeding.

SUMMARY

The role of the school nurse as a fulcrum point for a student's interdisciplinary health care team for the delivery of care and maintenance of health in the school setting is essential. There are a growing number of children and youth—from all racial and ethnic backgrounds as well as from a wide range of family constellations that attend school in a variety of environmental settings—that have been or will be diagnosed with a special health care need and/or disability. A number of federal laws and initiatives have been written and revised to describe the appropriate and mandated health care and services that must be available and accessible to these children in the school setting. National organizations, such as those serving nurses, school nurses specifically, and other health care providers have written position statements and briefs that detail the health care that is needed in the school setting and the scope and standards of practice for nurses serving in this setting. For children and youth with special health care needs and disabilities, there are several plans, depending on qualifications for service, that are completed on an annual and as-needed basis to instruct school personnel on the best practices for providing the optimal school environment for academic and developmental success. These have been detailed in this chapter, and additional information on aspects of these features can be found in other chapters in this book. Costante (2001) called for the consideration of subspecialization within school nursing, and the care of children and youth with special health care needs and disabilities may be one needed subspecialization in consideration of the continuing rise in numbers of children and youth with these conditions.

My Story   Pinal "Pinky" Patel

Talk about a zigzag life. I have a progressive disorder called Fredreich's ataxia (FA), which affects the nervous system and balance. My symptoms began showing at age 6, but I was diagnosed at around age 11. I was born in India, moved to the United States when I turned 4 years old, toured different states in the United States, moved back to India at age 11, and came back from India to the United States at age 16 in 1998.

When I moved back to the United States (to Bloomington, IL), I did not want to go back to school because I had not been in the classroom for the past three years. Indian schools do not have individualized education plans (IEPs) or any disability accommodations; thus, I had to drop out of school in India since my FA had progressed to the point where a wheelchair was needed for mobility.

However, with a push from a relative, I approached the school system and they placed me at Bloomington High School, determined by my age.

The school started an IEP as many of the American schools I attended. Meetings were held once every 2 months with my parents, faculty, occupational and physical therapist, and me. Six months left in the school year, they put me in fundamental math, English, history, and biology freshman classes. They provided a personal attendant to help me in note-taking, scribing for tests, transferring to the commode from wheelchair and vice versa, and maneuvering me on my manual wheelchair from class to class. They involved me in physical and occupational therapy primarily to help my aide and me in restroom transfers. Since physical education is required in Illinois, they also substituted occupational therapy (OT) and physical therapy exercises with physical education credits for me. For the first semester, I went to school from 8 a.m. to 12 p.m. instead of 8 a.m. to 3 p.m. I asked for that shortened day because I was afraid of fatigue. Next semester, they added more than an hour and a health class to the schedule with my consent. And the year went on, but I had to move at the end of the year.

After moving to Paducah, KY, from Bloomington, IL, in the summer of 1999, I enrolled in Paducah Tilghman High School. This school began a different IEP, following the Kentucky laws. However, the basics of the IEP were similar with exception of OT. The IEP meetings were frequent in the beginning. I had to repeat my freshman year because class-credits did not transfer. Remembering the boredom I felt during classes at Bloomington High School, I pleaded not to have to take any more remedial classes. I had an aide, and she assisted me in everything that the attendant at Bloomington had helped me with. The physical therapist helped me obtain a chest belt to attach to my new electric wheelchair I brought from Illinois. This belt was for the bus rides. My school day started at 7:25 a.m. and ended at 1:20 p.m. for the first semester; then I began to stay the full day to 2:20 p.m. The year went by quickly.

My sophomore year began at Paducah Tilghman High School. The IEP meetings were held at the beginning and end of each semester. The physical therapist evaluated me again, as she always did during IEP meetings. My strength was weaker and I lost weight, but the attendant was strong enough to help me in the restroom without any drastic changes to the routine we used to transfer. About 3 months into the first semester, I fell ill. I spent 13 days at the hospital and was diagnosed with Type I diabetes. I was home-schooled for the rest of the semester with a tutor who worked with me following the assignments my teachers sent. The school also issued a laptop, so I could work on the assignments during the home-school session. I needed to wear leg braces from that point on, but the therapist did not make any more changes in transfer routine. The second semester of the year went by and school ended.

The summer of that year went by in pondering. I was dissatisfied with my aide, and I knew she was going to be taking care of me until my graduation unless I did something. I was not trying to whine about my aide; I was grateful for her assistance. She took care of me as if I was her daughter, but that was the problem. I already had a mother to nag and mollycoddle me. I just wanted someone who would let me make friends, mistakes, and just be a normal high schooler. For example, she even ate with me! Thus, I approached my IEP handler.

After several IEP meetings with an extra member from the education board, I started working with a different person. She was around the same age as my previous aide, but she let me have more freedom and classmates began to befriend me. Since this aide was not able to lift and I was weaker, the physical therapist designed a new transfer routine. Two special education teachers helped me during the transfer. The teachers and I had to schedule bathroom trips. Scheduling was hard to deal with for me because I was used to going whenever I wanted with my prior aide. The therapist also put me on an exercise program and to do this, I had to miss a class each week. Dealing, the year ended.

I entered my senior year, looking forward to end my 5 years of high school. The IEP meetings were held as usual. The physical therapist designed another transfer routine with the same teachers and a sliding board. Since the therapist observed I did not get any stronger from the exercise program, I was taken off of it. I fell ill and spent the last 4 days of the first semester of this year at the hospital. I was diagnosed with Bradycardia (slow heart beat) and a pacemaker was planted. Luckily, I did not have to have any change in my academic and physical schedule when I went back for the last semester. A couple months before graduation, my IEP manager set a meeting with the vocational rehabilitation (VR) counselor. VR helps in funding for aides, part tuition and books at colleges because most colleges do not provide anything except for professors and accommodated buildings. And it was time to graduate!

I walked in the graduation ceremony with my peers—a teacher pushed my wheelchair. I had taken the ACT three times during high school and received a 26 composite score. My school made special arrangements for me to take them with my aide in a separate room instead of the regular times when the ACTs were given. My IEP team told me I did not need to take the SAT, living in Kentucky, so I did not push them because I knew it would just be a hassle to make the arrangements if I did not need it. Yes, I took harder classes at Paducah Tilghman High School than the ones I started out with at Bloomington High School, but I did not have a complete say in choosing. The IEP team did not let me take desired classes such as Advanced Placement English, American History, and Literature because they did not want me to get overstressed and sick.

Extremely satisfied with my IEP, I graduated high school. I am a senior at Murray State University, completing a baccalaureate in integrated studies in journalism. Additionally, I have Associates of Arts degree from West Kentucky Community College.

RECOMMENDED READINGS

American Academy of Pediatrics, Committee on School Health. (2001). The role of the school nurse in providing school health services. *Pediatrics, 108,* 1231–1232.

American Academy of Pediatrics, Committee on School Health. (2004). Guidelines for the administration of medication in school. *The Journal of School Nursing, 20*(2), 65–68.

National Association of School Nurses. (2001). *Issue brief: School health nursing services role in health care: Inclusion.* Retrieved April 4, 2006, from http://www.nasn.org/ Default.aspx? tabid=273

National Association of School Nurses. (2001). *Position statement: Medical services vs. health services in the school setting.* Retrieved April 4, 2006, from http://www.nasn.org/Default.aspx? tabid=229

National Association of School Nurses. (2002). *Issue brief: School health nursing services role in health care: School nurses and the Individuals with Disabilities Education Act (IDEA).* Retrieved April 4, 2006, from http://www.nasn.org/Default.aspx?tabid=274

National Association of School Nurses. (2002). *Position statement: Case management of children with special health care needs.* Retrieved April 4, 2006, from http://www.nasn.org/Default. aspx?tabid=208

National Association of School Nurses. (2002). *Position statement: The school nurse and specialized health care services.* Retrieved April 4, 2006, from http://www.nasn.org/Default.aspx?tabid= 249

National Association of School Nurses. (2003). *Position statement: Individualized health care plans.* Retrieved April 4, 2006, from http://www.nasn.org/Default.aspx?tabid=226

National Association of School Nurses. (2003). *Position statement: Medication administration in the school setting.* Retrieved April 4, 2006, from http://www.nasn.org/Default.aspx?tabid=230

National Association of School Nurses. (2004). *Position statement: Do not resuscitate.* Retrieved April 4, 2006, from http://www.nasn.org/Default.aspx?tabid=217

National Association of School Nurses. (2005). *Issue brief: School health nursing services role in health care: Section 504 of the Rehabilitation Act of 1973.* Retrieved April 4, 2006, from http://www.nasn.org/Default.aspx?tabid=280

National Association of School Nurses. (2005). *Position statement: Environmental impact concerns in the school setting.* Retrieved April 4, 2006, from http://www.nasn.org/Default.aspx?tabid= 293

Selekman, J. (Ed.). (2006). *School nursing: A comprehensive text.* Philadelphia: F.A. Davis.

REFERENCES

American Academy of Pediatrics, Committee on School Health. (2001). The role of the school nurse in providing school health. *Pediatrics, 108,* 1231–1232.

American Nurses Association. (1994). *Registered professional nursing and unlicensed assistive personnel.* Washington, DC: Author.

American Nurses Association. (2005a). *Consent action report to the board of directors on the delivery of care in schools for children with disabilities.* Washington, DC: Author.

American Nurses Association. (2005b). *School nurses: Providing safe health supervision and care for children in the school setting: Position statement.* Washington, DC: Author. Retrieved June 1, 2006, from http://www.ana.org/practice/SchoolNurseFinal1.doc

American Nurses Association and National Association of School Nurses. (2005). *School nursing: Scope and standards of practice.* Silver Spring, MD: American Nurses Association.

American Nurses Association and the American Association on Mental Retardation. (2004). *Intellectual and developmental disabilities nursing: Scope and standards of practice.* Silver Spring, MD: American Nurses Association.

Betz, C.L. (2001). Use of 504 plans for children and youth with disabilities: Nursing application. *Pediatric Nursing, 27*(4), 347–352.

Betz, C.L. (2003). Life after high school. In N. Keene (Ed.), *Educating the child with cancer: A guide for parents and teachers* (pp. 241–258). Kensington, MD: Candlelighters Childhood Cancer Foundation.

Betz, C.L., & Sowden, L. (in press). *Mosby's pediatric nursing reference* (6th ed.). St. Louis, MO: Mosby Yearbook.

Bloom, B., & Dey, A.N. (2006). Summary health statistics for U.S. children: National Health Interview Survey, 2004. *Vital and Health Statistics, 10*(227). Washington, DC: Centers for Disease Control and Prevention, National Center for Health Statistics.

Cedar Rapids Community School District v. Garrett F. (96-1793) 526 U.S. 66 (1999)

Centers for Disease Control and Prevention, National Center for Health Statistics. (2001). *National survey of children with special health care needs.* Retrieved December 22, 2006, from http://eshndata.org/anonymous/Dataquery

Centers for Disease Control and Prevention. (2004). *Addressing asthma in schools.* Center for Disease Control/Division of Adolescent and School Health. Retrieved August 18, 2006, from http://www.cdc.gov/HealthyYouth/asthma/pdf/asthma.pdf

Centers for Disease Control and Prevention, National Center for Health Statistics. (2006). Summary health statistics for the U.S. population: National Health Interview Survey, 2004. *Vital and Health Statistics, 10*(229), Washington, DC: Author.

Child and Adolescent Health Measurement Initiative. (2005). *National survey of children's health data resource center.* Retrieved December 6, 2006, from http://www.nschdata.org

Family Educational Rights and Privacy Act of 1974, PL 93-380.

Federal Interagency Forum on Child and Family Statistics. (2003). *America's children: Key national indicators of well-being 2003.* Vienna, VA: National Maternal and Child Health Clearinghouse.

Hazinski, M.F., Markenson, D., Neish, S., Geradi, M., Hootman, J., Nichol, G., et al. (2004). Response to cardiac arrest and selected life-threatening medical emergencies: the medical emergency response plan for schools. A statement for healthcare providers, policymakers, school administrators and community leaders. *Circulation, 109,* 278–291.

Health Insurance Portability and Accountability Act of 1996, PL 104-191, 42 U.S.C. §§ 201 *et seq.*

Healthy and Ready to Work National Center. (n.d.). *NFI: Delivery on the promise.* Retrieved May 11, 2006, from http://www.hrtw.org/systems/deliver.html

Heller, K.W., & Turnlin, J. (2004). Using expanded individualized health care plans to assist teachers of students with complex health care needs. *The Journal of School Nursing, 20*(3), 150–160.

Hootman, J., Houck, G., & King, M. C. (2003). Increased mental health needs and new roles in school communities. *Journal of Child and Adolescent Psychiatric Nursing, 16*(3), 93–101.

Individuals with Disabilities Education Act Amendments of 1997, PL 105-17, 20 U.S.C. §§ 1400 *et seq.*

Individuals with Disabilities Education Improvement Act of 2004, PL 108-446, 20 U.S.C. §§ 1400 *et seq.*

Kimberly, M.B., Forte, A.L., Carroll, J.M., & Feudtner, C. (2005). Pediatric do-not-attempt-resuscitation orders and public schools: A national assessment of policies and laws. *The American Journal of Bioethics, 5,* 59–65.

McCarthy, A.M., Kelly, M.W., & Reed, D. (2000). Medication administration practices of school nurses. *Journal of School Health, 70,* 371–376.

Moses, M., Gilchrest, C., & Schwab, N.C. (2005). Section 504 of the Rehabilitation Act: Determining eligibility and implications for school districts. *The Journal of School Nursing, 21,* 48–59.

National Association of Pediatric Nurse Practitioners. (2003). *Resolution: Access to a school nurse.* Retrieved April 2, 2006, from http://www.napnap.org/index.cfm?page=54

National Association of Pediatric Nurse Practitioners. (2004). *School-based and school-linked centers.* Retrieved April 8, 2006, from http://www.napnap.org/index.chm?page=108&sec=54&ssec=74

National Association of School Nurses. (2002a). *Issue brief: School health nursing services role in health care: Role of the school nurse.* Castle Rock, CO: Author.

National Association of School Nurses. (2002b). *Position statement: The school nurse and specialized health care services.* Retrieved April 4, 2006, from http://www.nasn.org/Default.aspx?tabid=249

National Association of School Nurses. (2005a). *Consensus statement: Clarification of the process of delegating in the school setting: Ensuring safe and effective care for students.* Retrieved May 10, 2006, from http://www.nasn.org/Portals/0/statements/consensusdelegation.pdf

National Association of School Nurses. (2005b). *Consensus statement: Safe delivery of care for children with diabetes in school.* Retrieved April 2, 2006, from http://www.nasn.org/Portals/0/statements/consensusdiabetes.pdf

No Child Left Behind Act of 2001, PL 107-110, 115 Stat. 1425, 20 U.S.C. §§ 6301 *et seq.*

North American Nursing Diagnosis Association (NANDA). (2004). *NANDA nursing Diagnoses: Definitions and classifications 2005–2006.* Philadelphia: NANDA International.

Rehabilitation Act of 1973, PL 93-112, 29 U.S.C. §§ 701 *et seq.*

Schulzinger, R. (1999). *Understanding 504: The role of state title V programs.* Gainsville, FL: Center for Policy and Partnerships.

Telljohann, S., Dake, J., & Price, J. (2004). Effect of full-time versus part-time school nurses on attendance of elementary students with asthma. *Journal of School Nursing, 20*(4), 189–196.

The Center for an Accessible Society. (1999). *Supreme Court upholds ADA "Integration Mandate" in Olmstead decision.* Retrieved May 11, 2006, from http://www.accessiblesociety.org/topics/ada/olmsteadoverview.htm

Thomas, S.B., & Hawke, C. (1999). Health-care services for children with disabilities: Emerging standards and implications. *The Journal of Special Education, 32*(4), 226–237.

U.S. Census Bureau. (2002). *Population profile of the United States: 2000.* Retrieved September 1, 2003, from http://www.censuslgov/population/www/pop-profile2000.html

U.S. Department of Education. (2004). *No child left behind: A toolkit for teachers.* Jessop, MD: Author. Retrieved June 1, 2006, from http://www.ed.gov/teachers/nclbguide/nclb-teachers-toolkit.pdf

U.S. Department of Education. (2005a). *Assessing students with disabilities: IDEA and NCLB working together.* Retrieved May 9, 2006, from http://www.ed.gov/admins/lead/speced/toolkit/idea-nclb.ppt

U.S. Department of Education. (2005b). *A decision framework for IEP teams related to methods for individual student participation in state accountability assessments.* Retrieved May 5, 2006, from http://www.ed.gov/admins/lead/speced/toolkit/iep-teams.doc

U.S. Department of Education. (2005c). *Proposed regulations on modified achievement standards.* Retrieved May 5, 2006, from http://www.ed.gov/policy/speced/guid/modachieve-nprm-summary.doc

U.S. Department of Education, Office of Special Education Programs. (2003a). *Racial/ethnic composition (number) of students ages 6-21 served under IDEA, Part B by disability, during the 2001-2002 school year–All disabilities.* Retrieved August 31, 2003, from http://www.ideadata.org/tables25th/ar_aa15.htm

U.S. Department of Education, Office of Special Education Programs. (2003b). *25th annual report to Congress on the implementation of the Individuals with Disabilities Education Act.* Washington, DC: Author.

U.S. Department of Education, Office of Special Education Programs. (2004). *Data tables for OSEP state reported data.* Washington, DC: Author.

U.S. Department of Health and Human Services. (2000). *Healthy people 2010: Understanding and improving health* (2nd ed.). Washington, DC: U.S. Government Printing Office. Retrieved June 1, 2006, from http://www.healthypeople.gov

U.S. Department of Health and Human Services. (2002). *Delivering on the promise. Self-evaluation to promote community living for people with disabilities.* Retrieved June 3, 2006, from http://www.hhs.gov/newfreedom/final/pdf/hhs.pdf

U.S. Department of Health and Human Services. (2003). *New freedom initiative.* Retrieved June 3, 2006, from http://www.hhs.gov/newfreedom/init.html

U.S. Department of Health and Human Services, Health Resources and Services Administration, Maternal and Child Health Bureau. (2004). *The National Survey of Children With Special Health Care Needs Chartbook 2001.* Rockville, MD: Author. Retrieved on August 18, 2006, from http://mchb.hrsa.gov/chscn/index.htm

U.S. Department of Health and Human Services, Office on Civil Rights. (2006). *HIPAA: Medical privacy-national standards to protect the privacy of personal health information.* Retrieved June 3, 2006, from http://www.hhs.gov/ocr/hipaa/

van Dyck, P.C., Kogan, M.D., McPherson, M.G., Weissman, G.R. & Newacheck, P.W. (2004). Prevalence and characteristics of children with special health care needs. *Archives of Pediatrics & Adolescent Medicine, 158*(9), 884–890.

Vought-O'Sullivan, V., Meehan, N.K., Havice, P.A., & Pruitt, R.H. (2006). Continuing education: A national imperative for school nursing practice. *The Journal of School Nursing, 22,* 2–8.

Witt, W.P., Kasper, J.D., & Riley, A.W. (2003). Mental health services use among school-aged children with disabilities: The role of sociodemographics, functional limitations, family burdens, and care coordination. *Health Services Research, 38,* 1441.

Zimmerman, B. (2006). Student health and education plans. In J. Selekman (Ed.), *School nursing: A comprehensive text* (pp. 177–203). Philadelphia: F.A. Davis.

CHAPTER 11

Developing and Implementing a 504 Plan

STANLEY D. HANDMAKER

U ntil the United States Congress passed the Rehabilitation Act of 1973 (PL 93-112, 29), there was essentially no recognition of the legal rights and privileges of individuals with disabilities in this country. Section 504 of the Rehabilitation Act of 1973 primarily addressed the employment training needs and job opportunities of adults with disabilities. However, the Act also recognized the educational rights and privileges of youth with special health care needs and disabilities, thus opening the door to these youth to receive a free appropriate public education (FAPE). These rights and privileges are realized through a 504 plan in which needed services in the areas of education, employment, and other activities (e.g., recreation, leisure, residential programs) are identified, planned, implemented, evaluated, and revised as needed. After a brief summary of current federal education acts, this chapter discusses the process for developing and implementing a 504 plan. The chapter concludes with one parent's advice to others on having a child with a 504 plan, as well as one student's journey with a 504 plan throughout high school.

FEDERAL EDUCATION ACTS FOR CHILDREN WITH DISABILITIES

As of 2006, there are three major federal laws that protect the rights and privileges of individuals with disabilities and prohibit discrimination based on that individual's disability. These laws include Section 504 of the Rehabilitation Act of 1973 (Section 504), the Individuals with Disabilities Education Improvement Act of 2004 (IDEA 2004; PL 108-446), and the Americans with Disabilities Act (ADA) of 1990 (PL 101-336).

Individuals with Disabilities Education Improvement Act of 2004

The law which most youth with special health care needs and disabilities and their families have experience with and are most familiar with is IDEA. IDEA is an educational act that governs special education and provides federal financial assistance to state and local school districts to guarantee special education and related services to eligible students with disabilities. Under IDEA, youth with special health care needs and disabilities are eligible to receive a FAPE including specialized instruction and related services from age 3 to 21 years of age. The federal mandate for FAPE requires that the individual educational needs of students with disabilities are met just as adequately as the educational needs of students in regular education. The FAPE mandate also requires that the local school district provide these services at no cost to youth with special health care needs and disabilities or their parents (IDEA, 2004).

Section 504 of the Rehabilitation Act of 1973

Section 504 is a civil rights law, which prohibits discrimination based on an individual's disability in any program or activity receiving federal financial assistance, and there is no age limit on eligibility. Failure to comply with Section 504 would threaten the loss of all federal funds to the school district. While there is no specific regulation under Section 504 regarding education per se, educational programs are almost all covered by Section 504. This is because there are in fact no public schools, and even many private secondary schools, and virtually no postsecondary schools that do not benefit from at least some federal funding. Further, the federal mandate for FAPE also applies to Section 504, so the educational needs of the student who qualifies for a 504 plan must be met as well as all other students. Also, there can be no cost to the child or his or her parents beyond what is charged for any child without a disability for any required accommodations under 504, including regular education as well as special education and related services (Rosenfeld, 2005).

Americans with Disabilities Act (ADA) of 1990

ADA is also a civil rights law, but it is not limited to organizations that receive federal funding. Under ADA, the prohibition of discrimination under Section 504 is broadened to include private businesses, state and local governments, and public accommodations—including accommodations and services, transportation, and telecommunications provided by entities that receive no federal funding (Henderson, 2001; Richards, 2000). Similar to Section 504, the definition of an eligible person with adisability under ADA also includes someone who does not meet the criteria for having a disability but is treated as if they have a disability; however, such individuals are not entitled to any special accommodations or services.

Differences between IDEA, Section 504, and ADA

There are some major differences between IDEA, Section 504, and ADA, such as: 1) the criteria for and determination of eligibility, 2) the nature of the instructional process and the services that can be provided, and 3) the allocation of funds. These differences are summarized in Table 11.1.

To begin, the definition of *disabilities* is much broader for Section 504 and ADA than it is for IDEA. Also, Section 504 and ADA eliminate barriers and provide access to activities and programs available to individuals without disabilities, while IDEA provides special programs and services in addition to those available to individuals without disabilities (Rosenfeld, 2005).

Regarding funding, the local school district receives federal funding to provide services to students under IDEA, but there is no such funding for Section 504

Table 11.1. Comparison of Rehabilitation Act of 1973 (Section 504) with Individuals with Disabilities Education Act (IDEA) and Americans with Disabilities Act (ADA)

Federal law	Section 504	IDEA	ADA
Type of law	Civil rights act	Educational act	Civil rights act
Assessment process	Not specified	Comprehensive formal evaluations by interdisciplinary team	Not specified
Ages of eligibility	All ages	3–21 years of age	All ages
Eligibility criteria	A physical or mental impairment that substaintially limits one or more major life activities (e.g., caring for one's self, learning, working), and the impairment need not adversely affect the student's educational performance.	Specific criteria for defined categories of disability, including mental retardation, hearing impairments (e.g., deafness), visual impairments (e.g., blindness), speech or language impairments, emotional disturbance, orthopedic impairments, autism, traumatic brain injury, specific learning disabilities, and other health impairments, and the disability must adversely affect the student's educational performance	A physical or mental impairment that substaintially limits one or more major life activities (e.g., caring for one's self, learning, working), and the impairment need not adversely affect the student's educational performance.
Educational services provided	Regular education setting with reasonable accommodations	Specialized instruction (i.e., special education services, and related services)	Regular education setting with reasonable accommodations
Settings	Elementary, secondary, and postsecondary and employment	Elementary and secondary education	Elementary, secondary, and postsecondary and employment
Funding	No funding provided	Federal and state funding	No funding provided

or ADA. If a student qualifies for modifications or accommodations under Section 504, it is the fiscal responsibility of the local school district to use general education funds to meet the student's needs, as IDEA funds may not be used to serve students under Section 504. Thus, there is a major disincentive to the schools to identify students who qualify for services under Section 504, whereas schools are more motivated to identify students for special education programs that receive fiscal support.

In the case of IDEA, eligible students must meet the criteria for one or more of the specific categories, and the determination of eligibility is by a defined interdisciplinary team. Also, under IDEA, the educational performance of the youth with special health care needs and disabilities must be adversely affected by the disability, and the student must require special education services (i.e., specialized instruction) in order to qualify.

Under Section 504 and ADA, there is no limit of specific disabilities, the disability does not have to affect the student's educational performance, and there is not a defined interdisciplinary team determining eligibility. Further, the youth with special health care needs and disabilities receives all instruction in a regular educational classroom without special education services.

However, any student who qualifies for services under IDEA will also meet the criteria for Section 504. Thus, even if a student has an individualized education program (IEP) under IDEA, he or she may also use a 504 plan to address some additional specific needs, such as health-related needs or other needs. However, health-related needs can be addressed in an IEP as well.

Students with disabilities and their families typically use a 504 plan primarily to address educational and health-related needs of youth with special health care needs and disabilities in elementary and secondary education. Consequently, most of what has been written about Section 504 in the public schools is regarding the use of a 504 plan for these purposes. However, Section 504 is not limited to these situations. A 504 plan can be used to address any program or activity receiving federal financial assistance, and, furthermore, there is no age limit to persons eligible.

The process of developing and implementing a 504 plan for youth with special health care needs and disabilities who are addressing their needs in planning their transitions is the same process as is used to address education and health-related needs. Thus, a 504 plan can serve as an excellent vehicle for adolescents with special health care needs and disabilities to address transition planning from secondary to postsecondary education, employment, or other activities or services, including residential programs and recreation and leisure activities.

If a student has a 504 plan in place for secondary education, the plan can be transferred with or without modifications and implemented in a postsecondary education or work setting (Betz, 2001). If the student has an IEP in place for secondary education, the IEP may need to be revised, but it can serve as the basis for developing a 504 plan that can then be used in a postsecondary education or work setting.

Furthermore, as described later in the chapter, the process of developing and implementing a 504 plan offers youth with special health care needs and disabilities multiple opportunities for self-determination in creating a meaningful plan and in assuring that the plan, as implemented, is meeting their needs.

However, as mentioned previously, there is no additional federal funding provided to support the 504 plans; thus, there is considerable resistance and increased scrutiny of 504 plans by postsecondary personnel, including questioning of the credentials of those who formulated the plans. This is where healthcare professionals, especially physicians and nurses, can use their clinical expertise and credentials in enhancing the credibility of the 504 plans that are developed.

ESSENTIAL FEATURES OF SECTION 504

It took 4 years of considerable action by individuals with disabilities and other advocates for disability rights after the Rehabilitation Act of 1973 was enacted before the federal government issued the Section 504 implementation guidelines (Jarrow, 1991; Rosenfeld, 2005). These specific regulations are found in Title 34 of the Code of Federal Regulations (C.F.R.), Pt. 104 (Rosenfeld, 2005).

Section 504 specifically prohibits any discrimination towards any "handicapped person" by any program or activity receiving federal funding. A "handicapped person" is defined as any "otherwise qualified individual" who has 1) either a physical or a mental impairment that results in a "substantial limitation" of one or more major life activities, 2) a record of such a disability, or 3) is regarded as having such a disability. Major life activities include a number of basic functions, such as caring for oneself, learning, or working (34 C.F.R. 104).

The "major life activity" that most frequently affects a student's performance in school is learning. However, the student does not need to have a disability limiting the major life activity of learning to qualify for Section 504. For example, the disability might substantially limit the major life activity of breathing (i.e., a student on a respirator or with severe asthma). Another relatively common condition for which a Section 504 plan has been used is diabetes.

Section 504 is subject to the federal mandate known as the "least restricted environment" (LRE). The LRE means that a student with a disability must receive his or her education alongside students without disabilities (i.e., in regular education classes) to the maximum extent possible. The only exception to the LRE rule is a situation in which the student with a disability cannot satisfactorily receive the needed services and supports. Section 504 also is subject to the federal mandate for FAPE, as stated previously (34 C.F.R. 104).

In addition to academic services and activities, Section 504 also applies to nonacademic and extracurricular activities, including recess periods, lunch periods, transportation, and health services. This means that a child with a disability should participate in these activities as much as possible with children who do not have disabilities. However, the local school district is allowed to offer separate and specialized physical education and athletic activities, as long as qualified students with disabilities are at least offered the opportunity to participate in the regular physical education program and compete for regular athletic teams (34 C.F.R. 104).

One regulation that is especially important regarding possible discrimination in nonacademic services for students with disabilities deals with the counseling services, in particular academic counseling and vocational counseling, guidance, or placement. This regulation requires the local school district to ensure that qualified students with disabilities are not directed towards more restricted placements or careers than their peers without disabilities but with comparable interests and abilities (34 C.F.R. 104.37 [b], 1973). This regulation obviously relates directly to counseling regarding postsecondary school transition planning.

DEVELOPING A 504 PLAN

Just as a student with a disability under IDEA must have a written IEP, a student with a disability who is entitled to accommodations under Section 504 also must have a written plan, known as a 504 plan. A 504 plan is similar to an IEP in that it is a legally binding document. A 504 plan 1) identifies and documents the student's disability and corresponding need for accommodation, and 2) describes the specific accommodations and modifications that will be implemented by the school. The 504 plan should be reviewed by the 504 committee at least annually to determine whether or not the student is still eligible and if there is a need for a change in modifications or accommodations.

Identifying Eligible Students

The first step in developing a 504 plan is identifying a student who might have a disability and who is eligible for specific accommodations or program modifications under Section 504. Under "Child Find," the local school district must make every effort to identify and evaluate any students suspected of having a disability. The school should identify such students based on their behavior in the classroom or poor academic performance or the student's performance in non-academic school activities (Richards, 2000).

In addition, the local school district should notify students and their parents or guardians of the district's obligation to provide youth with special health care needs and disabilities with a free and appropriate public education. Students also have the opportunity for self-direction in that students and their parents or guardians may also make self-referrals if they are concerned that the student may have a disability that requires special accommodations or program modifications (Richards, 2000).

Health care professionals are often the most likely to recognize those students who meet the qualifications for and are most likely to benefit from a 504 plan. This is a golden opportunity for the health care professional, either the school nurse or the child's physician, to provide students and families with the information needed to request a 504 plan. Alternatively, the school nurses can make the referral themselves (Betz, 2001).

Under Section 504, students with disabilities may include students who have been evaluated for special education and who either have been dismissed from or do not qualify for special education services under IDEA because they do not meet or no longer meet the criteria for eligibility for special education. Other students with disabilities who may qualify for a 504 plan are students with a health condition not covered by special education but that could interfere with learning, such as being respirator-dependent or having severe asthma, diabetes, or a life-threatening allergy. Some school districts have considered a temporary disability, such as a broken bone, to be an impairment that substantially limits a major life activity, thereby meeting the requirements of Section 504 (Richards, 2000).

Intervention

If a student has been identified as having a possible disability, the next step is for the school to implement appropriate intervention strategies to address the identified concerns. If the strategies are successful, they will establish that the student can benefit from the regular education curriculum. If the strategies work, but the teacher is still concerned that the student has a possible disability, then the strategies may serve as reasonable modifications and accommodations. If the strategies do not work and the child appears to have a disability, the student might require some further modifications and accommodation, or the student may need to be referred for special education or related services (Richards, 2000).

Referral to the 504 Coordinator

Each public school should have a person (usually an administrator, i.e., an assistant principal, or a guidance counselor, but not a special educator) who serves as the school's 504 coordinator. The 504 coordinator is responsible for coordinating the development, maintenance, and implementation of the 504 plans. The 504 coordinator must first review the documentation, including the student's response to the initial intervention strategies, and determine whether or not referrals are warranted. If a referral is warranted, then the 504 coordinator should call together a 504 committee meeting (Richards, 2000).

504 Committee Meeting

Unlike regulations under IDEA, which specify the membership of the review committee, Section 504 regulations do not specify who must be members of the 504 committee. However, the regulations do require that the 504 committee consist of a group of people. The regulations also require that the group includes 1) individuals who are knowledgeable about the student, 2) individuals who understand the meaning of the evaluation data, and 3) individuals who are aware of the placement options (§104.35 [c][3], 1973). A school nurse could serve any or all of these functions. Clearly, the student with a disability and her or his parent(s) or guardian(s) are certainly individuals "who are knowledgeable about the student" (Betz, 2001, p. 349). Individuals who understand the meaning of the evaluation data could be the student's teacher or therapist, an educational diagnostician, or a special educator. Individuals who are often aware of the placement options include the student's teacher and the 504 coordinator.

While not specifically designated by the federal regulations, a 504 committee may consist of the following members: 1) the student, 2) the student's parent(s) or guardian(s), 3) the student's teacher(s), 4) the school nurse, 5) the student's counselor, 6) the 504 coordinator, 7) other service personnel (e.g., speech/language pathologist, occupational therapist, physical therapist), as appropriate, and 8) a special educator in an advisory capacity. There is no maximum number of individuals required, and the regulations do not specify the level of knowledge required of the members (Richards, 2000).

Review and Determination of Eligibility by the 504 Committee

The 504 committee must determine whether or not 1) the student has a physical or mental impairment, 2) this physical or mental impairment affects one or more of that student's "major life activities," and 3) there is a "substantial limitation" in a major life activity affected by the impairment. Although the language of Section 504 also includes a person who has a record of such an impairment, or is regarded as having such an impairment as an eligible person who cannot be discriminated against, such a person is not entitled to any other special treatment (Richards, 2000).

Section 504 regulations give no specific guidance regarding what constitutes a "substantial limitation" in a major life activity. However, federal regulations under ADA defines an individual with a "substantial limitation" as being:

1. Unable to perform a major life activity that the average person in the general population can perform.

2. Significantly restricted as to the condition, manner, or duration under which the average person in the general population can perform the same major

life activity (29 U.S.C. § 1630.2[j][1], 1973; Moses, Gilchrest, & Schwab, 2005, p. 50).

A student and/or his or her parents or guardians may already have obtained an evaluation by an independent evaluator who has determined that the student has such a disability. Either way, the 504 committee may seek additional evaluation data. The evaluation data may, but not necessarily, be specific cognitive and/or achievement tests (Richards, 2000).

Once the 504 committee is satisfied that it has all of the necessary data, the committee then determines the student's eligibility for a 504 plan. If the student is indeed eligible for a 504 plan, then the committee develops the plan. If the committee believes the disability is too severe for a 504 plan, the student is then referred to special education for further evaluation under IDEA. If the committee determines that the student is not eligible, then the case is dismissed.

If the student's case is dismissed, the student and/or his or her parents may appeal the decision. They can appeal the decision to the local school district according to whatever due process procedures are in place. They also can appeal the decision to the U.S. Department of Education, Office of Civil Rights (OCR) within 60 days of a decision at the local level. Finally, they have the option of challenging the decision in the federal courts.

Creating the 504 Plan

The 504 committee first identifies and documents the student's disability, giving whatever background information is necessary to enable those who are implementing the plan to understand the student's disability and what needs to be done. The 504 committee then identifies the student's corresponding needs and the placement and specific accommodations and program modifications that will be implemented by the school. In determining the appropriate placement and accommodations, the committee must decide if the student requires in-class services or related services, such as tutoring, peer mentoring, and so forth (Richards, 1998). Specific accommodations and modifications may include physical, behavioral, and/or instructional accommodations (refer to Chapter 6). The placement decision must meet the provisions of the LRE (Richards, 2000; Rosenfeld, 2005). All of the information is prepared in a written document, known as the 504 plan.

Some Examples of Specific Accommodations for a 504 Plan

The following are some specific physical, instructional, and behavioral accommodations written into 504 plans (Blazer, 1999).

- Student will be given an assigned seat in each classroom nearest to and facing the teacher.

- Student will be provided a quiet area for study in study hall.

- All classroom and homework assignments will be given in written form.

- The volume of homework assignments will not exceed more than two hours per night.

- Student will be provided an extra set of textbooks to keep at home during the school year.

- Student will be allowed 1½ time to take tests, and all tests will be given in an area that is free from auditory and visual distractions.

- All teachers will communicate with the student's parents by telephone calls or e-mail on at least a weekly basis to notify the parents of the student's progress and to inform them as soon as possible of any problems that are occurring at school.

The effectiveness of accommodations can be derived from the student, his or her family, and the student's teachers. Self-direction has been found to be most helpful in identifying which specific accommodations are most likely to address the specific needs of the individual student. Therefore, the student and his or her family need to be given an opportunity to identify which accommodations best address their needs. The classroom teachers often can also provide helpful insight regarding which accommodations are currently working best for the student and what needs still have to be addressed (Blazer, 1999). The 504 committee also needs to identify and specify the knowledge and training needs of the school personnel, including all of the student's teachers, support staff, and/or school nurse, who will be responsible for implementing the 504 plan.

However, the services and supports as outlined in the 504 plan or IEP do not automatically carry over to postsecondary education but end with high school graduation. While postsecondary programs are covered by Section 504, colleges and universities are bound by Subpart E, which has significantly different requirements than Subpart D, which applies to secondary schools (Madaus, 2005). Thus, a new 504 plan needs to be developed for transition planning.

Implementing a 504 Plan

Implementation of a 504 plan requires the cooperation and collaboration of multiple school personnel, the student, and the student's parents or guardians. In the case of a 504 plan for postsecondary transition, it is critical to involve personnel from both the secondary level and the postsecondary programs—such as postsecondary educational programs, employment placements, and the Division of Vocational Rehabilitation (DVR)—in developing and implementing the plan.

It is imperative that there be a system in place, including both the teacher(s) and parents or guardians, monitoring the progress of the youth with special health care needs and disabilities and his or her response to the placement and specific accommodations provided. It is the responsibility of the school, and specifically the 504 coordinator, to assure that all relevant school personnel are held accountable for their compliance with the requirements of the 504 plan.

Review and Reevaluation by the 504 Committee

The 504 plan should be reviewed at least annually by the 504 committee to determine whether or not the student is still eligible for the plan and if there is a need for a change in modifications or accommodations. The 504 committee may request additional evaluation data to make the determination.

The procedural safeguards under Section 504 are not as extensive as they are under IDEA. Procedural safeguards provided to parents or guardians under Section 504 include the following: 1) notice, 2) an opportunity to examine relevant records, 3) an impartial hearing with opportunity for participation including representation by counsel, and 4) a review procedure (34 C.F.R. 104.36, 1993, Richards, 2000). The right to notice includes notice of child find (identification, evaluation, and educational placement), notice of parent rights, prior notice of evaluations and meetings, and notice of results/actions taken at 504 committee meetings. The relevant records include all of the documents that form the basis of any decisions being made regarding the student with disabilities. The impartial hearing must be requested by the child's parent or guardian. The review procedure involves an examination of the student's progress and whether any changes need to be made (Blazer, 1999).

SUMMARY

The Rehabilitation Act of 1973 was the first federal law passed that recognized the educational rights and privileges of students with disabilities. Under Section 504 of this Act, the specific services and supports (accommodations) a person with a disability needs to succeed are assured in a 504 plan. Section 504 applies to individuals of all ages, and thus a 504 plan remains as one of the best vehicles for adolescents with special health care needs and disabilities to address transition planning from secondary to postsecondary education, employment, or other activities or services, including residential programs and recreation and leisure activities.

My Story   Rebecah MacMurray

As a parent of a student with ADHD and with some years of experience with a 504 plan in place, I feel that I can offer some advice to other parents and youth facing the same situation. Therefore, the following points are offered from someone with experience with this federal law:

1. To begin with, it really helps for you and your family to find out everything that you can about what a 504 plan is and how it works. Many people find the quickest and most efficient way is to get on the Internet using the search term "504 plan(s)." This will let you know everything you need to know about Section 504 and will give you examples of 504 plans that others have used.

2. Also, your family really needs to understand what you are experiencing at school, at home, with your friends, and other places. When they understand, then they can do what they have to do to help you. Also, it will help them and you to understand and realize that you are going to be okay.

3. If you or your family believe you might qualify for and would be helped by a 504 plan, then your family should write the school and tell them that you should be considered for a 504 plan.

4. When requesting a 504 plan, it often works best if you are prepared with written documentation to reinforce your reasons for your request. This may be a doctor's letter or report explaining your diagnosis, results of testing that you have already had done, or reports from your teachers, therapists, and others. Often it helps to have a personal letter from your family explaining what they have noticed and why you and they, as parents, are requesting that you have a 504 plan in place.

5. You and your family need to contact the school to find out who is the 504 coordinator. This person is often an assistant principal or another person at the school who is responsible for making sure that everything regarding a 504 plan is done properly. The 504 coordinator is the most important person for you and your family to interact with so that everything goes smoothly regarding your 504 plan. This is also the main person in the school for you to go to when you need help with your 504 plan.

6. Once you have contacted the 504 coordinator with your written request, the 504 coordinator needs to decide if you appear to qualify for a 504 plan. If so, then the 504 coordinator needs to call together a 504 committee to meet.

7. The 504 committee typically includes you and your parents or guardians in addition to teachers, counselors, the school nurse, and others. The 504 committee needs to include people who know you best, people who are familiar with your disability and understand the evaluation data, and people who understand what can be put in a 504 plan to help you.

8. When the 504 committee meets, everyone will introduce themselves and sign a paper that lists everyone present.

9. The meeting typically lasts from 1 to 3 hours. The 504 coordinator is in charge of the meeting.

10. First, the committee needs to decide if you qualify for a 504 plan. They will usually begin by asking your parents or guardians questions, as to what your disability is, when you were diagnosed, and so forth. They will usually review the documentation, such as a letter or report from your doctor. Once they decide that you qualify for a 504 plan, the committee next needs to decide what your needs are and what accommodations will be provided to help you.

11. They will usually ask you questions and ask for your opinion on all that is said and done and how you feel. It's important to let them know what you think and how you feel about their suggestions. The 504 coordinator will also ask your teachers to say what they have noticed in the classroom regarding your academic performance and your behavior. You and your family will also have a chance to tell them what you think and ask them questions. It's also okay to ask people to talk slower or to explain what they mean.

12. Sometimes people will say things you or your family does not like, but you need to not get upset and to stay focused on your goals.

13. The 504 coordinator will usually take lots of notes, and its okay for you and your family to take notes, too.

14. After the meeting, the 504 coordinator will prepare a rough draft of your 504 plan. Once the rough draft is written, you and your family will receive a copy of it to look over and to make changes until both the school and you and your family agree.

15. Once agreed, then you and your family will get a copy of your final 504 plan and a copy of the Procedural Safeguards. These are what you can do in case the accommodations are not working well or your teachers or others are not doing what they are supposed to do according to your 504 plan.

16. Once you have a 504 plan in place, the 504 coordinator needs to make sure that, even if they were not at the meeting of the 504 committee, everyone understands what they need to do and that they all do what they are supposed to do for your 504 plan. This information includes all of your teachers and others at the school, including the school nurse. Sometimes they need to have training to understand your disability and what they need to do to help you.

17. In order for the 504 plan to work and for you to achieve your goals, it takes the school personnel and you and your family working together. This includes really good communication between the school and you and your family.

REFERENCES

Americans with Disabilities Act (ADA) of 1990, PL 101-336, 42 U.S.C. §§ 12101 *et seq.*

Betz, C.L. (2001). Use of 504 plans for children and youth with disabilities: Nursing application. *Pediatric Nursing, 27,* 347–352.

Blazer, B. (1999). Developing 504 classroom accommodation plans. A collaborative systematic parent-student-teacher approach. *Teaching Exceptional Children, 32,* 28–33.

Henderson, K. (2001). *An overview of ADA, IDEA, and Section 504: Update 2001.* Arlington, VA: The ERIC Clearinghouse on Disabilities and Gifted Education, The Council for Exceptional Children.

Individuals with Disabilities Education Improvement Act of 2004, PL 108-446, 20 U.S.C. §§ 1400 *et seq.*

Jarrow, J. (1991). Disability issues on campus and the road to ADA. *Educational Record, Winter,* 26–31.

Madaus, J.W. (2005). Navigating the college transition maze: A guide for students with learning disabilities. *Teaching Exceptional Children, 37,* 32–37.

Moses, M., Gilchrest, C., & Schwab, N.C. (2005). Section 504 of the Rehabilitation Act: Determining eligibility and implications for school districts. *The Journal of School Nursing, 21,* 48–58.

Rehabilitation Act of 1973, PL 93-112, 29 U.S.C. §§ 701 *et seq.*

Richards, D.M. (1998). *Section 504 committee decision-making chart.* Austin: Richards Lindsay & Martin, L.L.P.

Richards, D.M. (2000). *An overview of Section 504.* Austin, TX: Richards Lindsay & Martin, L.L.P.

Rosenfeld, S.J. (2005). *Section 504 and IDEA: Basic similarities and differences.* Retrieved December 6, 2006, from http://www.ldonline.org/ld_indepth/legal_legislative/edlaw504.html

CHAPTER 12

Working with Job Developers and Employers

ROBERTA ROSS AND WENDY M. NEHRING

Children, at varying ages, aspire to vocational goals in life. Whether to emulate a parent, relative, or television or movie personality, young people identify what they want to be when they grow up and more or less fashion their lives after those objectives. These aspirations continue to be developed and shaped by those in their immediate environments during their younger years and furthered by others as they reach adulthood.

All of us have vocational strengths and limitations. Our choices are guided by our interests, our self-knowledge, our abilities, what we know about employment environments, and luck in the ability to access that which will bring us vocational satisfaction. This statement holds true for all youth, including youth with special health care needs and disabilities. Youth with special health care needs and disabilities want to learn how to get a job, how to get to what they want and dream about, and how to become vocationally productive, as being employed can add meaning, generate a level of satisfaction, and provide financial stability in their lives.

This chapter is about having a vocation and developing plans for future employment by taking advantage of the job preparation and training opportunities offered in high school. Beginning in high school, job preparation and training experiences are initiated for students with special health care needs and disabilities using the individualized education program (IEP). A major goal of IEP transition planning is to make certain that students with special health care needs and disabilities are sufficiently prepared to seek and obtain employment. This chapter provides information on the job training opportunities available in high school, including the joint programs with state vocational rehabilitation departments and the federally funded Workforce Investment Act (WIA) job training programs, to name a few. This chapter also addresses the role of job developers in working with high school students and how educators, job developers, and health care professionals can work more effectively with each other.

EMPLOYMENT SNAPSHOT OF YOUTH AND ADULTS WITH SPECIAL HEALTH CARE NEEDS AND DISABILITIES

Youth

Instructive sources of data gathered from the National Longitudinal Transition Studies (NLTS) in 1987 and (NLTS2) in 2003 on the postschool outcomes two years following high school completion and graduation are available to gauge the effectiveness of IEP transition planning (Cameto, Levine & Wagner, 2004). The findings of these national surveys revealed that substantial progress has been made to better prepare young adults who were enrolled in special education for postschool employment, although further postschool employment improvement is needed.

In 2003, 70% of individuals with disabilities reported having a job during the two years following high school completion compared with 55% of individuals with disabilities in 1987. At the time that the 2003 NTLS2 was conducted, 39% of individuals with disabilities reported being currently employed. Closer examination of the postschool employment outcomes revealed a number of demographic characteristics associated with improved outcomes. Older youth were more likely to be employed and to be working in higher skill jobs. Youth from higher socioeconomic strata were more likely to have been employed compared with youth from lower socioeconomic strata. The employment status of girls improved dramatically from 1987 to 2003, nearly doubling from 35% to 67%, thereby eliminating much of the gender differences originally observed in 1987. Similarly, the employment gap between white and black students noted in 1987 diminished to 12% in 2003, with 74% of Caucasian students and 62% of African American students reporting employment.

Researchers found that youth whose parents were involved in their education performed better in school and had higher postsecondary ambitions. Improved employment outcomes and higher paying jobs were associated with students who had prevocational training and work experience in high school (U.S. General Accounting Office [GAO], 2003). NTLS2 revealed that 60% of students with disabilities had paid employment and 24% had vocational training (Wagner, Newman, Cameto, & Levine, 2005).

Student outcomes varied according to special education categories. Students with visual and hearing impairments had the highest rates of postschool employment (62%). Youth with other health impairments had the highest high school dropout rates (40%).

Patterns of jobs types held by youth with disabilities were noted between the 1987 and 2003 NLTS surveys. No differences in patterns were noted with the following job types: childcare, food service, routinized (assembly), and service positions. A decrease from 16% to 6% was noted in clerical jobs, whereas an increase of 16% was found for retail positions. In general, students with disabilities had low-wage, low-skill, and blue collar jobs (Wagner et al., 2005).

The number of individuals with disabilities who were employed or enrolled in postsecondary programs increased four times in 2003 when compared with the 1987 sample. These increases were most evident in youth with learning disabilities and with visual, hearing, and orthopedic impairments. A significant increase of 16% was noted in students who both worked and were enrolled in postsecondary programs from 1987 to 2003. The dropout rate of students decreased considerably from 1987 to 2003. Lower drop out rates were associated with students who had prevocational training and work experience in high school (Wagner et al., 2005). Only one quarter of students who dropped out later enrolled in GED programs. Students who dropped out were more likely to be employed in lower paying jobs as compared with students who did not drop out of high school (Wagner et al., 2005).

Adults

The employment gap between individuals with and without disabilities is significant. Thirty-two percent of adults ages 18 to 64 years of age with disabilities compared with 81% of adults without disabilities were employed full or part time. Employment rates for culturally diverse individuals were less than 40%. However, 75% of individuals surveyed reported they wanted to work. Employment rates varied considerably according to the individual's level of disability severity. Eight percent of individuals with more severe types of disabilities were employed compared with 64% of individuals with less severe disabilities (National Organization of Disability/Louis Harris and Associates, 2000; Stodden, Jans, Ripple, & Kraus, 1998).

Job patterns of adults with disabilities differed from individuals without disabilities. Adults with disabilities chose self-employment twice as often compared with individuals without disabilities. More than 50% of individuals with disabilities indicated that their jobs were obtained through personal contacts (Thornton & Lunt, 1997).

Healthy People 2010 (*HP* 2010; 2004) has recognized this serious employment disparity as a public health concern. In response, *HP* 2010 contains several objectives related to employment and employment-related concerns, including the following:

- Eliminate employment disparities between working-aged (18 to 62 years) adults with and without disabilities.

- Reduce the proportion of people with disabilities who report not having the assistive devices and technology they need.

- Reduce the proportion of people with disabilities who report encountering environmental barriers to participating in home, work, or community activities.

Updates on whether these objectives are being met will be assessed through future national surveys, such as the NLTS.

THE HIGH SCHOOL EXPERIENCE: YOUTH EMPLOYMENT PROGRAMS IN SCHOOL SETTINGS

Various employment programs are available to secondary students with special health care needs and disabilities. These programs include the educational supports available through the Individuals with Disabilities Education Act (IDEA), the joint programs of the Vocational Rehabilitation and educational programs, youth employment options through the school-to-work programs and the WIA, the Carl D. Perkins Vocational and Technical Education Act, the High School/High Tech program, and Independent Living Centers.

IDEA

The School to Work Opportunities Act of 1994 (PL 103-239) helped to stimulate the development of school-to-work programs for all youth. However, prior to that, IDEA mandated that all children with IEPs have transition plans that included vocational goals. School districts were mandated to provide youth with disabilities vocational experiences that included voluntary and paid tryouts in employment settings. Each state has developed programs that provide these opportunities. In California, for instance, youth are introduced to Project Workability, a joint program with the California Department of Rehabilitation, where they are placed in subsidized jobs with operating businesses and industry.

In the IDEA reauthorization of 1997 (PL 105-17), the IDEA transition plan originally stipulated that transition planning begin at age 14; the most recent reauthorization in 2004 (PL 108-446) changed the initiation of transition planning to 16 years of age or earlier as appropriate. According to child labor laws, paid employment can start only at 16 years of age, but other types of vocational access can be developed earlier to introduce the youth to the world of work. For example, volunteer and job shadowing positions can be developed with various organizations and businesses. As mentioned previously, state special education and school-to-work funding should be available for either subsidized opportunities or direct placement of youth in vocational venues.

Youth enrolled in special education have the option of staying in school until 21 years of age. After 18 years, these students may include working as part of their curriculum and attend school on a part-time basis. Students and their families may choose to enroll in sheltered workshops or organizations such as Goodwill, Volunteers of America, or Salvation Army that offer employment to individuals with disabilities. As advocates strive for greater independence, these programs have suffered a lapse in reputation; however, job placement in these environments continues to be appropriate and satisfactory for certain individuals and predicated on youth and family choice and the abilities of the youth. For others, participating in these programs can be a stepping stone to supported or competitive employment. The definition of supported employment includes a job coach to assist the worker with a disability in completion of the work assignment. Some students who have been in subsidized high school programs are able to continue in their same jobs as regular hired employees.

Vocational experiences are vitally important for youth in the development of self-image, planning for future employment, career and vocational choices, and clarification of their abilities. Such experiences are especially necessary for youth with special health care needs and disabilities—those who may have received a message that they are severely limited in achievement of vocational aspirations. Health care professionals can have a vital role in counseling youth with special health care needs and disabilities as to the appropriate parameters for employment based upon their special needs/disabilities.

Joint Vocational Rehabilitation and Educational Programs

State vocational rehabilitation departments are mandated to provide services and supports to individuals with disabilities to maximize their opportunities and enhance their potential for becoming independent and productive members of their community of choice. Contracts are written with various high school districts to serve adolescents with special health care needs and disabilities who will soon be transitioning for adult services follow-up. A partnership is formed between DR counselors and school personnel who work most closely with students with special health care needs and disabilities. As members of youth transition IEP teams beginning at age 16 in high school, vocational rehabilitation counselors can offer a wide array of job training experiences that assist youth in achieving IEP objectives. Youth and adult consumers who are enrolled as vocational rehabilitation clients have an individualized plan for employment (IPE) developed that contains the individual's goals for employment, identification of objectives to achieve those goals, and the services and supports needed to attain the IPE goals and objectives. Again, consultation with health care professionals in developing the transition IEP and/or IPE will be useful to determine what accommodations are needed due to the individual's physical limitations that affect work performance.

Services provided by vocational rehabilitation include job development and placement, provision of medical services, technological aids and devices, transportation assistance, training for learning job search skills, supported employment, vocational training, on-the-job training, job coaches, referral to other community programs, tuition stipends, purchase of work clothes/uniforms/licenses/equipment, and tutorial and notetaking aides. Individuals who apply to vocational rehabilitation must have documentation of their disability to receive services. In many states, vocational rehabilitation services are impacted, meaning that eligible potential recipients are placed on a waiting list for services, as the vocational rehabilitation resources are limited and cannot serve all eligible clients.

School-to-Work Programs

During the Clinton Administration, a nationwide effort was initiated through the School to Work Opportunities Act of 1994. This time-limited legislation directed the Departments of Education and Labor to oversee and administer federal funds to the states to develop and implement system partnerships between the schools, private industry, and the community to introduce students in both general and special education programs to the world of employment. The philosophy of school-to-work (STW) programs embraces a life-span perspective based on the premise that preparation for career and work begins in the early school years rather than later in high school when most students are getting ready to graduate. STW activities can be thought of as a three-legged stool consisting of work-based learning (e.g., job shadowing, apprenticeships), school-based learning obtained through classroom instruction, and the connecting activities that create the linkages between the schools, work settings, and communities. STW experiences focus on career awareness and preparation and include an array of instructional and work-based activities besides those already mentioned, such as mentorships, internships, career exploration, and the integration of academics with vocational experiences. An objective of this program is to ensure that students with disabilities are fully included rather than excluded with their schoolmates in general education (deFur, 2002; School to Work Project, Institute on Community Integration, University of Minnesota, 1998).

Workforce Investment Act
Youth Employment Programs

The passage of the Workforce Investment Act (WIA) of 1998 reorganized the job training and placement service system enabling the development of one-stop employment centers and the expansion of youth employment services to a year-round program statewide. The goal of WIA one-stop employment centers is to locate many job training and support programs receiving governmental support under one roof, enabling improved access to employment services. One-stop employment centers enable job seekers to obtain training for job skills, learn how to interview for a job, learn to access computer databases for locating jobs, and obtain assistance with developing a resume.

There are many comprehensive youth services that are offered year round. These services include on-the-job training, alternate secondary programs for obtaining a GED, training to learn study skills, one-to-one tutoring, strategies to prevent high school drop out, alternative secondary school programs, paid and unpaid work experiences that include job shadowing and internships, summer youth employment programs, counseling and guidance programs including those for substance abuse, leadership training, participation in adult mentor programs, and 12-month follow-up programs.

The General Accounting Office (GAO, 2003) reported that participation in WIA youth programs was limited. It concluded that participation was limited due to lack of information youth and families had about WIA programs, lack of programmatic linkages between school settings and job training and placement agencies, limited work-based training activities youth had while in school, and misinformation youth and parents had about possibly losing benefits if employed.

The Carl D. Perkins Vocational
and Technical Education Act

The Carl D. Perkins Vocational and Technical Education Act (1984), which was first authorized in 1984 and has had subsequent reauthorizations, pro-vides funding for secondary and postsecondary vocational education. This legislation authorizes the funding of state Tech Prep programs for secondary schools and programs at the postsecondary level. The Perkins Act stipulates that special populations, including high school and college students with disabilities, are to be served through these programs. The purpose of the Perkins Act is to support academic and technical education enabling students to obtain good paying jobs leading to an occupational certificate or college degree. Funds are used for furnishing equipment in classrooms, supporting infrastructure costs for teachers' salaries, creating apprenticeships for students, developing curricula, and supporting career guidance and counseling for students. For more information on the programs available in local high schools and colleges, contact the high school special education counselors or the campus Disabled Student Services, if available.

High School/High Tech Program

The High School/High Tech program is an initiative of the Office of Disability Employment Policy within the U.S. Department of Labor. This program is designed to encourage students with disabilities to explore career opportunities in science, technology, and mathematical science. This enrichment program provides students with career awareness and preparation activities. These activities include summer jobs in hi-tech firms, visits to science laboratories and businesses, job shadowing with a scientist or technology specialist (e.g., aerospace scientist, meteorologist), and mentoring by professionals in science and technology fields. School-based activities are focused on academic advisement, career counseling, and computer and career preparation classes. More information on this program can be obtained by accessing the High School/High Tech web site at http://www.dol.gov/odep/pubs/hsht00/chapter1.htm.

Independent Living Centers

Independent Living Centers (ILCs) offer a variety of services and supports for youth and adults with disabilities with the purpose of enhancing their independence, productivity, and inclusion in the community. Although ILC services are primarily directed to serving the adult population, youth 16 years and older can contact their local ILC to inquire about the type of services available to transitioning youth. Services provided by ILCs include advocacy, housing assistance, attendant registry and referrals, peer counseling and mentoring, and referrals to community resources. Some ILCs may offer job training programs in specialized areas such as computer training. ILCs can offer assistance in searching for and obtaining jobs. ILCs are directed and staffed by individuals with disabilities.

EMPLOYMENT EXPERIENCES IN HIGHER EDUCATION

Accessing Disability/Health-Related Supports for Employment Training Programs

Many adolescents with special health care needs and disabilities are choosing to attend community colleges or universities after completing high school. Some, adolescents plan to graduate from high school prior to age 21 and then complete their education at a community college as assured through IDEA (2004). These students often complete coursework in life-skills and community living skills, such as cooking and using public transportation, as well as coursework focusing on acquiring job-related skills (Hart, Mele-McCarthy, Pasternack, Zimbrich, & Parker, 2004).

Adolescents with special health care needs and disabilities who continue on to higher education—whether it is at a university, community college, or vocational school—should have a 504 plan. As with K-12 schools, all higher education programs that receive federal funding have an office or program, often called the Office of Disability, which services individuals with special health care needs and disabilities and can be instrumental in helping develop the 504 plan.

Adolescents with special health care needs and disabilities who do not require special education services while in high school are still eligible for a 504 plan in college or the university that delineates their medical or physical condition as it relates to the services they will require while in that school, work, or community setting, if they choose to disclose their special health care need or disability.

The 504 plan may outline the type of accommodations that are required at a work site, whether for a course requirement or for a work-study job (see next section). For example, a student may require special assistance carrying materials to or at the job or carrying books to a classroom, or the student may need time away from work or class for medical treatments. It should be noted that it is sometimes difficult to transfer assistive technology devices from the school to work setting. Due to the difficulties that may arise in this transfer, plans for this transfer needs to be included in the 504 plan (United Cerebral Palsy, 2006). For additional information about accommodations, see Chapter 6.

Employment Services in Postsecondary Settings

Most higher education programs also have an office that deals with employment or work-based learning for its students. These offices often provide job shadowing, workplace tours, apprenticeships, service learning, workplace mentoring, informational interviews, on-the-job training, and internships for students who are matriculating in areas where job training and/or work experiences are part of the curriculum. Benefits of these planned experiences include identification of support needs, skills, career interests and goals, and an understanding of the connection between school and work (Luecking & Gramlich, 2003). These offices should also be able to conduct a vocational evaluation to assist adolescents with special health care needs and disabilities to identify their career interests and goals (Pacer Center, n.d.).

Campus job centers will vary in terms of the range of services available. Some campuses may have centers with vocational rehabilitation counselors to assist students who are enrolled in joint college-vocational rehabilitation career and job training programs. Other campus job centers may have a WIA one-stop employment center enabling students to access a variety of state and federally funded job training programs in this location. Community colleges will offer a number of vocational and trade programs providing students opportunities to learn skills in many fields, including manual arts, auto mechanics, fashion design, and licensed vocational nursing.

These schools also receive college work study funds from federal funding sources. Access to these programs is available to students with special health care needs and disabilities and should be used as an additional part of the necessary exposure to employment that has already been discussed. Whatever the route of acquiring work-related experiences, adolescents with special health care needs and disabilities, the personnel from the Office of Disability, and the employer should determine clear expectations of what is expected of the student at the work site; what roles the teacher, job coach, and/or work supervisor have in relation to assisting the adolescent; and the plan for feedback to the adolescent on his or her performance and the value and success of provided supports and accommodations. Appropriate education and training on assistive technology devices is needed for the other workers and supervisors interacting with the adolescent with special health care needs and disabilities, in addition to a feedback mechanism for them.

This and other services described below can be obtained through the benefits of various programs provided by federal and state agencies, such as Impairment Related Work Expense (IRWE), Plan for Achieving Self-Support (PASS), Student Earned Income Exclusion (SEIE), and new rules and regulations regarding Social Security Disability Insurance (SSDI). Counselors and other officers in higher education venues should be available to provide this linkage to students with special health care needs and disabilities (Gramlich, Crane, Peterson, & Stenhjem, 2003). However, it is important for these students to know that they exist and contact SSA for additional information if they cannot obtain this information through their postsecondary program.

EMPLOYMENT IN THE REAL WORLD

The following federal government agencies administer employment programs designed to assist individuals with special health care needs and disabilities: the Office of Special Education and Rehabilitation Services (OSERS), the Department of Labor (DOL), and the Social Security Administration (SSA). The first two agencies fund state offices that are also supported by state revenues; however, guidelines for administration are largely based on federal laws. The SSA remains a federal agency, primarily serving the elderly with benefits such as pensions and Medicare; however, a division of SSA does service individuals with disabilities through Social Security Disability Insurance (SSDI) for workers who have a disability and Social Security Income (SSI) for individuals younger than 18 years, those who have never worked and were born with or acquired a disability before the age of 18 years.

Social Security Administration

The SSA has gotten into the employment business in a very different way. For one, individuals with special health care needs and disabilities must be receiving SSDI or SSI to be eligible for services. Those receiving SSI benefits as described above are provided with financial incentives when they go to work.

SSI benefits are received monthly. When a recipient becomes employed it is very important to keep records of income, as income is deducted from SSI benefits. An incentive for working, SSI does not deduct the first $50 that is earned monthly, then only one-half of the remaining income earned during the month is deducted from the SSI check. This incentive usually means that financial eligibility for SSI continues and the medical benefits provided remain intact. In addition, when an individual goes to work there are needs that do require added income, such as transportation, food and clothing, and incidental work expenses. These and other expenses can be made for attendant care, job coaches, and architectural modifications that are needed for an individual's home and any vehicles can be deducted from the name reported to the SSI administrator.

Although these initial costs are often funded by the other mentioned agencies, SSI recognizes that they continue throughout employment and therefore provides the incentive by continuing eligibility for SSI payments. This work incentive program is referred to as the Impairment Related Work Expenses (IRWE) program.

Sections 1619(a) and 1619(b) offer other alternatives for individuals who want to work and still have the security of SSI benefits. Section 1619(a) enables the beneficiary to continue to receive SSI cash benefits and Medicaid although earning income above substantial gainful activity levels. Section 1619(b) enables a beneficiary to continue to receive Medicaid benefits even though the individual's work income exceed the limits for receiving SSI payments.

A major difficulty with this effort is that benefits are adjusted after the fact and the reduction in the SSI check is not made until after income is reported. It is therefore incumbent upon the recipient to save part of his or her check for the time when deductions are made.

The SSA can also fund a PASS for employment that will cover expenses for college tuition and other needs, such as the costs of an automobile and housing. These are plans written by specialists and can be accessed through contacting local offices of the SSA.

Individuals receiving SSDI must carefully assess returning to work since their benefit is based on total disability. Any effort to return to employment can be interpreted as evidence that they have fully recovered from the disability and are able to resume employment. For a summary of SSI work incentives programs, refer to Table 12.1.

Department of Vocational Rehabilitation

State offices of the Department of Vocational Rehabilitation (DVR) have services for adolescents with special health care needs and disabilities who are still in high school, as mentioned previously. They are mandated to provide employment services and programs to increase independence for individuals with cognitive, emotional, physical, and sensory disabilities. During postsecondary education, the DVR can further assist in setting up apprenticeship programs in collaboration with the DOL, job training, and career education as part of the student's financial aid (deFur, 2002). Hopefully adolescents with special health care needs and disabilities and their families are fully involved in the decision-making process.

DVR services are more likely to be available to individuals who are out of school. An adolescent with special health care needs and disabilities is required to document the condition that motivates the application for services. Medical reports, both past and current; reports from previous employers; and school records are necessary for this requirement. The DVR will then order a current medical report and other medical, educational, or social follow-up reports to determine the applicant's status and eligibility for services. Eligibility consists of having a documented disability and the consideration that with the receipt of DVR services the applicant will go to work. When all documents are compiled, a mutual decision is made between the counselor and the applicant regarding the steps necessary for employment.

The DVR can help in a variety of ways to secure a job for an applicant. For those who require assistance to learn various skills while working on a job, there is a program called "supported employment." A job coach is hired to work with the employee and then gradually fade services as the skills are learned. The DVR will pay for the services of the coach and thus make employment possible for those who otherwise would not be able to perform the requirements of a job.

Table 12.1.   Social Security Administration (SSA) work incentive programs

Program name	Description
Impairment Related Work Expense (IRWE)	The cost of impairment-related services, supplies, and equipment may be deducted from an individual's gross income. IRWE deductions can be taken if costs 1) enable the person to work, 2) are not reimbursed by another program, 3) correspond to the community standard, and 4) are incurred during a month when the individual worked. Examples of deductions include medical services, work-related equipment, transportation costs, attendant care services, and medical supplies.
Plan for Achieving Self-Support (PASS)	The PASS plan enables individuals with disabilities to set aside money to pay expenses for education, vocational training, or starting a business related to achieving their work goal. Income that is set aside in the PASS plan is not counted as income when the SSI payment is calculated. A PASS can help an individual establish or maintain SSI eligibility and can increase the SSI payment amount. A PASS does not affect the Substantial Gainful Activity (SGA) determination for the initial eligibility decision. The PASS plan needs to be 1) based on an individual's needs, 2) documented in writing, 3) have a specific work goal and timeline, 4) demonstrate what money and resources will be used and how they will be used to reach the goal, 5) approved by SSA, and 6) reviewed periodically. Anyone can assist with the development of the PASS plan, including vocational counselors, social workers, benefits specialists, or employers. More information on PASS plans can be obtained by calling 1-800-772-1213 (toll free). Copies of PASS plans can be obtained from the SSA web site or from any PASS expert.
Earned Income Exclusion	Earned Income Exclusion is used when calculating earned income when the SSI payment amount is determined. The calculation is based on the first $50 of monthly income plus one-half of the remaining earned income.
Student Earned Income Exclusion	Student Earned Income Exclusion is specifically designed for students who are younger than 22 years and attend school regularly. Up to $1,410 of early income per month or up to $5,670 per year is excluded when the SSI payments are calculated. Students must be 1) attending high school (grades 7–12) at least 12 hours per week (if home schooled, the home school must be in accordance with the law of the state or jurisdiction in which the beneficiary resides), 2) in a training course to prepare for employment for at least 12 hours a week (15 hours a week if the course involves shop practice), or 3) attending college or university for at least 8 hours a week. The time requirements indicated may be lowered for reasons beyond the student's control, such as illness.
1619 (a)	SSI cash payments can be continued even when earned income (gross wages and/or net earning from self-employment) is at the SGA level. This provision eliminates the need for the trial work period or extended period of eligibility under SSI. This provision does not apply to individuals with visual impairments, however, as the SGA requirement

(continued)

Table 12.1.   *(continued)*

	does include individuals with visual impairments. If the state provides Medicaid to individuals on SSI, the Medicaid benefit continues.
1619 (b)	Medicaid coverage can continue even if earnings alone or in combination with other income becomes too high for an SSI cash payment. Individuals must have gross earned income that is insufficient to replace SSI, Medicaid, and any publicly funded attendant care. The "threshold amount" is the measure that is used to decide whether earnings are high enough to replace SSI and Medicaid benefits. The threshold amount is based on the amount of earnings which would cause SSI cash payments to stop and the annual per capita Medicaid expenditure in the state. If gross earnings are higher than the threshold amount for the state, the individual may still be eligible if the individual has 1) impairment-related work expenses, 2) blind work expenses, 3) a PASS plan, 4) publicly funded attendant or personal care, or 5) medical expenses higher than the state per capita amount.

The SGA 2005 amount is $850 for individuals with disabilities and $1380 for individuals with visual impairments.

Adapted from Social Security Administration Red Book (2005).

The DVR is an agency that can assist individuals with special health care needs and disabilities throughout their working lives. It is always a goal that those who are launched into the world of employment when they complete education will be able to continue on their own. Rehabilitation services including counseling, designing and providing workplace accommodations, telesensory devices, sign language interpreters, guide trainers for individuals with visual impairments, training and college tuition, and purchase of work supplies and uniforms are available for those who need assistance in maintaining employment or entering new employment (see Chapter 6).

The Americans with Disabilities Act (ADA) of 1990 (PL 101-336) specifies that individuals can not be denied employment on the basis of disability and that reasonable accommodations must be made to enable an individual to obtain employment. Thus, the DVR should be equipped to provide such services. If an individual has a physical or sensory limitation, specialists within the department should be equipped to design a workplace modification. Some of these ideas are developed while individuals are still in school. For example, there are organizations dedicated to rehabilitation engineering and development of telesensory devices for individuals with hearing and visual impairments. These resources are used by the rehabilitation agencies to provide contacts and funding for individuals entering employment.

The DVR may also assist individuals with finding employment. It will often refer clients to services/agencies that provide job seeking and job keeping skills. These programs will also provide placement services. The Ticket to Work and Self Sufficiency Program, for example, is an employment program designed to provide eligible individuals more choices in selecting assistance with getting a job. The program is based on the concept that an individual can decide to use and apply a ticket provided by this program for services provided by the state Vocational Rehabilitation program or another employment provider that is part of the state's employment network. If the individual is not satisfied with the services provided, then he or she can find another provider (Social Security Administration, n.d.).

Other Federal Agencies and Information Sources

Federal agencies also provide funding to support national clearinghouses for information and referral to resources for adolescents and young adults with special health care needs and disabilities who desire employment. Examples include the National Center on Secondary Education and Transition, the Disability and Business Technical Assistance Centers, the Job Accommodation Network, the National Collaborative on Workforce and Disability, and the Healthy & Ready to Work National Center. Web pages for each of these and other centers are found in Appendix A at the end of the book. Of special note is the Office of Disability Employment Policy, which was formerly the President's Committee on Employment of People with Disabilities.

Special Employment-Related Services

Intermediaries

As would be expected, the myriad of agencies and personnel involved in assisting adolescents with special health care needs and disabilities to be successful in employment can be great. Intermediaries, or third-party brokers, can assist in coordinating this process. Intermediaries can assist adolescents with special health care needs and disabilities to identify realistic career goals, connect classroom learning to eventual work responsibilities, obtain needed accommodations, identify job opportunities, and serve as advocates for the adolescent. In turn, intermediaries can help employers to identify qualified potential employees, design work-based learning, provide and arrange for needed accommodations, provide feedback among all individuals involved in the work experience of the adolescent, and work to improve the workplace setting through the identification of trends and solutions. Intermediaries can also help educators through better planning for work-related skill and knowledge acquisition (Mooney & Crane, 2002).

Mentors

Mentors are a service support provided by many employment programs (e.g., School-to-Work Opportunities Act) and can take many forms. For example, a mentor can be a peer (same age) without disabilities or can be older in age and have similar special health care needs and disabilities. Mentoring sessions can take place in person in a group setting or on a one-to-one basis, or sessions can take place via letters and e-mail (Sword & Hill, 2002; U.S. Department of Labor, 2005). Mentoring also can be informal or formal. The focus of mentoring programs is usually to build relationships and provide a social and/or academic connection. Unfortunately, research on the success of mentoring programs has found that there has been a lack of focus for mentoring programs for adolescents with special health care needs and disabilities (Sword & Hill, 2002).

Mentoring provides many benefits for both the adolescent receiving services and the mentor. For the adolescent, benefits can include increased self-esteem, decreased risk for alcohol or drug use, and increased academic achievement. Mentor benefits include increased self-esteem and greater feelings of accomplishment (Sword & Hill, 2002).

Mentors must remember that adolescents with special health care needs and disabilities are individuals and, therefore, interesting activities and topics of conversation may be different for different people. Mentors may also receive privileged information and must be able to keep this confidential, unless in rare instances, it is necessary to disclose what is said during a session. Mentors need to be instructed on how to use any needed accommodations, including assistive technology devices. Therefore, mentors need initial and periodic training and education opportunities, as well as opportunities to discuss their experiences with program staff (Sword & Hill, 2002).

Workplace Issues

Concerns with Employers

Integrating adolescents and adults with special health care needs and disabilities into the workplace has occurred for a number of years; yet, even though employers have stated that they are willing to hire a person with special health care needs and disabilities, the actual hire rate is rather low. Much work is still needed to assist and support employers to hire individuals with special health care needs and disabilities. This can be accomplished through a) matching the strengths and skills of the adolescent or adult with special health care needs and disabilities to a workplace that may require job carving and/or a new job description, b) identifying a plan for the institution of accommodations for the benefit of both the employer and employee, c) developing training and education programs for both employers and employees to work more successfully with a person with special health care needs and disabilities, and d) identifying optional work hours or job sharing arrangements (Anderson, Boone, & Watson, 2003; Luecking & Mooney, 2002; Rogan, Banks, & Herbein, 2003; U.S. Department of Labor, 2006). These steps can assist in diminishing or eliminating negative attitudes of employers and fellow employees (Shaw, MacKinnon, McWilliam, & Sumsion, 2004).

Personal Assistance in the Workplace

Medicaid currently provides funding for personal assistants in the home. Several states are now planning to extend this funding to the workplace. This would be a very important step to assist more individuals with special health care needs and disabilities to obtain gainful employment (Hinton, 2003). This change would have great meaning for individuals with multiple and more severe special health care needs and disabilities, as research has shown that employment has assisted individuals with special health care needs and disabilities to increase their level of adaptive skills—this is a trend that is reversed when the person is not working (Stephens, Collins, & Dodder, 2005).

Cultural Concerns

Little has been written about employment success and individuals with special health care needs and disabilities from different cultures. It is important to ascertain what value the culture the individual belongs to has on employment, but remember that acculturation can affect traditional values. In the case of individuals with special health care needs and disabilities, employment may not be expected or encouraged by the family (Blue-Banning & Turnbull, 2002).

Stodden and colleagues (2003) discussed a number of barriers for individuals from minority cultures with special health care needs and disabilities, including a lack of cultural knowledge and sensitivity of others, and a lack of knowledge of social mores and language used by the majority culture. These authors noted that a triple jeopardy could exist for women with special health care needs and disabilities who are members of a minority culture. A great need for these individuals is education to acquire self-advocacy skills.

Condition-Specific Issues for the Workplace

Often, an individual with special health care needs and disabilities is identified as such, and the differences prescribed by the specific condition are not discussed. Recently, these specific characteristics have been discussed in the literature as they relate to employment. For example, Muller, Schuler, Burton, & Yates (2003) spoke about the employment support needs for individuals with autism spectrum conditions who have unique problems with habit formation and social skills. For these individuals, job coaches must have specific knowledge and skills in assisting the person with these conditions to work successfully. Scheid (2005) spoke about the misconceptions of employers and other employees about working with someone with a mental illness. Berry (2000) wrote about the severity of health problems and their relationship to successful employment. Finally, Martz (2003) wrote about the correlation between employment status and the invisibility of the special health care needs and disabilities; if the special health care needs and disabilities were invisible, then the person was most likely employed. This, of course, brings up the issue of whether or not to disclose a special health care need and disability when applying for work.

SUMMARY

Employment is a possibility for any individual who wants to work, regardless of disability, age, or gender. Many federal and state supported programs are available to assist adolescents and adults with special health care needs and disabilities. There are also a number of clearinghouses (see Appendix A) that provide information and resources concerning employment needs and supports. Professional assessments of aptitudes and other abilities are also available. Individuals who want to know what they can do and what additional training is necessary to achieve reachable employment objectives can readily access such services, but there is unevenness of services across and within states. Having a special health care need or disability should not be a deterrent to employment. We are in need of national models of "best practices" (Smits, 2004). A good support system, a positive attitude, and motivation provide initial steps to approach the world of employment. In the literature concerning the employment of adolescents and adults with special health care needs and disabilities, the role of health care professionals are rarely mentioned, if at all—in order to provide an individual with the highest quality of life, it is important that all systems of care for the individual are coordinated and fluid.

REFERENCES

Americans with Disabilities Act of 1990, PL 101-336, 42 U.S.C. §§ 12101 *et seq.*

Anderson, G.B., Boone, S.E., & Watson, D. (2003). Impact of federal legislation and policy on VR services for consumers who are deaf or hard of hearing: Perspectives of agency administrators and program specialists. *American Annals of the Deaf, 148,* 315–322.

Berry, H.G. (2000). The Supplemental Security Income program and employment for young adults with disabilities: An analysis of the National Health Interview Survey on Disability. *Focus on Autism and Other Developmental Disabilities, 15,* 176–181.

Blue-Banning, M., & Turnbull, A.P. (2002). Hispanic youth/young adults with disabilities: Parents' visions for the future. *Research & Practice for Persons with Severe Disabilities, 27*(3), 204–219.

Cameto, R., Levine, P., & Wagner, M. (2004). *Transition planning for students with disabilities: A special topic report of findings from the National Longitudinal Transition Study-2 (NLTS2).* Menlo Park, CA: SRI International. Retrieved January 30, 2006, from http://www.nlts2.org/pdfs/transitionplanningcomplete.pdf

Carl D. Perkins Vocational Education Act of 1984, PL 98-524

deFur, S.H. (2002). Transition planning: A team effort. *Transition summary, 10,* 1–24. Retrieved February 1, 2006, from http://www.nichcy.org

General Accounting Office. (2003). *Government auditing standards: 2003 revision.* Washington DC: Author.

Gramlich, M., Crane, K., Peterson, K., & Stenhjem, P. (2003). Work-based learning and future employment for youth: A guide for parents and guardians. *NCSET Information Brief, 2*(2), 1–6. Retrieved February 1, 2006, from http://www.ncset.org.

Hart, D., Mele-McCarthy, J., Pasternack, R.H., Zimbrich, K., & Parker, D.R. (2004). Community college: A pathway to success for youth with learning, cognitive, and intellectual disabilities in secondary settings. *Education and Training in Developmental Disabilities, 39,* 54–66.

Healthy People 2010. (2004). *Healthy people with disabilities.* Retrieved January 30, 2006, from http://www.cdc.gov/ncbddd/factsheets/DH_hp2010.pdf

Hinton, D.M. (2003). Personal assistance services on the job. *Info Brief, 6,* 1–2. Retrieved February 1, 2006, from http://www.ncwd-youth.info

Individuals with Disabilities Education Act Amendments of 1997, PL 105-17, 20 U.S.C. §§ 1400 *et seq.*

Individuals with Disabilities Education Improvement Act of 2004, PL 108-446, 20 U.S.C. §§ 1400 *et seq.*

Luecking, R.G., Crane, K., & Mooney, M. (2002). Addressing the transition needs of youth with disabilities through the WIA system. *NCSET Information Brief, 1*(6), 1–4. Retrieved February 1, 2006, from http://www.ncset.org

Luecking, R., & Gramlich, M. (2003). Quality work-based learning and postschool employment success. *NCSET Issue Brief, 2*(2), 1–6. Retrieved February 1, 2006, from http://www.ncset.org

Luecking, R.G., & Mooney, M. (2002). Tapping employment opportunities for youth with disabilities by engaging effectively with employers. *NCSET Research to Practice Brief, 1*(3), 1–6. Retrieved February 1, 2006, from http://www.ncset.org

Martz, E. (2003). Invisibility of disability and work experience as predictors of employment among community college students with disabilities. *Journal of Vocational Rehabilitation, 18,* 153–161.

Mooney, M., & Crane, K. (2002). Connecting employers, schools, and youth through intermediaries. *NCSET Issue Brief, 1*(3), 1–4. Retrieved February 1, 2006, from http://www.ncset.org.

Muller, E., Schuler, A., Burton, B.A., & Yates, G.B. (2003). Meeting the vocational support needs of individuals with Asperger syndrome and other autism spectrum disabilities. *Journal of Vocational Rehabilitation, 18,* 163–175.

National Collaborative on Workforce and Disability. (2003). Serving youth with disabilities under the Workforce Investment Act of 1998: The basics. *Info Brief.* Retrieved February 1, 2006, from http://www.ncwd-youth.info

Pacer Center. (n.d.). *Mapping your dreams: Making the transition team work.* Retrieved February 1, 2006, from http://www.pacer.org/tatra/MYD-Employment.pdf

Rogan, P., Banks, B., & Herbein, M.H. (2003). Supported employment and workplace supports: A qualitative study. *Journal of Vocational Rehabilitation, 19*, 5–18.

Scheid, T.L. (2005). Stigma as a barrier to employment: Mental disability and the Americans with Disabilities Act. *International Journal of Law and Psychiatry, 28*, 670–690.

School-to-Work Opportunities Act of 1994, PL 103-239, 20 U.S.C. §§ 6101 *et seq.*

School to Work Project, Institute on Community Integration, University of Minnesota. (1998). *School to Work is. . .* (Fact Sheet). Accessed February 7, 2006, from http://ici.umn.edu/schooltowork/factsheet.html

Shaw, L, MacKinnon, J., McWilliam, C., & Sumsion, T. (2004). Consumer participation in the employment rehabilitation process: Contextual factors and implications for practice. *Work, 23*, 181–192.

Smits, S.J. (2004). Disability and employment in the USA: The quest for best practices. *Disability & Society, 19*, 647–662.

Social Security Administration. (2005). *2005 Red Book: A summary guide to employment support for individuals with disabilities under the Social Security Disability Insurance and Supplemental Security Income programs.* Baltimore: Social Security Administration, Office of Disability and Income Security Programs.

Social Security Administration (n.d) *Ticket to work.* Retrieved February 10, 2006, from http://www.yourtickettowork.com/program_info

Stephens, D.L., Collins, M.D., & Dodder, R.A. (2005). A longitudinal study of employment and skill acquisition among individuals with developmental disabilities. *Research in Developmental Disabilities, 26*, 469–486.

Stoddard, S., Jans, L., Ripple, J., & Kraus, L. (1998). *Chartbook on work and disability in the United States, 1998. An InfoUse Report.* Washington, DC: U.S. National Institute on Disability and Rehabilitation Research. Retrieved January 30, 2006, from http://www.hsl.creighton.edu/CINAHL-PDF/99046045.pdf

Stodden, R.A., Stodden, N.J., Kim-Rupnow, W.S., Thai, N.D., & Galloway, L.M. (2003). Providing effective support services for culturally and linguistically diverse persons with disabilities: Challenges and recommendations. *Journal of Vocational Rehabilitation, 18*, 177–189.

Sword, C., & Hill, K. (2002). Creating mentor opportunities for youth with disabilities: School to Work programs issues and suggested strategies. *NCSET Issue Brief, 1*(4), 1–6. Retrieved February 1, 2006, from http://www.ncset.org.

Thornton, P., & Lunt, N. (1997). *Employment policies for disabled persons in eighteen countries: A review of the 'United States'.* A University of New York, Social Research Unit paper. Ottawa, Can.: Global Applied Disability Research and Information Network on Employment and Training (GLADNET) Research (NIDRR).

U.S. General Accounting Office (GAO). (2003). *Special education: Federal actions can assist states in improving postsecondary outcomes for students.* GAO-03-773. Retrieved January 30, 2006, from http://www.gao.gov/new.items/d03773.pdf

U.S. Department of Labor. (2005). *Cultivating leadership: Mentoring youth with disabilities.* Retrieved February 1, 2006, from http://www.dol.gov

U.S. Department of Labor. (2006). *Customized employment: Principles and indicators.* Retrieved February 1, 2006, from http://www.dol.gov/odep/pubs/custom/indicators.htm

United Cerebral Palsy. (2006). *Employment: Transferring assistive technology from school to work.* Retrieved February 1, 2006, from http://www.ucp.org

Wagner, M., Newman, L., Cameto, R., & Levine, P. (2005). *Changes over time in the early postschool outcomes of youth with disabilities: A report of findings from the National Longitudinal Transition Study and National Longitudinal Transition Study-2.* Menlo Park, CA: SRI International.

Workforce Investment Act of 1998, PL 105-220, 29 U.S.C. §§ 794 *et seq.*

CHAPTER 13

Forming Interagency Partnerships

ROBERTA ROSS AND JUDY REICHLE

Interagency partnerships refer to the formalized relationships created by service agencies for a common service purpose and serve as the linking mechanism for bringing together agencies that typically do not work together because they serve disparate age groups. An interagency partnership enables youth and adult-oriented agencies to work together with the youth and family to create an individualized transition plan based on the youth's goals for achieving competencies associated with becoming an adult and is the model recommended for comprehensive transition planning (Bang & Lamb, 1997). Interagency transition partners can include representatives from child and adult health care organizations, secondary and postsecondary educational settings, vocational rehabilitation, Workforce Investment Act (WIA) job development and placement agencies, Independent Living Centers, transportation organizations, social services, disability organizations, Social Security, Housing and Urban Development (HUD), youth and family advocacy organizations and community living agencies, and leisure and recreational organizations, among others.

The challenges youth with special health care needs and disabilities face transitioning to adulthood have been well documented as evidenced by the research conducted demonstrating limited success in postsecondary and employment settings and living in the community (Wagner et al., 1991; Wagner, Newman, Cameto, & Levine, 2005). In an effort to address these concerns, a number of strategies have been suggested to improve the outcomes for youth with special health care needs and disabilities—one of these strategies is interagency collaboration. Although, there is a limited amount of research that supports interagency partnerships for the purposes of service delivery or system change (Hasazi, Furney, & DeStefano, 1999), anecdotal accounts find interagency partnerships to be positive when effective. Most of the literature on interagency partnerships is predicated on anecdotal accounts of models developed at the local, regional, or state levels, or on the opinions of experts and policy makers (Johnson, Stodden, Emanuel, Luecking, & Mack, 2002).

This chapter begins by providing background information about the influences leading to the development and implementation of interagency partnerships as an innovative approach to address the growing needs for postsecondary services and supports of youth with special health care needs and disabilities. These needs include but are not limited to accessing adult health care services, learning job skills, participating in community activities, and developing leisure and recreational interests. A description of the interagency partnerships developed in the educational and health care systems will be provided. The interagency partnership models will be compared and contrasted to illustrate the challenges in facilitating linkages between them. A process for developing and implementing interagency partnerships to create a seamless system of service between disparate systems also will be provided, beginning with a needs assessment and concluding with identification of methods to evaluate the outcomes.

INTERAGENCY PARTNERSHIPS IN EDUCATION

Beginning with the deinstitutionalization movement in the 1960s, advocated by consumers and families and coupled with the longer lifespans of individuals with special health care needs and disabilities, new service approaches were required to address the new array of consumer needs. Consumers needed new and different services and supports to assist them in becoming as independent as possible as adults, unlike the services of the past that, according to advocates, covertly fostered dependency. For example, prior to the deinstitutionalization movement, the SSI program provided income support programs and health insurance coverage to individuals with disabilities predicated on the requirement of no or limited employment, thereby forcing individuals to forego employment opportunities for fear of losing health insurance coverage. The SSI program was retooled to adjust to the mounting needs of consumers to enjoy the benefits of employment and the security the rescue net of SSI benefits provides until paid employment to adequately sustain an independent lifestyle with health care benefits is achieved.

As a result, advocates worked with legislators, policy makers, and experts to create the legislation needed to effect systemic changes and service innovations. These legislative efforts produced laws and regulations in education, rehabilitation, employment, and disability services. Although federal and legislative efforts to provide children with disabilities a free and appropriate public education (FAPE) began in the 1960s, later legislation such as the Education for All Handicapped Children Act of 1975 (PL 94-142) and the Individuals with Disabilities Education Act (IDEA) of 1990 (PL 101-476) enlarged the scope of services provided.

Individuals with Disabilities Education Act

The Individuals with Disabilities Education Act Amendments of 1997 (IDEA 1997; PL 105-17) and subsequent amendments, including the most recent in 2004 (the Individuals with Disabilities Education Improvement Act of 2004 [IDEA 2004], PL 108-446), specified the implementation of a variety of services designed to direct educators to focus increased attention on transition planning beginning early during the high school years and to include interagency partners as members of the youth's individualized educational program (IEP) team (IDEA, 1997, 2004). IDEA 1997 and IDEA 2004 mandate educational agencies to develop interagency partnerships to create, plan, implement, and/or evaluate the programs needed to support transition-age students to develop the knowledge and skills necessary to enter the postsecondary world of lifelong learning, employment, community living, and citizenship.

This legislation also stipulates that large-scale programmatic evaluations be conducted to assess effectiveness at the state and local levels. A nationwide survey, known as the Study of State and Local Implementation and Impact of the Individuals with Disabilities Education Act (SLIIDEA), was developed to address this requirement. One of the areas assessed by SLIIDEA was transition planning for high school students with disabilities, including the extent to which interagency agreements and guidelines were implemented at the state and local levels, as interagency planning was a new transition requirement of IDEA 1997.

According to the *Final 2nd Interim Report (2002–2003 School Year)* (Schiller, Bobronnikov, O'Reilly, Price, & St. Pierre, 2005), 94% of states had written interagency agreements and 84.3% had written guidelines for implementing interagency agreements. At the school district level, 54.6% had written interagency agreements and 79.4% had written interagency guidelines. The report revealed significant differences at both the state and district levels in having written interagency agreements in contrast to implementing interagency partnerships. The levels of involvement reported reflect the differences that would be anticipated as some partners—such as vocational rehabilitation, developmental disability agencies, and juvenile justice programs—have mandates to coordinate services with education. Other partners, such as social service, mental health, and health care, have no such requirements. States reported that they were "very involved" with vocational rehabilitation (51%), public developmental disability agencies (36%), public juvenile justice programs (32%), public social services agencies (25%), and public mental health agencies (24%). At the school district level, being "very involved" with other agencies in the delivery of services was considerably less. The highest percentages of being "very involved" in interagency partnerships were Title 1 (37.3%), public vocational rehabilitation agencies (17.2%), vocational/technical schools (14.3%), and public mental health agencies (11.9%). No data were reported for health care agencies (Schiller et al., 2005).

Mandated and Non-Mandated Interagency Services

Unlike educational agencies, many noneducational agencies do not have a legislative mandate for interagency involvement. Other systems of service such as Vocational Rehabilitation and the Workforce Investment Act (WIA) network have program-specific mandates, for example, fiscal responsibilities to provide services that may be identified in the student's IEP, such as job training or the purchase of uniforms or equipment needed for employment, and whether the agency representative attends or does not attend IEP meetings. To date, no comparable mandates or fiscal responsibilities exist related to the provision of health care services.

Health care partners or members of the school staff who are health personnel (e.g., physician, school nurse) are rarely identified as interagency members of the student's IEP team, although they should be considered. Health care partners could also include the service coordinator or members of the youth's specialized health care team located in a medical center wherein the student receives services. Other health care partners can include a member of the primary health care team, personnel from the State Title V Children with Special Health Care Needs Program (the actual name of the state program varies), a representative from the public or private health insurance plan, and/or a medical equipment vendor (Kosciulek, 2004). The potential productive roles health care professionals could have as a member of the IEP interagency team, however, has yet to be realized (Johnson et al., 2002).

INTERAGENCY PARTNERSHIPS IN HEALTH CARE

Historically, the delivery of health care to youth with special health care needs and disabilities involved the pediatrician making all of the decisions about the youth's health. Health care was also primarily delivered in segregated, institutional pediatric settings where youth with special health care needs and disabilities often resided. Deinstitutionalization and advances in medicine and technology, which extended the survival rates of youth with special health care needs and disabilities, resulted in the need for new systems of health care delivery for the transition of youth to adult health care delivery systems existing in the community.

Today, health care delivery to youth with special health care needs and disabilities has largely been based on an interdisciplinary framework that recognizes that youth with special health care needs and disabilities have a myriad of biopsychosocial needs requiring the expertise of not only medical specialists but also a team of professionals who can address the physical, learning, and psychosocial needs of the youth and his or her family. The membership of interdisciplinary teams vary depending on the service needs of the youth, but interdisciplinary teams for youth with special health care needs and disabilities are typically composed of pediatric primary and specialty practitioners, advanced practice and registered nurses, social workers, psychologists, speech and language specialists, dieticians, physical and occupational therapists, dentists, and audiologists. Health care professionals working with youth with special health care needs and disabilities recognize that improved comprehensive services are needed to assist youth in making the transition to adulthood in the community, including the transfer of care from pediatric to adult health care providers. Health care transition planning also includes uninterrupted access to health insurance and instructing the youth in learning to become more self-reliant in managing his or her daily treatment regimen, making his or her own health care decisions, and obtaining workplace and/or classroom accommodations. One strategy to address these needs is to use an interagency framework of care, not unlike the interagency education models, in the provision of health care transition planning services.

Traditionally, transition service models for youth with special health care needs and disabilities have been largely confined to interdisciplinary teams composed of pediatric and adult physicians. Models of interdisciplinary teams for transition-aged youth have been described to include both pediatric and adult specialty practitioners in an effort to facilitate the transfer to adult health care providers (Hagood, Lenker, & Thrasher, 2005; Sawin et al., 1999). There have been few examples of interagency teams evident in health care settings unlike the interagency teams in educational settings (Betz & Redcay, 2002).

Child health and pediatric health care providers, including case managers, are typically unfamiliar and uninformed about the accessible transition and adult health and related services for youth with special health care needs and disabilities as well as the array of public and nonprofit social, educational, employment, community, disability, rehabilitation, housing, and transportation services. Therefore, knowing where to start is a major challenge. There are a number of obstacles that child health and pediatric providers have to overcome to develop interagency partnerships in their local communities. These obstacles include the lack of information about adult services previously mentioned, limited time allocated to form partnerships, competing demands of time within the acute and primary care health care settings to attend to the immediate services of clients seen, and the lack of reimbursement for health care transition planning by third party payers (Geenen, Powers, & Sells, 2003; McDonagh, Foster, Hall, & Chamberlain, 2000; Scal, 2002; Scal, Evans, Blozis, Okinow, & Blum, 1999).

As mentioned previously, interagency partnerships for the delivery of health care is not a model upon which services have been developed for youth with special health care needs and disabilities. In health care settings, the interdisciplinary team has been the service model used, a model similar in concept but different in scope. For pediatric and child health care professionals, the adult service world is an unknown, unlike the experience of educators working with transition-aged youth. The following section on national findings presents data on the outcome of efforts in education to improve the quality of services provided to youth with special health care needs and disabilities.

INTERAGENCY TEAMS: NATIONAL FINDINGS

Advocating for the implementation of interagency partnerships with noneducational agencies and actually implementing interagency partnerships according to the spirit of IDEA is comparable to the age-old adage of "saying and doing," as these are two entirely different processes. Data from the National Longitudinal Transition Study (NLTS) revealed that only 29% of interagency representatives invited to participate in a student's IEP did so. In revamping the proposed regulations for IDEA 2004, experts estimated a savings of $6.3 million by dropping the requirement to repeatedly contact interagency representatives absent at the student's transition meeting, illustrating the challenge of forging interagency partnerships (Assistance to States for the Education of Children with Disabilities, 2005; IDEA, 2004).

However, findings from NLTS2 in 2001 demonstrated improvements in the number and type of support services youth with disabilities received as compared to the NLTS survey completed in 1987. In 2001, parents reported that nearly 75% of students with disabilities received at least one of eight support services as compared with students with disabilities in 1987 (SRI International, 2003). One quarter of the transition-aged students in special education received vocational services and speech therapy, making these the most commonly received services (Levine, Marder, & Wagner, 2004). The services least likely to be used by students in this survey were health and health-related services. Less than 1% of students with disabilities accessed nursing services on school campuses; 11% received occupational services, and 4% received physical therapy services. Approximately 25% of students with disabilities received diagnostic or evaluation medical services (Levine, Marder, & Wagner, 2004). These findings highlight the underutilization of health care professionals in transition planning for students with disabilities.

An important question left unanswered were the amount of services general education students with special health care needs received during this important period of transition. Although data are not available as to level of health care services general education students with special health care needs require, the level of need will be dependent on the prevalence of special health care need conditions and the consequent health needs. Some students with special health care needs will require minimal to no assistance in addressing health care needs with transition planning, whereas other students' needs will involve significant planning.

Youth with special health care needs and disabilities have made impressive strides in achieving improved postsecondary outcomes. However as the NLST-2 data and the body of research on youth with special health care needs and disabilities indicate, this population continues to need support and services to ensure that greater numbers of individuals achieve postsecondary outcomes comparable to youth without disabilities. Conspicuous gaps in the array of interagency services accessed by transition-aged students are health and health-related services. The following chapter sections on creating interagency partnerships will address strategies for developing and implementing a seamless transition system of services with other partners including those from the health care system.

CREATING INTERAGENCY PARTNERSHIPS

This section describes the steps involved in creating interagency partnerships— including preplanning, conducting a community needs assessment, and implementation—which can be applied to other settings.

Preplanning

Preplanning is necessary to determine the selection of agencies and/or individuals to be involved in students' transition processes. The preplanning process described here is based on two interagency models: 1) the California School to Work Interagency Transition Partnership (CA SWITP), which was funded by the U.S. Department of Education and demonstrates both statewide and local interagency models for transition planning purposes in educational settings, and 2) an adaptation of the CA SWITP interagency model titled Creating Healthy Futures, which was a pilot project funded by the Maternal Child Health Bureau (Betz & Redcay, 2002). Preplanning steps include 1) determining the interagency partnership goals, 2) preplanning for recruiting interagency partners, and 3) forming the work group task force. Depending on the size of the agency and available funding, these steps can be modified to accommodate to agency needs and resources.

Determining the Interagency Partnership Goals

Determining the goals for developing and implementing an interagency partnership to create a seamless system of transition services for youth with special health care needs and disabilities is essential, as local communities have different needs and resources. Achieving a seamless service system results in a myriad of outcomes including, but not limited to, improved consumer satisfaction, reduction in the duplication of services, creation of integrated services, elimination of barriers that impede access to services including health care services, improved service coordination and referrals, interagency goals, cost reductions, and improved communication between agencies (U.S. General Accounting Office [GAO], 1996). The structure and function of the interagency team is dependent on the composition of the membership, designated roles and responsibilities of members, level at which the partnership operates (e.g., state, regional, local levels), and amount of authority for allocating fiscal resources. Interagency teams organized at the state or regional levels are primarily oriented to policymaking and systemic change issues. For example, the CA SWITP established a state-level interagency board composed of the directors of eight California state agencies and one federal agency; the California Departments of Education, Rehabilitation, Mental Health, and Developmental Services; the Employment Development Department; community colleges; Workforce Investment Act agencies; state universities; coalition of parents, families, and consumers; and the Social Security Administration (SSA) (CA SWITP, 1996; GAO, 1996). Four coalitions based upon this interagency model were created in local communities to form partnerships to improve the quality of transition services offered to special education students.

The Creating Healthy Futures (CHF) interagency team was based on the CA SWITP model with important differences: the CHF team was composed of nearly the same membership but with the addition of health care professionals, the CHF team was situated in a health care setting rather than in the typical educational or community setting, and CHF members provided consultation on issues pertaining to transition service coordination and referrals of youth who received health care transition planning. For example, the CHF team was asked to consult on issues pertaining to accessing health care insurance, locating adult primary and specialty care physicians, and finding a job (Betz & Redcay, 2002).

Interagency partnerships formed in local communities are focused more on the provision of direct services and/or the development of interagency programs to improve services provided to transition-aged youth. Local programmatic issues can intersect with system issues, such as agency fiscal responsibility for services and service barriers related to burdensome eligibility requirements, illustrating the complexity of attempting to facilitate change. For example, issues pertaining to what agency is responsible for paying for transportation to an after school program can be a contentious issue between the local school district and the disabilities program. Also, the purchase of an appropriately sized wheelchair becomes a timely issue as the youth is transitioning out of the Title V Program for Special Health Care Needs and the Department of Rehabilitation.

The programmatic issues that are embedded within the larger state system present significant challenges. Effecting systemic changes statewide are time consuming, convoluted, and complicated and not easily achieved, as in many circumstances, these changes can only be effected by federal or state legislation. Issues at the state level can include statute requirements for determining eligibility for services and departmental cost sharing for services and equipment.

California School to Work Interagency Transition Partnership

In 1991, the Office of Special Education and Rehabilitation Services (OSERS) initially provided funding to 20 states, including California, to effect systemic change within special education, based on the intent of IDEA for transition-aged students with disabilities. The California project, titled SWITP, was designed to improve transition partnerships at the state and local levels among interagency personnel, representatives and advocates from the community, youth, and families. At the state and in four local communities, partnerships were formed among the following state agencies:

- Department of Rehabilitation

- Department of Education, Division of Special Education

- Community colleges

- California State Universities

- Employment Development Department (now known as the California Labor and Workforce Development Agency)

- Developmental services

- Mental health

- State Job Training Coordinating Council (now known as Workforce Investment Agency [WIA])

Other partners included:

- Social Security Administration

- Consumer and family organizations

- Advocacy organizations

At the conclusion of this project in 1996, the state level partners signed a Memorandum of Understanding (MOU) to sustain the partnership and advance the goals of the project. (Refer to section on Creating Interagency Agreements.)

Preplanning for Recruiting Interagency Partners

Preplanning is needed prior to engaging in formal recruitment of interagency partners for the purpose of developing and implementing a seamless transition system of services. This involves conducting a review of the literature and program materials to develop an informed understanding of the issues, examples of models previously developed, and available evidence. Perusal of the literature on interagency partnerships will be found primarily in the education, disability, and rehabilitation fields. There is very little written on interagency partnerships in the health care literature, and most of the content is on topics pertaining to early intervention services for infants and toddlers at risk for and with disabilities (Harbin, 1996; Reiss, Cameon, Matthews, & Shenkman, 1996). For those with time and resource constraints, contacting other professionals who have developed interagency partnerships to discuss their experiences can provide an expedient route to obtaining information.

Reviewing information detailing the experiences of other colleagues in forming interagency partnerships is helpful in terms of understanding the issues and process. More relevant materials pertaining to interagency partnerships with health care partners will be found via Internet searches and on transition web sites. Manuals describing the "how to's" of implementing a community needs assessment, recruiting tips for convening workforce task members, and developing interagency agreements or memorandum can be obtained by using the search terms *interagency partnerships, interagency collaboration,* and so forth, on the web. There are a number of web sites and electronic databases that can be accessed for obtaining scholarly articles and program information on interagency partnerships.

Convening a work group of colleagues who share the vision and values of interagency partnering and a seamless transition system of services is needed to provide input on the development of a workplan for conducting a community needs assessment. Some experts have also referred to the community needs assessment as *community resource mapping, asset mapping,* or *environmental scanning*

(Crane & Mooney, 2005; Crane & Skinner, 2003; Tindle, Leconte, Buchanan, & Taymans, 2005). This small workgroup of colleagues can also provide input on programmatic strategies, offer nomination recommendations for interagency representatives, and contribute transition-related and community resources, including health and health-related resources that may not be well known to educators and other nonhealth interagency partners.

Ultimately, the purpose of this workgroup task force is to provide direction and support for conducting the community needs assessment and developing and implementing interagency partnerships for transition planning that will ultimately be based on formalized interagency agreements. For example, the CHF workgroup consisted of a rehabilitation specialist who was the executive director of the Southern California Transition Coalition (SCTC), one of the local CA SWITP transition coalitions and a health care professional with experience in working with youth with special health care needs and disabilities in hospital and community settings (Betz & Redcay, 2002). Given the rich experience of the SCTC executive director, the workgroup was limited to these individuals. The SCTC executive director served as the champion for the CHF program and was extremely helpful in providing recommendations for recruiting interagency partners.

Recruiting colleagues for the task force known to have expertise with community partnerships is a priority. Colleagues who are familiar with community resources that intersect with agencies providing transition-related or adult services can quickly provide a "roadmap" for navigating unfamiliar territory. Finding health care professionals who are involved in health care transition planning for youth with special health care needs and disabilities may be a challenge, as they typically have not "been at the table" as members of IEP teams. School nurses and related services personnel may be helpful in providing suggestions as they often develop relationships with members of the youth's specialized interdisciplinary team to coordinate service needs.

It is important to incorporate into the recruitment process interagency partners who represent geographic, cultural, age span, disability, and interdisciplinary diversity. Members of the workgroup task force are expected to contribute and be actively involved in supporting the efforts of the leader or chairperson. Active involvement includes attending meetings convened in person or electronically, responding appropriately to requests for input, or answering questions and reviewing document drafts. If a task force member is found to be remiss or unable to fulfill commitments, then a frank conversation about the participation problems is needed.

In many instances, these community experts can provide the names, contact information, and organizational synopsis needed to get started. Keeping a record of phone conversations in terms of the individual contacted, date of contact, and a summary of the conversation is essential to maintaining an organized and productive approach to achieving program goals and objectives for developing and implementing interagency partnerships and the vision of the seamless transition service system.

During this initial stage of introduction, it is easy to feel overwhelmed by the amount of new information being collected, new contacts being made, and exposure to the unfamiliar cultures of health care organizations and other community-based programs. Additionally, during this preplanning stage, documents will begin to be developed that include contact lists, descriptions of membership roles and expectations, descriptions of community resources and agency visits, meeting agendas, and minutes to name a few. It is also during this time, that a spirit of collegiality and sense of common purpose begins to develop among the fledgling group members.

Forming the Workgroup Task Force

This initial stage of preplanning serves as the foundation for all subsequent interagency activities. The level of effort, time expended, and critical and reflexive thinking devoted to this early phase of development cannot be underestimated. Building bridges with new partners takes time, patience, and receptivity to new information and ideas. At the beginning, the meetings with community representatives, especially those from health care settings, may feel awkward, stilted, and perhaps even feel as though something is amiss, as the professional context may be entirely unfamiliar. However, a useful educational resource to consult with as questions arise and issues surface is the school nurse or physician or other related services personnel. These individuals may be able to provide contextual information about a question or issue related to health care, ranging from terminology used or the health care provider's interpersonal style encountered during the needs assessment process to enhance insight and understanding.

Conducting the Community Needs Assessment

The process for conducting a community needs assessment will vary depending on the personnel and fiscal resources available. The needs assessment may involve a fairly manageable focus group of 10 to 15 interagency professionals and key stakeholders such as youth, family members, and advocates who provide the input. With additional extramural funding, a more extensive needs assessment may be conducted that includes focus group meetings with several groups of community members, interviews with key informants, and information from community public records.

There are a number of methods that can be used to conduct a needs assessment. Data can be collected using the interview method. One can apply this method to a number of different approaches, such as interviewing people individually or together as in the focus group approach.

Predetermined criteria should be considered when selecting people to be interviewed individually. Interviews may be conducted with key informants who are considered to be highly knowledgeable about the subject matter. For example, the medical director of the State Title V Program for Children with Special Health Care Needs may be an ideal choice to interview about transition planning, as this expert would have an expansive understanding of the agency, its regulations and service mandates, and the composition of its workforce. It is important to include individuals who are from diverse geographic areas within the community and are diverse in terms of their cultural beliefs, age range, disability and discipline.

A focus group interview format and the process for recording, transcribing, and analyzing the interviews will need to be developed if interviewing several people together. Professionals who have the experience and expertise to conduct focus groups, analyze the data, and produce a report of findings will be needed. In addition, it will be necessary to ensure that the needs assessment is in compliance with the Institutional Review Board (IRB) and the Health Insurance Porta-bility and Accountability Act (HIPAA) of 1996. Any questions or issues should be directed to the IRB director who is the resource expert for providing guidance and direction regarding compliance issues.

The SCTC used a focus group format to collect data from the targeted com-munity about the local resources and needs before initiating its coalition of part-ners (Betz & Ross, 1997). This same methodology was used to gather data on the health-related transition planning needs of students and their families and on in-teragency training and resource needs pertaining to health care transition plan-ning. The data from both of these projects provided the basis for subsequent pro-gram planning and development. The data enabled project staff to develop services and informational resources and to provide training specific to identified needs. For example, community members who participated in the SCTC needs assessment indicated that they wanted more information about transition-related and adult community agencies in order to make appropriate referrals for youth.

Other helpful strategies in collecting needs assessment data are to gather materials from municipal, county, and state governmental entities and advocacy groups. In today's environment, access to legislation, population statistics, and topical reports is easily accomplished. Substantial information can be obtained electronically to buttress the analysis of needs for program planning purposes. Actually using more than one method to share resource information is prefer-able as it increases the validity and the reliability of information collected (Burns & Grove, 2005).

The outcomes of the needs assessment process should result in the following:

- Assessment of service needs of the targeted group of youth with special health care needs and disabilities and their families, including cultural con-siderations.

- Determination of the community resources available to address the needs of youth with special health care needs and disabilities and their families.

- Support and commitment from interagency representatives and key stake-holders to participate.

Determining Community Resources

One of the outcomes of the needs assessment is the identification of available community resources. Identification of community resources can be thought of as a bifurcated process, as information will be gathered for later use in providing services and technical assistance as well as for recruitment of interagency repre-sentatives to participate as transition partners. Decisions as to the selection of in-teragency partners for transition planning will be predicated on the partnership goals, extent of participation availability, and characteristics of agency represen-tatives, such as level of commitment, interpersonal style, and professional exper-tise. It is also important to recruit interagency representatives who have a level of organizational authority to effect changes whether at the local, regional, or state levels, which will be discussed in more detail in the section on implementation.

Potential interagency members include youth, family members, representa-tives from community-based transition and adult agencies, business executives, and government representatives. Of particular importance is the recruitment of health care professionals from settings wherein youth with special health care needs and disabilities are served, such as tertiary health organizations (hospitals) where specialized interdisciplinary services are provided, the Title V Program for Children with Special Health Care Needs, or academic scholars with knowledge of health care transition planning for youth with special health care needs and disabilities from the nearby medical or nursing schools, or if in the vicinity, the University Center for Excellence in Developmental Disabilities (UCEDD). The 61 UCEDDs located in university settings provide training, research, and technical assistance in the field of developmental disabilities. As mentioned previously, the criteria to ensuring diversity will be important in this process as well. These outcomes will be the outgrowth of a comprehensive and deliberate needs assessment process that was enhanced with the involvement of community task force members.

Pragmatically, information gathered on available community resources is only useful if it is relevant for consumer needs and it can be retrieved easily in response to consumers' queries. Ideally, organizational information can be gathered and organized for easy retrieval. Relevant agency profiles should contain the following information:

- Type of services provided, such as diagnostic assessments/evaluations, treatment services, and therapy services, in thematic areas related to health care transition planning, postsecondary education, community living, and so forth

- Location(s) of where services are provided

- Profile of service providers to include discipline and professional licenses

- Eligibility criteria for obtaining services

- Appeal process for denial of eligibility and services

- Costs of services

- Enrollment process involving in-person appointments or fax/telephone/ e-mail applications

- Contact information including phone and fax numbers and web site and e-mail addresses

Analyzing the Results

Depending on the type of data collected, whether it is qualitative information gathered by interviewing key informants or focus groups or quantitative data extracted from public records, the findings need to relate to the original purpose of the needs assessment. Producing findings that do not address the purpose originally intended with conducting the needs assessment is counterproductive. Obtaining assistance from an expert in qualitative analysis and/or a statistician for quantitative analysis can help the needs assessment team with generating the findings and with the interpretation of findings for application to practice. Producing a report of the needs assessment findings will be helpful in disseminating results to interagency colleagues, key stakeholders, and members of the target community. Dispersing results to a broad constituency will assist in generating support and resources for the goal of implementing a seamless transition system of services.

Acting on the Results

There could be a temptation by the interagency partners to review and discuss the needs assessment findings, develop both strategic and operational plans, and then fail to follow through on the recommendations of the plans. Both plans, if used as they were designed to be used, provide the template for implementing interagency partnerships. This template can facilitate the development process of creating a seamless system of comprehensive transition services for youth with special health care needs and disabilities and their families to improve the quality of their lives as demonstrated by improved postsecondary outcomes. Alignment with the project plans will require not only strong leadership of one or a few, but also the strong commitment from all interagency partners. Assessing the progress of the partners toward meeting the goals and objectives of the strategic and operational plans is warranted on a periodic basis. Programmatic adjustments may be necessary to continue forward movement with the plans.

Conducting a community needs assessment is an involved but worthwhile process. Interagency partners can use the findings of the needs assessment to develop a strategic vision and operational plan that has credible substance and is responsive to the unique local needs of the community. A plan developed by interagency partners to address the existing obstacles and create new and possibly innovative strategies has the potential to succeed when other past attempts have been unsuccessful. The potential for success is greater under these circumstances, as the range and scope of barriers and issues have been finally "flushed out" to implement a plan for change.

Implementing Interagency Partnerships

As opportunities increase in transition for youth with special health care needs and disabilities, so does the necessity for implementing interagency partnerships. The complexity of navigating various agency systems can be daunting for those who are providing service to consumers. Participation in a partnership will not only help them to be more efficient in their own provision of service, but allow them to learn about what other services are available.

Creating the Environment for Interagency Partnerships

What actions are necessary to engage interagency partners to work collaboratively together? What is needed to realize the goal of a seamless transition system of services? There are a number of strategies that can be used to both initiate and sustain the commitment of partners. However, sustaining the participation commitment of interagency partners does not guarantee that the goal of a seamless transition system of services will be achieved. Creating a collegial environment is pivotal wherein interagency partners are respected and appreciated. Respect for other colleagues involves not only the customary formalities associated with professional interactions but also the recognition of the value of their contributions as partners. Engagement and commitment of interagency partners will be facilitated if their time is well spent and their effort is fruitful, as they will encounter their own organizational constraints in terms of work responsibilities, fiscal accountability, and the agency's mission.

What can be done to ensure that interagency partners' time and efforts are productive? Sensitivity to colleagues' time will be demonstrated by carefully constructing meeting agendas for maximizing productivity. Conducting meetings that integrate the latest technological advances will be helpful as well. A balance of flexibility and structure will be needed to assure interagency partners that rigidity is not paramount nor is a feckless approach.

Recruitment and Confirmation of Members

Interagency members that were previously identified as candidates will be re-contacted to confirm their participation in the interagency partnership. During the reconfirmation contact/visit, the mission and goals of the interagency partnership are reviewed, contact information is verified, available meeting dates are identi-fied, length of term served is settled, and information is provided about methods used to maintain communication amongst group members (e.g., use of a Listserv, mailings, telephone). It is important that accurate information is given about the amount of time that will be required for participation. Information on members who have been reconfirmed can be shared with others as it becomes available.

In both the SCTC and CHF experiences, over the course of their interagency partnerships, the turnover of representatives was fairly constant. Interagency repre-sentatives resigned due to position and job changes and alterations of work respon-sibilities with new supervisors, to name a few explanations for the constant changes in membership. These changes required an orientation for each new representative involving the aforementioned information. Oftentimes, representatives with longer periods of membership informally served as mentors to newer members.

One of the leaders of the interagency partnership from the host agency, with assistance from advocates from youth organizations or youth leaders, can set up additional time to orient youth members, as it may be their first leadership expe-rience of this type. During the initial orientation meeting, the following topics can be covered: 1) an overview of the interagency partnership, 2) information on the roles/responsibilities of interagency members, 3) background information on the members themselves, and 4) methods that the youth might find helpful for en-hancing communication skills to assure full interaction during meetings. It is likely and appropriate that ongoing technical assistance be provided to youth including debriefing as needed following meetings to support their development as youth leaders and partnership members. The inclusion of youth leaders is essential in in-teragency partnerships, as their input is needed to assure that youth perspectives are heard and integrated into the activities of the partnership. Yet, inclusion of youth leaders, particularly those who are still in high school, can be a challenge, as their school schedule may prevent them from participating in partnership meet-ings during their school day. After school or weekend meetings may be other op-tions; however, this meeting time may be inconvenient for interagency partners. Other arrangements such as scheduling separate meetings for both interagency and youth groups may be a realistic option.

Creating Interagency Agreements

Findings suggest that interagency agreements are essential to promoting intera-gency partnerships at the local level for transition-aged youth. A positive associa-tion was found between school districts with interagency agreements and positive transition experiences (Haszai et al., 1999). As the findings from the 2002–2003 SLIIDEA survey indicate, most states, and to a lesser degree school districts, have interagency agreements; however, the level of involvement in providing services is substantially less (Schiller et al., 2005). Content of effective interagency agreements were identified as having statements of common purpose, recommendations for facilitating group cohesiveness, the recognition of the need for cross-training, coordination as an integral component of services, and the development of a transition and adult resource database (Betz & Redcay, 2002; CA SWITP, 1996; Crane, Gramlich, & Peterson, 2004; Johnson et al., 2002).

The CA SWITP developed a memorandum of understanding (MOU) with eight goals. The MOU contained both values and goals related to transition planning and are listed below:

- Focus on who the system is for—individuals in transition.

- Include the individual and family as partners.

- Eliminate barriers to interagency transition planning.

- Reduce duplication by improving collaboration.

- Provide incentives for participation on local teams.

- Utilize a common transition planning process and document.

- Provide interagency cross training.

- Become a resource for the California Workforce Preparation System (CA SWITP, 1996).

The MOU effected between the eight state partners and SSA stated the following:

> We agreed in 1991 to work together to improve existing transition services for youth with disabilities and the results of those services. This agreement was formalized with the awarding of a federal grant, California School to Work Interagency Transition Partnership. Four local interagency teams were supported with grant funds to develop, recommend, and facilitate interagency systems for providing transition services for youth with disabilities. Through this agreement, we support their recommendations . . . and seek statewide implementation of this collaborative system for individuals with disabilities. (CA SWITP, 1996)

For additional information on constructing interagency agreements, see various resources listed at the end of this book.

Strategies for Implementation

Any implementation of a partnership involves some communications between the partners. Preferably a face-to-face meeting should occur, although conference calling, electronic options such as e-mail, and other communications have also been effective. Whatever the option, it is necessary to have some common objectives and references for communication.

Electronic Options

Virtual meetings have become more prevalent as they enable a level of flexibility not possible with traditional meetings or audioconferencing. If interagency partners have video conferencing equipment and ISDN lines to support distance technology for distance conferencing, this meeting format could be a viable option. If hosting virtual meetings are not technically or economically feasible, then other locations could be found to enable access to videocasting. Webcasting is another option for convening meetings among interagency partners enabling them to participate from their office computers, provided they have the technologic capacity.

In conceptualizing the possibilities of electronic usage, a number of programmatic enhancements are available. If interagency partnership meetings were convened via videocasting or webcasting, agenda items could be posted two to three weeks prior to meetings on a closed web page of the host agency enabling members to post additional items for the agenda. The finalized meeting agenda together with supplemental materials such as transition informational resources, governmental reports, project materials developed by staff, and articles could be sent to interagency members prior to meetings. Meeting follow up and requests for information from members could be more easily accomplished using electronic communication. Another possibility includes the use of a closed distribution Listserv for members to facilitate ongoing communication amongst themselves, share information concerning the partnership, monitor progress in meeting goals, and provide news updates.

However, face-to-face meetings are preferable in terms of hosting meetings, as this format encourages interpersonal interactions that cannot be entirely captured using the electronic format. Electronic communication can be used as a supplemental tool to facilitate communication among members as has been previously described.

Promoting Equal Partnerships

A number of recommendations have been offered to promote "equal partnership" amongst interagency members. The CA SWITP recommendations were based on the collective experience of interagency transition teams designed to provide individualized services to students with disabilities (CA SWITP, 1996). The list of recommendations to encourage equal partnership is presented below.

- Hold equality as a team value.

- Avoid the use of acronyms, jargon, bill numbers, and so forth.

- Use meeting processes that promote equality.

- Use consensus as the decision-making model.

- If not enough people can attend a meeting, cancel it.

- Rotate meeting places among agencies.

- Set meeting agreements by consensus.

- Define everything in group functioning.

- Ask each individual for his or her opinion.

- Use name tags.

- Develop team stationary.

- Use alphabetical order when listing agencies or members.

- Allow equal access to the budget process (assuming your team has a budget).

- Give people access to the decision-making process early.

- Give each member equal access to training opportunities and other special resources (CA SWITP, 1996).

Coupled with the concept of "equal partnerships" is the recognition that agencies are different from one another. Agencies differ in terms of their mission, purpose, and structure. The type of agency—whether it is a governmental, nonprofit, or for profit agency or an educational institution—is another factor to consider. Recognition and appreciation of differences is another means of promoting the concept of "equal partnership," as no one agency is designated or treated as being superior to the others (Stodden, Brown, Galloway, Mrazek, & Noy, 2005).

Conducting Productive, Inclusive Meetings

A key to creating and maintaining viable interagency partnerships is to ensure that meetings are perceived as having value by the membership. If representatives believe that meetings are a "waste of time," their attendance will drop off. Although it is beyond the scope of this chapter to discuss strategies for conducting effective meetings, there are a number of suggestions that can be briefly reviewed. Perhaps the most difficult decision interagency partners will make is when to meet if having in-person meetings. Determining a consistent time and day of the month will facilitate members' participation as the likelihood that the meeting will become a routinized activity is increased. Meeting times can be included on the meeting agendas sent to interagency partners as a monthly reminder. Announcements sent one and two weeks ahead of monthly meetings is yet another prompt for members.

It is helpful to send agendas and accompanying materials ahead of time with a sufficient amount of time for members to review. As mentioned in the section on electronic options, two to three weeks is suitable. Agendas may need to include time frames to ensure that all items are covered during the meeting. It will be the leader's responsibility to ensure that the meeting adheres to the time allotted to each item on the agenda. When starting the meeting, a brief review of the agenda to determine any last minute revisions is a method of keeping the agenda relevant and timely.

The responsibility for chairing meetings can be rotated based on the value of "equal partnerships." Some members may be more vocal than others and may have a tendency to dominate the meetings, requiring the group leader to involve the participation of other members. A portion of the meeting time can be allotted for interagency updates such as scheduled events, personnel changes, program resources, and new service mandates. When the time allotted for agenda items allows it, an interagency partner can provide an overview of the agency or a more detailed explanation about a particular agency program.

Conflict resolution strategies can be used when tense situations arise during meetings reflecting conflicting views of interagency members. A leader with the skill to extract input from all members is needed when disagreements arise, particularly in circumstances when there is conflict regarding fiscal responsibility.

The physical environment has been identified as an important meeting feature. Rooms with adequate ventilation, good lighting, comfortable seating and meeting supplies/equipment will be conducive to hosting meetings (Saskatchewan Industry and Resources, Business and Co-operative Services, 2003).

It is important that meetings end with an assessment of "how we are doing." That is, an ongoing assessment of progress is a method of providing members feedback about the performance of the group. A sense of shared purpose and achievement will generate a collective spirit of enthusiasm and ownership about the interagency partnerships. Additionally, a list of tasks assigned to be completed prior to the next meeting can be reviewed. This summary of tasks to be performed is an effective strategy of concluding the meeting (Hawkins, 2005; Ohio State University, 2003).

Containing Costs

In today's environment, operating on a tight budget is not unusual. Certainly the question of how to contain costs is an operational and strategic concern. There are a number of ideas that can be considered such as sharing the costs for mailings between each of the interagency partners. As mentioned previously, a paperless approach would not only solve the problem with mailing costs but also the indirect or in-kind costs of personnel time, as hardcopy mailings are more time consuming than electronic mailings over an extended period. Meeting sites could be rotated between agencies. Rotation of meeting sites also has the advantage of exposing colleagues to another agency environment and culture, thereby enlarging their understanding of that agency.

SUMMARY

There are various service system approaches between education and health care in forming interagency partnerships. Educators are mandated to create interagency partnerships for IEP transition planning to ensure that youth in special education achieve their goals as they reach adulthood and leave the school system. Developing and implementing interagency partnerships are more of a challenge for health care professionals as they have less experience in working with community-based transition and adult agencies as their focus has been oriented almost exclusively on pediatric and child health issues. For educators, developing interagency partnerships with community health care professionals is an atypical experience as well. However, interagency partnerships developed in educational and health care settings can facilitate the transition of youth with special health care needs and disabilities.

REFERENCES

Assistance to States for the Education of Children with Disabilities, 70 Fed. Reg. 35, 670 (June 21, 2005) (to be codified at 34 C.F.R. pts. 300, 301, and 304)

Bang, M.Y., & Lamb, P. (1997). *Impacts of an inclusive school-to-work program.* Paper presented at the 75th Annual Convention of the Council for Exceptional Children. Salt Lake City, Utah.

Betz, C.L., & Redcay, G. (2002). Creating Healthy Futures: An innovative nurse managed clinic for adolescents and young adults with special health care needs. *Pediatric Nursing, 29*(1), 25–30.

Betz, C.L., & Ross, R. (1997). Creating healthy futures for adolescents with special health care needs and disabilities: A monograph for consumers, families, professionals and service providers. Los Angeles: California Healthy and Ready to Work Project (Project MCJ-06HRW9B).

Burns, N., & Grove, S.K. (2005). *The practice of nursing research: Conduct, critique, & utilization* (5th ed.). St. Louis: Saunders.

California School to Work Interagency Transition Partnership (CA SWITP). (1996). *Breaking through: Best practices for building interagency teams.* Sacramento, CA: CA SWITP.

Crane, K., Gramlich, M., & Peterson, K. (2004). Putting interagency agreements into action. *NCSET Information Brief, 3*(1). Retrieved December 9, 2005, from http://www. ncset.org/publications/viewdesc.asp?id=1689

Crane, K., & Mooney, M. (2005). Essential tools: Community resource mapping. Retrieved August 29, 2006, from http://www.ncset.org/publications/essential tools/mapping/default.asp

Crane, K., & Skinner, C. (2003) Community resource mapping: A strategy for promoting successful transition for youth with disabilities. *NCSET Information Brief, 2*(1). Retrieved December 9, 2005, from http://www.ncset.org/publications/viewdesc.asp?id=939

Education for All Handicapped Children Act of 1975, PL 94-142, 20 U.S.C. §§ 1400 *et seq.*

Geenen, S.J., Powers, L.E., & Sells, W. (2003). Understanding the role of health care providers during the transition of adolescents with disabilities and special health care needs. *Journal of Adolescent Health, 32*(3), 225–233.

Hagood, J.S., Lenker, C.V., & Thrasher, S. (2005). A course on the transition to adult care of patients with childhood-onset chronic conditions. *Academic Medicine, 80*(4), 352–355.

Harbin, G.L. (1996). The challenge of coordination. *Infant and Young Children, 8,* 68–76.

Hasazi, S.B., Furney, K.S., & DeStefano, L. (1999). Implementing the IDEA transition mandates. *Exceptional Children, 65*(4), 555–566.

Hawkins, C. (2005). *Conducting effective meetings: The four "F" words.* Retrieved January 9, 2006, from http://www.sideroad.com/Meetings/conducting-effective-meetings.html

Individuals with Disabilities Education Act (IDEA) of 1990, PL 101-476, 20 U.S.C. §§ 1400 *et seq.*

Individuals with Disabilities Education Act Amendments of 1997, PL 105-17, 20 U.S.C. §§ 1400 *et seq.*

Individuals with Disabilities Education Improvement Act of 2004, PL 108-446, 20 U.S.C. §§ 1400 *et seq.*

Johnson. D.M., Stodden, R.A., Emanuel, E.J., Luecking, R., & Mack, M. (2002). Current challenges facing secondary education and transition services: What research tells us. *Exceptional Children, 60,* 519–531.

Levine, P., Marder, C., & Wagner, M. (2004). *Services and supports for secondary school students wtih disabilities. A report from the National Longitudinal Transition Study-2 (NLTS2).* Menlo Park, CA: SRI International. Retrieved December 10, 2005, from http://www.nlts2.org/pdfs/servicesupport_execsum_standalone.pdf

McDonagh, J.E., Foster, H.E., Hall, M.A., & Chamberlain, M.A. (2000). Audit of rheumatology services for adolescents and young adults in the UK. British Paediatric Rheumatology Group. *Rheumatology, 39*(6), 596–602.

Reiss, J., Cameon, R., Matthews, D., & Shenkman, E. (1996). Enhancing the role public health nurses play in serving children with special health needs: An interactive videoconference on Public Law 99-457 Part H. *Public Health Nursing, 13*(5), 345–352.

Saskatchewan Industry and Resources, Business and Co-operative Services. (2003). *Conducting effective meetings.* Retrieved January 9, 2006, from http://www.cbsc.org/servlet/ContentServer?pagename=CBSC_ON%2Fdisplay&lang=en&cid=1081945277203&c=GuideFactSheet

Sawin, K.J., Cox, A.W., Metzger, S.G., Horsley, J.W., Harrigan, M.P., Deaton, A., et al. (1999). Transition planning for youth with chronic conditions: an interdisciplinary process. *National Academies of Practice Forum: Issues in Interdisciplinary Care, 1*(3), 183–196.

Scal, P. (2002). Transition for youth with chronic conditions: Primary care physicians' approaches. *Pediatrics, 110*(6 Pt 2), 1315–1321.

Scal, P., Evans, T., Blozis, S., Okinow, N., & Blum, R. (1999). Trends in transition from pediatric to adult health care services for young adults with chronic conditions. *Journal of Adolescent Health, 24,* 259–264.

Schiller, E., Bobronnikov, E., O'Reilly, F., Price, C., & St. Pierre, R. (2005). *Final 2nd interim report (2002-2003 school year).* Bethseda, MD: Abt Associates, Inc. Retrieved December 15, 2005, from http://www.abt.sliidea.org/Reports/complete%20Interim%20Report%2003-05%20for%20web.pdf

Stodden, R.A., Brown, S.E., Galloway, L.M., Mrazek, S., & Noy, L. (2005). *Interagency transition team development and facilitation.* Retrieved December 1, 2005, from http://www.ncset.org/publications/essentialtools/teams/default.asp

Tindle, K., Leconte, P., Buchanan, L., & Taymans, J.M. (2005). Transition planning: Community mapping as a tool for teachers and students. *NCSET Research to Practice Brief, 4*(1). Retrieved December 9, 2005, from http://www.ncset.org/publications/viewdesc.asp?id=2128

U.S. General Accounting Office (GAO). (1996). *People with disabilities: Federal programs could work together more efficiently to promote employment.* (No. GAO/HEHS-96-126). Washington, DC: Author.

Wagner, J., Newman, L., Cameto, R., & Levine, P. (2005). *National longitudinal transition study 2: Changes over time in the early post-school outcomes of youth with disabilities: A report of the findings from the national longitudinal transition study and national longitudinal study 2.* Menlo Park, CA: SRI International.

Wagner, J., Newman, L., D'Amico, R., Jay, E., Butler-Nalin, P., Marder, C., et al. (1991). *Youth with disabilities: How are they doing? The first comprehensive report of the national longitudinal transition study.* Menlo Park, CA: SRI International Department of Education.

CHAPTER 14

Care Coordination

KATHRYN SMITH

F amilies of youth with special health care needs and disabilities face serious challenges in identifying and accessing needed services. The service system can be confusing, with varying eligibility requirements, difficult application processes, or services that are not clearly evident. Oftentimes, families can benefit from the assistance of a care coordinator, someone educated to facilitate access to and navigation of the service system, ensuring that the youth and family have necessary supports and services.

This chapter focuses on the process of care coordination and its components. Specifically, the chapter covers definitions of care coordination, its history, the role of the care coordinator, the elements of the care coordination process, outcomes for care coordination, care coordination tools, and the issues around financing care coordination.

PROCESS OF CARE COORDINATION

Care coordination is a process that facilitates the linkage of children and their families with appropriate services and resources in a coordinated effort to achieve good health outcomes, and can lead to increased quality of life, fewer hospitalizations, and decreased costs (Blaum et al., 2001). Care coordination can be carried out by a variety of individuals; both trained professionals and lay staff. In the care coordination process, strengths and needs are identified, goals are set, a plan for meeting those goals is established, resources are identified and the plan of care is evaluated and revised as needed, on behalf of or in collaboration with youth with special health care needs and/or disabilities. Care coordination for youth with special health care needs and disabilities is often complicated because there is no single point of entry into the multiple systems of care, and complex criteria frequently determine the availability of funding and services among public and private payers.

Economic and sociocultural barriers to coordination of care exist and affect families and health care professionals. Families often bear the burden of coordinating care for their child, even though they may not have the necessary experience or knowledge of the resources. Thus, coordinating care can be a time consuming, trial-and-error activity for family members. This is a national problem for many families coordinating services for a loved one with an illness or disability. The cost of care coordination in lost work and income for family members was conservatively estimated at $115 billion in 1997 (Blaum et al, 2001). Access to care coordination can reduce the burden on families and the impact on the U.S.

economy. Yet, breakdowns in care coordination can lead to poor cost and quality outcomes, such as missed or delayed diagnoses, missed appointments or treatments, repeated or unnecessary testing, preventable hospital use, fragmented health care, lack of communication between providers, poor referral completion, and family and provider frustration (Blaum et al., 2001; Forrest et al., 2000).

In their important role of providing a medical home for all children, primary care physicians have a vital role—in concert with the family—in the process of care coordination. Hospital and agency-based care coordinators are often nurses or social workers, although members from other disciplines, such as psychology or occupational therapy, may serve in this role. Community-based agencies may use lay case managers who are specially trained to carry out care coordination activities.

Often parents of youth with special health care needs and disabilities have served as their children's care coordinators, with or without support from professionals. Parents are often the de facto care coordinator since they know their children best, provide consistency, and are ultimately responsible for their children's care. Youth themselves can and should begin to participate in the care coordination process, as they begin to assume responsibility for their own care. It is important for both youth and their parents to understand how care coordination is defined by the agencies serving them, as there is variability that can cause confusion or unmet expectations.

Defining Care Coordination

Different service systems may have differing definitions of *care coordination*, and may use different terminology that is often established in legislation. For instance, the Social Security Act, Title V statute that provides legislative authority for federal maternal and child health programs, including those for children with special health care needs, defines care coordination as "services to promote the effective and efficient organization and utilization of resources to assure access to necessary comprehensive services for children with special health care needs and their families" (Maternal and Child Health Services Block Grant, 1935). The Case Management Society of America defines case management as a "collaborative process which assesses, plans, implements, coordinates, monitors and evaluates options and services to meet an individual's health needs through communication and available resources to promote quality cost-effective outcomes" (Powell, 2000). Part C, the Early Intervention Program for Infants and Toddlers with Disabilities, of the Individuals with Disabilities Education Improvement Act (IDEA) 2004 defines service coordination as "the activities carried out by a service coordinator to assist and enable a child eligible under this part and the child's family to receive the rights, procedural safeguards, and services that are authorized to be provided under the State's early intervention program" (IDEA, 2004). Medicaid defines case management as an "activity that assists individuals in gaining access to needed waiver and other state plan services, as well as needed medical, social, educational, and other appropriate services, regardless of the funding source for the services to which access is gained" (4442.3.13; Centers for Medicare and Medicaid Services, n.d.). The responsibility for these activities rests with a specific person or organization.

Care coordination is also known by other terms, such as *service coordination* and *case management*. While there are similarities among these terms, they are not the same. While care coordination and service coordination both share some common goals with case management related to coordinating services and meeting client needs, case management typically does so in the context of one organization, with a narrow scope, and will be discussed below. Care and service coordination typically have a broader scope, and cross multiple agencies in seeking appropriate services for youth and their families.

Case Management

Specifically, the use of the term *case management* has a slightly different connotation than care coordination, often referring to some kind of gate keeping (limiting access to services), or cost containment goals. Case management programs often rely on a medical model focusing on health, while care coordination tends to use a broader social service model considering other patient needs as well. Case management programs tend to coordinate services internally, coordinating only covered services, while care coordination coordinates a full range of health and related services within and outside of an organization (Rosenbach & Young, 2000). An insurance company, for instance, may use a case manager to determine the necessity of a procedure and then provide authorization if it finds the procedure to be appropriate, medically necessary, and a covered benefit of the youth's policy.

Case management services may be used to locate, coordinate, and monitor necessary and appropriate services, and may be used to encourage the use of cost-effective medical care by referral to appropriate providers, and discourage over-utilization of costly services such as emergency room care for routine procedures. Case management services may also serve to provide necessary coordination with providers of nonmedical services, such as local education agencies or departments of vocational rehabilitation, when the services provided by these entities are needed to enable the individual to function at the highest attainable level or to benefit from programs for which he or she might be eligible (4442.3.13, Centers for Medicare and Medicaid Services, n.d.).

Many children and youth who are currently receiving Medicaid do so through managed care organizations. Typically, managed care plans provide some level of coordination of services, most often in the form of case management, and typically, only for youth with expensive, significant, long-term needs. The case management often focuses on authorizing services, controlling costs, and moving clients to less-expensive care options. The emphasis is often on managing the use of health plan resources to contain costs. There are some health plans that have comprehensive youth and family-friendly care coordination programs in which they coordinate care across service systems, but they may be the exception. One reason for this is the cost of care coordination, as coordination typically requires someone with extensive knowledge of community resources, experience in working with youth and their families, and knowledge of the health care issues the youth faces. In addition, the care coordination process, done correctly, is time consuming, although it may yield cost savings in the end by preventing complications or providing access to previously unavailable services. Case management may be provided through the health plans using health plan staff, it may be delegated to a medical group or individual provider, or it may be carried out through specialized "carve-out" organizations that are not part of the health plan and that contract with the plans to provide this service (Kastner & The American Academy of Pediatrics Committee on Children with Disabilities, 2004).

Case management, in the context of authorization of services, has been sub-ject to criticism, with providers arguing that they, and not the case manager, know best what their clients need, and that the primary motive of the case mana-ger is cost containment on behalf of the payer. One of the reasons for the nega-tive connotation associated with case management is that it is associated with ensuring that clients get only what is absolutely essential, and not what they need (Sofaer, Kreling, & Carmel, 2000). For the purposes of this chapter, we will focus on the broader concept of care coordination.

HISTORY OF CARE COORDINATION

Care coordination is not a new concept—it was the basis of delivering services through charity programs in large urban areas at the beginning of the last century—and has long been a focus of public health nursing (Association of Maternal and Child Health Programs [AMCHP] Working Group on Care Coordination, 2000). The term *case management* appeared in the 1970s, and in the 1980s insurers used case management to coordinate care and manage costs (AMCHP, 2000). From that time, care coordination has evolved to a comprehensive, cross-agency process aimed at improving access and services for the target population.

Role of the Care Coordinator

The scope of practice of care coordination can vary widely, depending on the agency and the goals of its programs. The care coordination position includes a number of different roles, including those of advocate, facilitator, provider, liai-son, coordinator, collaborator, broker, educator, negotiator, evaluator, communi-cator, risk manager, mentor, consultant, and researcher (American Nurses Asso-ciation [ANA], 2005). Individual care coordinators are likely to be more skilled in some of the roles than others, and the roles that will be carried out will in part be dictated by the agency or program in which the care coordinator works.

Powell (2000) includes the following roles in the definition of scope of prac-tice: patient advocacy; protector of privacy and confidentiality; coordinator of care, assessment, and reassessment; facilitator in level of care changes; negotia-tor; clinical expert; critical thinker; problem solver; team player; coach; docu-menter; educator; and liaison.

Nehring and colleagues (2004) use the following measurement criteria for the coordination of care: making referrals, supervising and/or providing direction to unlicensed personnel, keeping the youth with special health care needs and disabilities and his or her family informed about the status of their health and available resources, and identifying strategies that promote health.

The AMCHP (2000) identifies the following principles of care coordination for children with special health care needs and their families:

- Care coordination is important to children with special health care needs and their families, and should be universally available to all children and youth with special needs and their families.

- Care coordination should look beyond health care needs and consider social, developmental, educational, vocational and financial factors as well.

- The complexity of the service system has created a strong need for care coordination.

- Families are at the center of the care coordination process, receive this service by choice, direct the goals of the process and serve as effective leaders and partners.

- Care coordination must serve to meet the unique goals and needs of the family.

- Youth and families have different needs for care coordination over time, and the care coordination system should be responsive to this.

- Partnerships between agencies, programs, families, providers and other supports are essential for effective care coordination. (pp. 4–5)

The Merck Manual (Berkow, Beers, & Burs, 1999) describes the elements of care coordination for the chronically disabled child as follows: assessing needs of the child and family; planning comprehensive care for medical and nonmedical services; coordinating services, including training community providers and monitoring services and patient and family progress; and counseling, educating, training, and supporting the patient and family. This description represents a simple and straightforward definition of activities that will help to ensure the receipt of appropriate services for the youth and his or her family.

Regardless of the definition of the scope of practice for care coordination, the primary elements of assessment, planning, coordinating, and assisting families to access services will remain constant. Guiding principles for care coordination within a successful transition program include services that are adolescent-focused, a transition manager to coordinate the transition across disciplines and institutions, and a forum for providers to discuss management and readiness issues (MacKenzie, 2004).

Who Assumes the Care Coordinator Role?

A number of individuals or organizations may assume the role of care coordinator. Entities that may coordinate services include developmental disabilities organizations; mental health organizations; health care organizations, which may be either a provider or a facility such as a hospital; the State Title V Program for Children with Special Health Care Needs; the special education program within a school, or family members themselves. Youth may have contact with a number of different care coordinators who may work together in a cohesive manner or may contribute to fragmentation of care. Most often, care coordinators will coordinate services only within their own agency or program, leaving the youth and his or her family to negotiate cross-agency/program relationships. Comprehensive care coordination, in which all elements of the youth's care are considered, is the ideal means by which to serve the youth and family. Whoever is responsible for care coordination must have a comprehensive knowledge of the service system and the services available in the youth's community. This requires gathering electronic and written program descriptions and establishing person-to-person contact with agency staff (Massachusetts Consortium for Children with Special Needs, Care Coordination Workgroup [MA Consortium], 2005). For additional information on coordinating services with interagency representatives, refer to Chapter 13.

Medical Home

A concept that includes comprehensive care coordination is that of the medical home. According to the American Academy of Pediatrics (AAP; 2005), "a medical home is not a building, house, or hospital, but rather an approach to providing comprehensive primary care." A medical home is defined as primary care that is accessible, continuous, comprehensive, family-centered, coordinated, compassionate, and culturally effective. In a medical home, a pediatric clinician works in partnership with the child and his or her family to ensure that all of the child's medical and nonmedical needs are met. Through this partnership, the pediatric clinician can help the child and his or her family access and coordinate specialty care, educational services, out-of-home care, family support, and other public and private community services that are important to the overall health of the child and his or her family (AAP, 2002). Care coordination is an essential element of the medical home. The physician may or may not be the person within the medical home who takes direct responsibility for care coordination; however, this function may instead be delegated to a nurse, social worker, specially trained office staff, or parent/professional (AAP, 2005). Regardless of who provides care coordination, the primary consideration should be the development of a partnership of mutual responsibility and trust between parents, youth, and providers.

In the 2001 National Survey of Children with Special Health Care Needs, approximately 50% of youth met all criteria for having a medical home (Lotstein, McPherson, Strickland, & Newacheck, 2005). This outcome was measured using the following five criteria: 1) a usual source of care, 2) a personal physician or nurse, 3) no problems in obtaining referrals when needed, 4) effective care coordination when needed, and 5) receipt of family-centered care (Lotstein et al., 2005). With only 50% of youth meeting all criteria for having a medical home, it is clear that additional work needs to be done to promote the concept. Lack of time, money, and staff are frequently identified as the reasons that physicians are not able to carry out all of the components of the medical home, such as attendance at care coordination meetings, specialized staff to perform care coordination activities, and practice changes to promote accessibility all necessitate additional resources. Insurers do not often pay for care coordination activities, despite the fact that they are of great value to youth and their families, and coordination activities can require extensive time on the part of providers. A system whereby providers are reimbursed for this vital activity would help to improve access to comprehensive care coordination and easier access to the myriad of services used by youth with special health care needs and disabilities.

An ideal goal of health care transition planning is to move a youth from a pediatric medical home provider to a new medical home within an adult health care setting. This move should seek to ensure continuity of medical and health care that is seamless, coordinated, based on the youth's developmental needs, community based, psychosocially appropriate, and comprehensive (MacKenzie, 2004). This is an area that is a particular challenge to youth with special health care needs and disabilities and their families, as they oftentimes have had a long-term relationship with their pediatric providers, they may have conditions that adult providers are unfamiliar with, and they may have funding issues that make locating appropriate providers difficult. Care coordinators within the youth's health plan, specialty pediatric setting, state Title V agency, or developmental disabilities or mental health system may be able to assist youth and families in locating appropriate providers. In addition, some large medical centers have clinics for adults that specialize in conditions once unique to children, such as congenital cardiac defects, cystic fibrosis, Down syndrome, and spina bifida.

COMPONENTS OF THE CARE COORDINATION PROCESS

While not thought of as a formal part of care coordination, it is important to introduce and explain the concept of care coordination to youth and families and define roles and expectations in order to engage the youth and parents as partners in the process and to avoid misunderstanding, conflicts, and disappointments resulting from unmet expectations. This is also an appropriate time to discuss the family's and youth's expectations of their roles in the process, in addition to the role of the care coordinator. Also, guidelines regarding frequency of contact and ways to reach the care coordinator can be defined.

Care coordination will be an integral part of the development and implementation of the health care transition plan, and the youth's care coordinator may assume primary responsibility for bringing the transition team together to begin the process, or may bring his or her own expertise or agency's resources to the planning process. Care coordinators can be located in a number of different agencies or programs, and, in fact, some youth may have more than one. For instance, the youth may have one care coordinator from the developmental disabilities system, another from the school district, and yet another from his or her specialty hospital clinic. While this is not an ideal situation, it is typical of how services are delivered. One care coordinator may be especially close to the youth and family, or may play a critical role in service delivery because of the youth's special needs. Some youth may simply have one care coordinator who works across service systems. One or more of these care coordinators may participate in the health care transition plan, weaving their care coordination plan into the health care transition plan.

The next several sections will describe the care coordination process. Although agencies and programs have their unique policies and procedures for this process, the basic elements are included here.

Assessment of Strengths and Needs

Care coordination ideally builds on the strengths of the youth and his or her family. Strengths may include family support, financial resources, church or community, and proximity to resources. For instance, good public transportation in a family's neighborhood is a strength, as the family will be able to travel about the community for services more easily. A large, local extended family can be a strength as well, as additional help for respite, transportation, and support may be available. After the care coordinator identifies youth and family strengths, needs are identified. The needs assessment should include all domains that affect the youth's health and well-being, including family support, school, health care, and employment. Too often, needs assessments focus solely on health care, yet other factors play a significant role in the youth's successful transition to adult services. The needs assessment may be carried out in the clinic, school, or youth's home, depending on the needs of the youth, family, and care coordinator. It can be very useful to the care coordinator to view the environment in which the family lives, both the resources in their home and community, and some of the challenges and limitations the environment presents.

Goal Setting

Goal setting should occur between the youth, the caregivers, and the care coordinators. No goal should appear in the plan without explicit agreement among the participants in the process. Goals should be based directly on the needs identified by the youth and family and should capitalize on their strengths. The use of the term *nonadherent* can be controversial, in that it implies noncooperation with a plan or set of recommendations. In fact, the goals and the plan may have been developed without full participation of the youth and family, and without consideration of the feasibility of suggested strategies.

Development of a Plan for Care Coordination

The plan flows from the goals developed by the youth, parents, and providers. The goals are reviewed and prioritized, specific activities are defined for meeting the goals, and information is provided by the care coordinator to the youth and family to facilitate completion of activities. Specific timelines should be established, as well as checkpoints to discuss progress toward completion of activities. The youth and family members should know how to reach the care coordinator should questions arise. In addition, they should be given specific details regarding referrals to specific agencies in terms of phone numbers, locations, what will be expected during an appointment, what supporting documents will be needed, and any other information the care coordinator has about the agency. It is also helpful to offer youth and parents practical tips to facilitate a referral, such as availability of public transportation, parking fees, area food establishments, and approximate length of time of an appointment.

If the youth or his or her parents maintain a notebook for the youth, this can be brought to any appointments, but parents and youth should be cautioned to never provide their original documents to an agency, but rather offer copies instead. Prior to any appointments, the care coordinator can offer any written material available about the program, agency, or service, and can help identify on-line resources for families with computer access. For those families without computers in their homes, the care coordinator can direct them to public libraries, schools, and family resource centers that have free computer access. The care coordinator can help the family formulate questions that they wish to ask during the application process, and should encourage the family to write the questions down, take them to the appointment, and plan to write out all answers.

Often, youth and family members can and should bring other individuals to provide support during meetings, help write or interpret information, ask or prompt questions, or simply provide emotional support. For instance, parents participating in an individualized education program (IEP) for the first time may find it overwhelming and intimidating. They may choose to invite their care coordinator, social worker, or other support person to take notes for them, or if the child has a complex medical condition, they may invite the clinical nurse specialist or nurse practitioner from the youth's specialty care center. Giving permission to bring support persons can be very helpful to the youth and family.

Care Coordination Tools

A number of care coordination tools exist, both to assist care coordinators and youth and families as they work through the care coordination process, as well as to enhance the professional's role as a care coordinator. The following list provides examples of such tools:

- American Nurses Association Credentialing Center: provides the basic eligibility requirements for nursing case managements (available at http://nursingworld.org/ancc/cert/eligibility/CaseMgmt.html)

- Center for Infants and Children with Special Needs, Cincinnati Children's Hospital and Medical Center, and the National Center for Medical Home Initiatives for Children with Special Needs: Care Coordination Toolkit; Proper Use of Coordination of Care Codes with Children with Special Health Care Needs (available at http://www.medicalhomeinfo.org)

- All About Me: a model notebook with various forms that can be used by parents and youth to organize and track health and related information (available at http://www.medicalhomeinfo.org)

- American Academy of Pediatrics: provides care coordination articles and resources (available at http://aappolicy.aappublications.org/cgi/content/full/pediatrics)

- The National Survey of Children with Special Health Care Needs: provides information about parents' perceptions and needs related to care coordination (available at http://www.mchb.hrsa.gov/chscn/pages/coordination.htm)

Assignment of Care Coordination Responsibilities

During the development of the plan, the youth, parents, and care coordinator need to determine who will take responsibility for which activity in the plan. This is a good opportunity to provide support to the youth to begin to make phone calls and appointments, and to ask for information and write it down. It may be difficult for parents to let go of some of these activities, but the transition process includes assuming more responsibility for self-care on the part of the youth. (For more information on self-care needs, refer to Chapter 4.) Parents may need additional support during this time to avoid feeling displaced, to reduce anxiety, and to assist the youth in self-care activities. It may be necessary for parents to rehearse phone calls to make appointments or calls to renew prescriptions with the youth. The care coordinator can work with the parents to identify ways to provide support to the youth during these activities, and at the same time, can provide support to the parents and congratulate them as they work with their youth toward transition, and ultimately independence.

The written plan should include specific details about which activities the youth, the care coordinator, and the parents will each take responsibility for, as well as any other professionals that are part of the planning process. Parents and youth should be given a copy of the plan to refer to. Some parents may wish to assume the role of care coordinator, and should be supported in doing so. They must be aware that they can call on the agency's care coordinator for support or information as needed, and that they may transfer care coordination activities back to the agency when they need to be relieved of the responsibility, for instance, during a period of time when a youth is experiencing a health crisis, or the family is dealing with other stressors.

Inherent in the activities of the care coordination process at this point is education of the youth and family. Families will need to be given information about the service systems with which they will interact and how to access them. In addition, youth and families may need an "update" in their basic knowledge of the youth's condition. The youth should be asked questions about his or her condition and plan of care to ascertain understanding. It is not uncommon for the family to have been given information at the time of diagnosis and not have had the information updated for a period of time, especially in the context of the youth transitioning to adult services. Families and youth may also need to be taught advocacy skills so that as they encounter barriers, they can work to resolve them.

Reassessment of Timelines and Activities/Monitoring

Once the initial plan is written, periodic reassessments must take place to determine progress toward the achievement of goals, obstacles encountered, and changes needed. Reassessment may take place daily, weekly, or monthly, depending on the urgency of the situation and the activities needing to be carried out. The youth and parents should be informed about when they should expect to hear from the care coordinator, and they should also be encouraged to call if problems occur. This allows for revisions to the plan as needed, with reassignment of responsibilities and timelines as appropriate. If the youth and family are encountering barriers in accessing services or completing referrals, the care coordinator assumes the role of advocate and works to intervene on the family's behalf. If the care coordinator has established relationships in the community, these relationships can be leveraged to obtain needed services for the youth and family. Timeliness is of the essence for the transitioning youth. Eligibility for programs may be ending as the youth reaches the period of 18–22 years of age, and time must be allowed to order necessary equipment, find new service providers, and perhaps even schedule surgeries while the youth still has insurance coverage. This process of planning prior to eligibility termination requires constant vigilance on the part of the care coordinator.

Evaluation

Evaluation occurs when the care coordinator, youth, and family meet together, perhaps every 6 months or annually, to assess overall achievement of the care coordination plan goals. This can be done face to face or by phone but is often more successfully done in person to allow adequate discussion of the successes and shortcomings in the plan. The plan is then revised, based on this discussion, for the next period of time, again following the same procedure of mutual agreement, assignment of responsibilities, and establishment of timelines. This is also an opportunity for the care coordinator to assess the youth's participation and transition to self-care activities, as they relate to the plan. (For information on evaluation of health outcomes, refer to Chapter 9.)

Outcomes of Care Coordination

Care coordination should result in satisfaction of the youth, family, and providers; enhanced well-being of the youth and the family; improved capacity of providers; and effectiveness and efficiency of the service systems. In addition, outcomes should result in achievement of identified youth and family health outcomes that include prevention of secondary complications; the maintenance or improvement of health status, functional status, independence, and community participation; and decreased family care giving burden (MA Consortium, 2005; Sofaer et al., 2000).

Smith and the Outcome Measures Workgroup (1998) identified the following outcomes of care coordination:

- Families are given information about care coordination services, and the process of care coordination, and receive services and make choices that best meet their needs.

- Families receive care coordination services that are consistent with their cultural beliefs and values, and in their preferred language.

- Families receive care coordination in their communities whenever possible.

- Families receive timely and responsive care coordination services.

- Families receive care coordination services that support the youth's and family's developmental needs.

- Families serve as their own care coordinators, with support, when they choose to.

- Families choose their goals for care coordination and revise their goals and plans as needed.

- Families participate in the development of a plan, based on their identified needs, that promotes optimal access to services.

- Families have access to appropriate services.

- Families experience continuity of care among health, education, and social service providers.

- Families receive information and support in planning for transitions.

- Families are supported while exercising their rights to appropriate services.

- Families are satisfied with their care coordination services.

Case Closure

When the relationship between the care coordinator, youth, and parents is to end—because the youth no longer needs services, is no longer eligible for services, or is moving to a different service system—it is essential to end the relationship in an orderly way so that the youth and parents are aware of next steps, future resources, and who to call should problems arise. If the care coordinator feels comfortable doing so, and if agency rules permit it, the youth and parent may be given permission to call the care coordinator as questions arise during the period following case closure. This continued contact allows for a smoother transition to the new services and prevents anxiety and lack of follow through on the part of the youth and parents.

The successes and pending activities of the care coordination plan (whether a component of the IEP and health care transition planning processes or part of another agency's or program's efforts), its successes, and pending activities should be summarized for the youth and parents, preferably in writing so that they can share this information with their new care coordination provider. This is an optimal time for the care coordinator to work with the youth and family to update a notebook that they may use and provide copies of key documents that are missing.

Whenever possible, and with the parents' and youth's permission, the care coordinator should introduce him- or herself and the youth and family to the new care coordinator or contact within the new agency or program. Care coordinators for adult services can be found in health plans, provider offices, mental health or developmental disabilities systems, and some special care centers focusing on conditions such as sickle cell disease or cystic fibrosis.

These case closure activities complete the loop that began with the introduction to the care coordination process and through the care coordination activities in which the youth and parents participated in, leading to a smooth transition to the next level of care for the youth—that of adult services.

SUMMARY

Care coordination is an essential service for youth with special health care needs and their families. It helps provide access to needed services, unravels the complicated service system for families, and reduces obstacles and barriers to care. Care coordination can be carried out by a variety of professionals and lay staff in different settings. The most important element of the process is skilled communication with parents, youth, and all of the members of the youth's team.

REFERENCES

American Academy of Pediatrics. (2005). *The National Center for Medical Home Initiatives for Children with Special Health Care Needs.* Retrieved December 15, 2005, from http://www.medicalhomeinfo.org/index.html

American Academy of Pediatrics, Council on Children with Disabilities. (2005). Care coordination in the medical home: Integrating health and related systems of care for children with special health care needs. *Pediatrics, 116,* 1238–1244.

American Academy of Pediatrics, Medical Home Initiatives for Children with Special Needs Project Advisory Committee. (2002). The medical home. *Pediatrics, 110,* 184–186.

American Nurses Association. (2005). *Nursing case management certification.* Retrieved January 1, 2006, from http://nursingworld.org/ancc/cert/eligibility/CaseMgmt.html

Association of Maternal and Child Health Programs Working Group on Care Coordination. (2000). *Care coordination for children with special health care needs and their families in the new millennium.* Washington, DC: Association of Maternal and Child Health Programs.

Berkow, R., Beers, M.H., & Burs, M. (Eds.). (1999). *Merck manual of diagnosis and therapy.* Hoboken, NJ: John Wiley and Sons.

Blaum, C., Douglass, B.A., Marion, L.N., Olivares, E., Prela, C.M., Scalettar, R.E., et al. (2001). *Mainstreaming care coordination for people with complex health care needs.* Retrieved November 19, 2005, from http://www.nonpf.com/lmpcfppr.htm.

Forrest, C.B., Glade, G.B., Baker, A.E., Bocian, A., von Schrader, S., & Starfield, B. (2000). Coordination of specialty referrals and physician satisfaction with referral care. *Archives of Pediatric and Adolescent Medicine, 154*(5), 499–506.

Individuals with Disability Education Improvement Act of 2004. PL-108-446, 20 U.S.C. §§ 1400 *et seq.*

Kastner, T.A., & American Academy of Pediatrics Committee on Children with Disabilities. (2004). Managed care and children with special health care needs. *Pediatrics, 114,* 1693–1698.

Lotstein, D.S., McPherson, M., Strickland, B., & Newacheck, P.W. (2005). Transition planning for youth with special health care needs: Results from the National Survey for Children with Special Health Care Needs. *Pediatrics, 115,* 1562–1568.

MacKenzie, R.G. (2004, Winter). The problem of transition—the challenges of success. *Los Angeles Pediatric Society,* 6–7.

Massachusetts Consortium for Children with Special Needs, Care Coordination Workgroup. (2005). *Care coordination: Definition and principles.* Boston: New England Serve.

Maternal and Child Health Services Block Grant, Maternal and Child Health Bureau, Health Resources and Services Administration, Title V of the 1935 Social Security Act. Section 501 (b)(3).

Nehring, W.M., Roth, S.P., Natvig, D., Betz, C.L., Savage, T., & Krajicek, M. (2004). *Intellectual and developmental disabilities nursing: Scope and standards of practice.* Silver Spring, MD: American Nurses Association and the American Association on Mental Retardation.

Powell, S.K. (2000). *Case management: A practical guide to success in managed care.* Philadelphia: Lippincott Williams &Wilkins.

Rosenbach, M., & Young, C. (2000). *Care coordination and Medicaid managed care: Emerging issues for states and managed care organizations.* Princeton, NJ: Mathematica Policy Research, Inc.

Smith, K.A., & the Outcome Measures Workgroup. (1998). *Care coordination outcomes for children with special health care needs.* Los Angeles: ACCESS-MCH.

Sofaer, S., Kreling, B., & Carmel, M. (2000). *Coordination of care for persons with disabilities enrolled in Medicaid managed care: A conceptual framework to guide the development of measures.* Washington, DC: Office of Disability, Aging and Long-Term Care Policy, Office of the Assistant Secretary for Planning and Evaluation, U.S. Department of Health and Human Services.

Transition
and Transition-
Related Web Sites

HEALTH CARE TRANSITION

Adolescent Health Transition Project

http://depts.washington.edu/healthtr/

The Adolescent Health Transition Project web site offers a number of useful re-sources. *Transition Timelines,* an excellent tool for displaying the major bench-marks for transition planning, can be accessed from this site. It is also available in Spanish, Vietnamese, Russian, and Chinese. Several PowerPoint slide programs are available for self-instruction on the topic of health care transition planning.

American Diabetes Association

http://www.diabetes.org/uedocuments/504-plan-2004.pdf

The American Diabetes Association web site contains a sample Section 504 plan and diabetes medical management plan for a student with diabetes.

American Medical Association

http://www.ama-assn.org

The American Medical Association web site has a number of web pages on health issues pertaining to adolescent health. The health topics include violence and bul-lying, nutrition and physical fitness, teen pregnancy, reproductive health, and the State Children's Health Insurance Program.

Bandaids and Blackboards

http://www.lehman.cuny.edu/faculty/jfleitas/bandaides/

The Bandaids and Blackboards web site provides the user with numerous vignettes that were submitted by children, youth, and adults with chronic dis-abilities and their parents as a way of enabling others to better understand what it means to live with a chronic condition. Tips are provided for teachers and health professionals who work with children with chronic conditions.

Bright Futures

http://www.brightfutures.org

The Bright Futures web site (developed in partnership with the Maternal and Child Health Bureau and American Academy of Pediatrics) provides age-specific guidelines on what is considered to be best practice pertaining to health care and developmental screening from infancy to adolescence.

Centers for Medicare and Medicaid Services

http://www.cms.hhs.gov/

The Centers for Medicare and Medicaid Services web site provides consumer information and both public insurance plans on the State Child Health Insurance Program. Information is provided on eligibility and benefits.

Health Care Transitions

http://hctransitions.ichp.edu/

Health Care Transitions is the web site of the Institute for Child Health Policy located at the University of Florida at Gainesville. This site offers a number of resources for health care transition planning such as service and training manuals, videos, and a bibliography. Of particular interest are the Health Care Transition Workbooks in PDF format for children and youth. Each of the three workbooks is targeted for a particular age group: 12–14 years, 15–17 years, and 18 years and older.

Healthy & Ready to Work National Center

http://www.hrtw.org

Healthy & Ready to Work National Center is one of the leading health care transition web sites funded by the Maternal and Child Health Bureau that provides extensive resources on transition resources for adolescents with special health care needs. The focus is on the health-related transition resources. The information and resources provided on the web site includes service guidelines, transition checklists, links to other transition web sites, youth resources, health and mental services, laws and legislation, and other resources.

Kentucky Commission
for Children with Special Health Care Needs

http://chfs.ky.gov/ccshcn/

Kentucky Commission for Children with Special Health Care Needs web site has a section titled *Transition Resources*. Located on this page are a number of youth and family resources that have been disseminated widely for use such as a section titled *Life Maps* that are meant to track the child's and youth's progress developmentally. State specific information on resources is available as well.

National Center on Secondary Education and Transition

http://www.ncset.org/

The National Center on Secondary Education and Transition (NCSET) web site is a clearinghouse on information pertaining to secondary education and transition of students with disabilities. The site contains publications such as *NCSET Briefs* on policies, National Longitudinal Transition Study findings, parent information, applied research findings, and current issues and trends pertaining to transition and secondary education. NCSET also sponsors activities nationally to disseminate information and provide technical assistance as a means of improving transition services in secondary educational settings.

National Organization of Rare Disorders

http://www.rarediseases.org/

The National Organization of Rare Disorders web site contains information on 1,150 rare disorders. A profile of the disorder is presented together with links to other web sites that are related to the disorder in terms of information about services, resources, and advocacy/consumer groups. Information about organizations associated with rare disorders is available as well. This site charges a fee for downloading files from the site.

Shriners Hospitals for Children

http://www.shrinershq.org/hospit.html

The Shriners Hospital for Children web site provides information about the national network of Shriners Hospitals for Children. Primarily burn and orthopedic services are provided to children and youth.

Society for Adolescent Medicine

http://www.adolescenthealth.org

The Society for Adolescent Medicine (SAM) web site is primarily for use by adolescent multidisciplinary health professionals. However, there is a feature on the web site that enables consumers to locate adolescent medicine specialists in their community who are members of SAM.

Teen Growth

http://www.teengrowth.com/

The Teen Growth web site offers comprehensive information on a wide variety of topics related to teen health: body, emotions, health, doctor, friends, sports, danger, school, family, and sex. Each of the sections provides basic information directed to teens followed by teen questions on particular topics. There is also a feature enabling teens to e-mail questions to physicians.

TeenHealth

http://www.kidshealth.org/teen/

The TeenHealth web site is sponsored by the Nemours Foundation and provides comprehensive information on health topics for youth. There is information on food and fitness, and diseases/chronic conditions commonly associated with youth such as asthma, infections (e.g., mononucleosis, colds), and sexually transmitted diseases. There is a section on safety tips and basic first aid, preventive health measures, sexuality, puberty, and mental health problems.

University of Illinois, Chicago, Division of Specialized Care for Children

http://internet.dscc.uic.edu/dsccroot/parents/transition.asp#interview

The University of Illinois, Chicago, Division of Specialized Care for Children web site contains a number of transition resources and worksheets for families and youth. Many of the resources are specifically geared for Illinois residents, although useful for out-of-state residents.

Western University Center for Disabilities and the Health Professions

http://www.westernu.edu/xp/edu/cdihp/about.html

The Western University Center for Disabilities and the Health Professions web site provides information about the array of programs available for individuals with disabilities. Goals of the center are to increase the number of individuals with disabilities in the health professions, provide informational resources on the provision of care to individuals with disabilities to health professionals, and empower individuals with disabilities to become better consumers.

Womenshealth.gov

http://www.4women.gov/wwd/

The Womenshealth.gov web site provides information on a variety of health-related topics for women with disabilities, care providers, health care professionals, and researchers. Information provided on the site includes access to issues such as health care, abuse, reproductive health, legislation, health problems associated with type of disability conditions, illness symptomology and resources, and services and support.

HEALTH INSURANCE

American Disabilities Administration, *Health Insurance for Disabled Individuals*

http://www.diabetes.org/advocacy-and-legalresources/healthcare/healthinsurance/disabled-persons.jsp

The American Disabilities Administration web site has a section titled *Health Insurance for Disabled Individuals,* which provides information for consumers on Supplemental Security Income, Social Security Disability Insurance, prescription assistance, individual health insurance policies, and state high-risk pools.

Healthinsuranceinfo.net

http://www.healthinsuranceinfo.net/

Healthinsuranceinfo.net of the Georgetown Health Policy Institute web site provides consumer guides on health insurance coverage guidelines/regulations for each state.

National Association of Insurance Commissioners

http://www.naic.org/state_web_map.htm

The National Association of Insurance Commissioners web site provides access to each state's insurance commissioner's web site, thereby enabling the user to obtain a profile of insurance options within a particular state. Also, the web sites provide users with information on how to report fraud or problems with insurance coverage.

MENTAL HEALTH

Anxiety Disorders Association of America

http://www.adaa.org

The Anxiety Disorders Association of America web site provides comprehensive information on all types of anxiety disorders as well as referral information. There is a web page on anxiety disorders affecting children and youth with some of the information directed for youth use.

Depression and Bipolar Support Alliance

http://www.dbsalliance.org/

The Depression and Bipolar Support Alliance is a consumer-oriented web site directed to assisting individuals with mood disorders and their families. Information is provided on accessing support groups in local communities. Informational resources and publications are provided as well.

Institute for Mental Health Initiatives

http://www.gwumc.edu/sphhs/imhi

The Institute for Mental Health Initiatives web site provides information on mental health issues for families, media, and professionals. The pages for parents contain practical information that they can use in dealing with their children such as anger management strategies, assisting their child through a crisis, and parental resources.

National Institute on Mental Health

http://www.nimh.nih.gov

The National Institute on Mental Health web site provides information about the programs and initiatives supported by this federal agency. Consumer information is also provided on the identification and treatment of mental health problems.

This site also contains information on the mental health problems of children and youth including bipolar and anxiety disorders, depression, and other mental health topics such as violence and the use of medications.

National Alliance on Mental Illness

http://www.nami.org/

The National Alliance on Mental Illness web site describes the organization that promotes self-help support for individuals with mental illness. Consumer information is provided on mental health problems, support groups, and effective treatments.

Research & Training Center
on Family Support and Children's Mental Health

http://www.rtc.pdx.edu

The Research & Training Center on Family Support and Children's Mental Health web site contains information on services for families and children with emotional, behavioral, and mental health problems. The web site also contains pages specifically for youth.

U.S. Department of Education Safe and Drug Free Schools

http://www.ed.gov/offices/OESE/SDFS

The Department of Education Safe and Drug Free Schools web site contains information on programs and initiatives pertaining to developing and implementing drug prevention programs in school settings.

SEXUALITY AND REPRODUCTIVE CONCERNS

MossRehab ResourceNet

http://www.mossresourcenet.org/sexuali.htm

MossRehab ResourceNet is a web site on sexuality and disability. This web site contains links to other organizations that have expertise in this field, publications on the topic, sexual aids for individuals with disabilities, and a listing of disability-related newsgroups.

Susan's Sex Support Site

http://www.sexsupport.org/

Susan's Sex Support Site is a web site on providing sexuality information and support for individuals with disabilities. There is an extensive amount of information and links to other sites pertaining to sexuality, such as adolescents and sexuality, gay and lesbian issues, and aging and sexuality, as well as professional issues. The adolescent and sexuality content covers a wide range of topics from definition of terminology used in discussing sexuality, information about reproductive and sexual organs for males and females, issues pertaining to being a gay or lesbian teen, date rape, sexual abuse, and pregnancy prevention.

EDUCATION

A World of Options . . . A Guide to International Educational Exchange, Community Service and Travel For Persons with Disabilities, Mobility International

P.O. Box 10767, Eugene, OR 97440, (541) 343-1284 (Voice/TTY), $35.00 non-member; $25.00 member

http://www.miusa.org/publications/books/worldofoptions

This web site provides information on international exchange programs for students with disabilities.

Council for Exceptional Children

http://www.ideapractices.org/

The Council for Exceptional Children web site's Idea Practices offers extensive information on educational practices designed to improve outcomes for students with disabilities and exceptionalities and those who are gifted. Although the web site is primarily directed to professional educators, there is information of interest to parents. There is a section of the web site devoted to college students, which may be of interest to individuals, who plan on entering the education profession with plans to work with exceptional, gifted students, or students with disabilities.

ERI Distance Learning Center, Employment Law

http://www.eridlc.com/index.cfm?FuseAction=hrlaws.main

The ERI Distance Learning Center, Employment Law web site contains copies of relevant employment legislation and regulations including provisions related to health care and insurance such as the Family and Medical Leave Act and the Health Insurance Portability and Accountability Act of 1995.

George Washington University HEATH Resource Center

http://www.heath.gwu.edu/

The George Washington University HEATH Resource Center web site is the national clearinghouse on postsecondary education for individuals with disabilities. It contains extensive information on topics of interest to students, professionals, and advocates such as financial aid programs for students with disabilities, disability policies, and procedures and educational programs.

Mobility International USA

http://miusa.org/ncde/tipsheets/strategiesinclusion/arrangingtravel/view

Mobility International USA is a web site for students with disabilities who are interested in studying abroad. It provides information on international exchange and development programs. The *Arranging Travel and Health Insurance* section provides the consumer with relevant information about health insurance coverage when traveling internationally as part of an exchange program. In addition, links to other web sites for obtaining insurance when studying abroad are available.

National Longitudinal Transition Study 2

http://www.nlts2.org/

The National Longitudinal Transition Study 2 web site provides comprehensive findings from the national survey conducted on students who were enrolled in special education 2 year postschool exit. The survey consisted of a national sample of 3,000 students (13–16 years old in 2000) and 6,000 parents and guardians. Information gathered included data on secondary school experience and postschool outcomes pertaining to education, training employment, and independent and community living. This is an excellent resource for obtaining statistics on a national sample of youth with disabilities.

Office of Special Education and Rehabilitative Services

Office of Special Education and Rehabilitative Services:
    http://www.ed.gov/about/offices/list/osers/programs.html

Office of Special Education Programs:
    http://www.ed.gov/about/offices/list/osers/osep/programs.html

Rehabilitation Services Administration:
    http://www.ed.gov/about/offices/list/osers/rsa/index.html

National Institute on Disability and Rehabilitation Research:
    http://www.ed.gov/about/offices/list/osers/nidrr/index.html?src=mr

The Office of Special Education and Rehabilitative Services web site links the user to the programs for students and people with disabilities within the U.S. Department of Education. The Office of Special Education Programs offers information on the projects and programs authorized by the Individuals with Disabilities Education Act and its amendments. These special education programs are designed to assist infants, children, and youth with disabilities. The Rehabilitative Services Administration (RSA) supports programs that assist individuals with disabilities to lead productive and independent lives. RSA administers the Title 1 program that provides federal funds to the state vocational programs. The National Institute on Disability and Rehabilitation Research (NIDRR) web site contains information on various research and related initiatives sponsored by this Institute. Research sponsored by NIDRR includes studies on full inclusion, employment, community integration, and independent living of people with disabilities across the life span.

Special Education Resources on the Internet

http://seriweb.com/

The Special Education Resources on the Internet web site is a compilation of links to web sites on special education and disability-related resources. For example, the page on mental retardation lists sites that are consumer-focused, those for professionals and academicians and for the general public.

TeenWorkers

http://www.osha.gov/SLTC/teenworkers/rights.html

The TeenWorkers web site provides information on labor rights and regulations such as the child labor laws, minimum wage laws, safety requirements, and health and safety regulations. This site has sections for youth, parents, educators, and employers specific to their needs. There is also information in Spanish for users.

The National Dissemination Center for Children with Disabilities

http://www.nichcy.org/

The National Dissemination Center is a national on-line clearinghouse of information pertaining to educational resources, as well as disability topics related to infants, children, and youth and their families. Information is available in both English and Spanish. A number of publications are available on a wide variety of topics related to each age group. This site is a useful resource for families as the information is reader friendly for individuals not familiar with the terminology used by professionals. Information is available at 1-800-695-0285 with TTY.

EMPLOYMENT

Career One-Stop

http://www.careeronestop.org

The Career One-Stop web site is a gateway site to jobs, training programs, resources for a large audience of users. This site has information for students in terms of findings jobs and assistance with resume development as well as selecting schools and obtaining financial aid. Employers can find information on industry resources such as labor market analyses and developing job descriptions. Additional information is provided on the workforce development system.

Disability Employment Guide

http://www.ed.gov/about/offices/list/osers/products/employmentguide

The Disability Employment Guide web site represents a joint effort between the U.S. Department of Education and the Chamber of Commerce to provide information to employers and business leaders on hiring of individuals with disabilities. This site contains a publication titled *Disability Employment 101*, which can be downloaded from this site.

Employer Assistance Referral Network

http://www.earnworks.com

The Employer Assistance Referral Network web site offers employers assistance with locating potential employees with disabilities. This web site is funded by the U.S. Department of Labor, Office of Disability Employment Policy. This site is considered to be a one-stop for obtaining information pertaining to finding applicants with disabilities, listing of jobs, tools, and resources.

Job Accommodation Network

http://janweb.icdi.wvu.edu/

The Job Accommodation Network web site is a free service to employers, educators, and individuals with disabilities who want to obtain information on accommodations for the work and school setting. Features on the web site include fact sheets, distance learning opportunities, links to other disability web sites, and technical assistance by phone, e-mails, mail, and fax. Technical assistance on the federal laws and regulations such as the American Disability Act is also provided.

National Association of State Workforce Boards

http://www.subnet.nga.org/workforcecouncilchairs/InternetResources.htm

The National Association of State Workforce Boards is a web site that provides links to numerous federal and state employment web sites. These links include U.S. Department of Labor, key employment sites (e.g., U.S. Job Bank), state universities, and workforce statistics.

National Center on Workforce and Disability/Adult

http://www.onestops.info

The National Center on Workforce and Disability/Adult web site originates at the University of Massachusetts Institute for Community Inclusion and is funded by the U.S. Department of Labor. This site provides an array of information pertaining to workforce development systems. This center offers training, technical assistance, information, and policy analysis for consumers, families, professionals, and providers. Areas of interest include use of accommodations, assistive technology, and assistance with finding jobs.

Rehabilitation Engineering and Assistive Technology Society of North America

http://www.resna.org

The Rehabilitation Engineering and Assistive Technology Society of North America web site contains information on assistive technology that would be of primary interest to other professionals. This organization is a professional association and contains information on professional issues such as training programs, research, professional publications (conference proceedings and journal), credentialing, and annual conference.

Technical Assistance on Transition and Rehabilitation Act

http://www.pacer.org/tatra/tatra.htm

The Technical Assistance on Transition and Rehabilitation Act web site, located at the Pacer Center, provides a listing of national conferences relevant to students with disabilities, links to other transition and disability-related national and Minnesota web sites, publications both free and for purchase, videos, listing of parent centers in each state, and consumer information in Spanish, Somali, and Hmong.

The National Collaborative on Workforce and Disability

http://www.ncwd-youth.info/index.html

The National Collaborative on Workforce and Disability web site provides an array of resources for youth with disabilities who want to work. Resource materials include information on One-Stops, disability legislation, a translation of acronyms used by workforce agencies that youth will access for services, information about disability disclosure, and practice standards. This web site is for youth, families, providers, professionals, and policy makers. This web site represents a joint effort of the Institute for Educational Leadership, Center for Workforce Development, Academy for Educational Development-Disability Studies & Services Center, National Association of Workforce Boards, National Center on Secondary Education and Transition, National Youth Employment Coalition and TransCen, Inc.

U.S. Department of Labor, Office of Disability Employment Policy

http://www.dol.gov/odep/

The U.S. Department of Labor, Office of Disability Employment Policy web site contains information on the employment laws affecting medical and disability leave, which includes explanation of the American with Disabilities Act (ADA), Workman's Compensation, FMLA, and JAN.

GOVERNMENT PROGRAMS

DisabilityInfo.Gov

http://www.disabilityinfo.gov

This web site serves as the portal of entry for all government services and programs for people with disabilities. The user can be directed to government sites on employment, education, housing, transportation, health, benefits, technology, benefits, community life, and civil rights.

Federal Citizen Information Center

http://www.pueblo.gsa.gov

Sponsored by the U.S. General Services Administration, this web site provides a wide array of consumer information about the federal government. The site is intended to assist consumers to better understand services and programs offered by the federal government. For example, there is information on resources in Spanish, consumer information on how to get assistance with malfunctioning products, how to self publish, and so forth. The page on health offers information minor illness, health insurance, exercise and diet, mental health, and medications.

GovBenefits.gov

www.govbenefits.gov

This web site provides a comprehensive listing of government benefit programs by federal and state listing. For example, information can be obtained about the health insurance programs available in a particular state for youth, by selecting choices on a screen display to create a listing of programs tailored to the request.

Social Security Administration

http://www.ssa.gov/SSA_Home.html

The Social Security Administration web site can be accessed for complete information on all social security programs that include Supplemental Security Income and work incentive programs.

FAMILY RESOURCES

Family Village

http://www.familyvillage.wisc.edu/index.htmlx

Family Village is a comprehensive resource web site on disability resources for families and consumers. The web site is designed in a family/consumer friendly format to enable family members and consumer to access information on a vast array of disability topics. In addition, on-line chat rooms and parent groups are listed.

Family Voices

http://www.familyvoices.org

Family Voices web site contains information on advocacy issues and resources that families who have children with special health care needs can use. The web site also contains information about its parent advocacy organization that is staffed and directed by families for families of children with special health care needs.

National Clearinghouse on Families & Youth

http://www.ncfy.com

The National Clearinghouse on Families & Youth web site provides information, resources, and links to other web sites to assist families, youth, and professionals on developmental concerns and challenges that today's youth face.

National Parent to Parent Network

http://www.netnet.net/mums/

National Parent to Parent Network web site provides information about this national family advocacy organization. Parents are connected with other parents whose children have the same diagnoses. For families whose children do not have a specific diagnosis, families are matched based on the symptomology the child/youth presents. The purpose of parent to parent matching is to assist parents with information and support from other parents who understand the life experience of raising a child with a disability/chronic illness.

Pacer Center

http://www.pacer.org

The Pacer Center web site contains disability information to assist families in raising a child with a disability. Numerous transition and health related resources are available on this site. Pacer Center, located in Minnesota, is one of the largest advocacy organizations for families in the nation. Their web site has numerous transition and family-center resources available.

TEEN RESOURCES

Kids as Self Advocates

http://www.familyvoices.org

Kids as Self Advocates (KASA) is a self advocacy organization for youth with special health care needs. KASA is a program of Family Voices, and information on it can be found on the Family Voices web site. An on-line newsletter for youth is distributed on a bimonthly basis.

Partners for Youth with Disabilities

http://www.pyd.org/how_to_help/volunteer.htm

This web site presents information about mentoring programs available for youth in Massachusetts. The Massachusetts mentoring program includes matching mentee with mentor with a disability or similar career interests, an on-line mentoring, and "Mentor for a Day" program. The National Mentoring Center for Youth with Disabilities is located on this site. Technical assistance is available nationally for agencies interested in developing mentoring programs in their own communities.

Youthhood.org

http://www.youthhood.org/youthhood/index.asp

The Youthhood.org web site, affiliated with NCSET, is specifically designed by and for youth with disabilities. This web site has interactive features enabling youth to keep a personal journal and use worksheets for transition planning either alone or with their teachers, parents, or mentors. Web site areas include high school, jobs, health care, living independently, advocacy, and social relationships.

HOUSING AND INDEPENDENT LIVING

Adatravelplus.com

www.adavacationsplus.com

This web site offers information on travel for individuals with disabilities. This travel agency provides a full range of services for interested travelers.

Beach Center on Disability

http://www.beachcenter.org/

The Beach Center on Disability web site contains disability-related information for families and consumers. The thrust of the site is to provide information that enables families and consumers to use that has practical application for daily living.

Easter Seals

http://www.easterseals.com/site/PageServer

The Easter Seals web site contains information about the range of services and programs offered by this organization nationwide for individuals with disabilities including developmental disabilities. Easter Seals agencies in local communities can be accessed through this site for additional information about the type of programs and services available for consumers.

Independent Living USA

http://www.ilusa.com/links/ilcenters.htm

This web site contains a complete listing of Independent Living Centers throughout the United States. Independent living centers are listed by state.

National Accessible Apartments Clearinghouse

http://www.accessibleapartments.org/website/article.asp?id=4

The National Accessible Apartments Clearinghouse web site maintains a database of more than 80,000 apartment units in each of the 50 states that are accessible. Users are encouraged to contact this organization via their web site/email (clearinghouse@naahq.org), fax (1-703-518-6191), or toll free phone number (1-800-421-1221). Services are free.

National Assistive Technology Technical Assistance Partnership

http://www.resna.org/taproject/about/index.html

The National Assistive Technology Technical Assistance Partnership web site is a gateway site that provides extensive links to other web sites pertaining to assistive technology. The information provided on this site includes information on regulations and legislation, practical information for application in home, work, educational and community settings, and research conducted in this field.

National Rehabilitation Information Center

http://www.naric.com/

The National Rehabilitation Information Center web site is gateway site for professionals, policy makers, consumers, and families. The pages for consumers contain practical rehabilitation tips for application in educational, employment, community, and home settings.

The Family Center on Technology and Disability

http://www.fctd.info/

The Family Center on Technology and Disability web site offers extensive information for parents, caregivers, and youth on written information on assistive technology (AT) and its applicability for individuals with disabilities. The site contains newsletters on selected topics of interests to consumers, on-line conferencing with AT, and links to other disability sites.

DISABILITY INFORMATION

Disability Resources

http://www.disabilityresources.org/

The Disability Resources web site is a gateway to numerous on-line disability resources on every topic of relevance to individuals with disabilities. Disability resources are also categorized by state.

Federation for Children with Special Needs

http://www.fcsn.org/

The Federation for Children with Special Needs web site is a family-oriented policy and advocacy group designed to inform and empower families and consumers with the aims of engaging families in the process and facilitating systemic change.

Internet Resources for Special Children

http://www.irsc.org/

Internet Resources for Special Children is a web site offering links to a number of disability-related web sites. There are links to employment, adaptive equipment, and resources (such as vehicle conversions and sports equipment) and condition-specific information. There are a multitude of links to resources on specific conditions such as autism spectrum disorder, cerebral palsy, Rett disorder, and visual impairments, to name a few. This information is useful for youth (with at least a high school reading level for many of the web sites), parents, educators, and health care professionals.

Untangling the Web

http://www.icdi.wvu.edu/Others.htm

This web site is a gateway to a multitude of disability web sites. The categories of links to other web sites include health care resources, various disability-specific sites, employment, education, community living, accommodations, legal issues, and assistive technology.

Youreable.com

http://www.youreable.com/

Youreable.com is a web site for individuals with disabilities. This web site contains information on products, disability-specific news stories, and chat forms of interest.

DISABILITY/CHRONIC ILLNESS SPECIFIC

Association of Retarded Citizens

http://www.thearc.org

Autism Society of America

http://www.autism-society.org

Braille Institute

http://www.brailleinstitute.org

Children and Adults with Attention Deficit/Hyperactivity Disorder
http://www.chadd.org

Learning Disabilities Association of America
http://www.ldanatl.org

National Association for Down Syndrome
http://www.nads.org/

National Attention Deficit Disorder Association
http://www.add.org

National Down Syndrome Society
http://www.ndss.org/

Spina Bifida Association of America
http://www.sbaa.org/site/PageServer?pagename=index

Tourette Syndrome Association, Inc.
http://www.tsa-usa.org/

United Cerebral Palsy
http://www.ucp.org/main.cfm/1

INTERAGENCY WEB SITES, RESOURCES, AND EDUCATION RESOURCES

Healthy & Ready to Work National Center

http://www.hrtw.org

Information is presented on topics related to health care transition planning. This web site is geared primarily for a health professional audience, although there is information for youth, families, and non–health providers.

National Center on Secondary Education and Transition

http://www.ncset.org/

This web site contains information on transition-related topics using an educational focus. Although this web site is primarily directed to educators, it is a useful resource for all professionals involved in transition planning for youth with special health care needs and disabilities.

Data Sources
for Tracking Youth
Transitioning to Adulthood

Measuring and monitoring youth transition experiences is important to determine if programming is effective. States and other agencies can use existing data sources to track the outcomes of their programming. This list of data sources with their web sites offers a sample of respected data sources.

DATA RESOURCES ON ALL
YOUTH AND YOUNG ADULTS

U.S. Census Bureau

http://www.census.gov

This web site contains information about the American population offered in a variety of ways, such as state-specific or age group-specific data, and is useful in comparing information on youth with special health care needs with their typically developing peers.

Current Population Survey

http://www.bls.census.gov/cps

Current Population Survey (CPS) is a monthly survey of about 50,000 households conducted by the Bureau of the Census for the Bureau of Labor Statistics. Estimates obtained from the CPS include statistics on employment, unemployment, earnings, hours of work, and other indicators. The population estimates are available by a variety of demographic characteristics including age, sex, race, marital status, educational attainment, occupation, industry, and class of worker. Supplemental questions to produce estimates on a variety of topics including school enrollment, income, previous work experience, health, employee benefits, and work schedules are also often added to the regular CPS questionnaire. The web site is a gateway to other related surveys.

Centers for Disease Control and Prevention

http://www.cdc.gov

The primary purpose of the Centers for Disease Control and Prevention is to prevent and control the outbreak of diseases, the occurrence of injuries, and disabilities. This purpose is achieved through surveillance activities, prevention research, development of health policies, and recommendations.

Healthy People 2000 Final Review

http://www.cdc.gov/nchs/products/pubs/pubd/hp2k/review/highlightshp2000.htm

This document provides an overview of the status of achievement of the Healthy People 2000 objectives. As this document indicates, progress was made in fully or partially achieving 62% of the objectives.

Healthy People 2010

http://www.healthypeople.gov

Healthy People 2010 documents can be accessed at this web site. The goals for the health of the U.S. population and various subgroups for the year 2010 that direct federal and state health funding and programming can be found on this web site.

Behavioral Risk Factor Surveillance System

http://www.cdc.gov/brfss/

The Behavioral Risk Factor Surveillance System (BRFSS) surveys are conducted through the Centers for Disease Control and Prevention and provide annual state-level data based on a randomized sample of the general adult population. Data collected from the survey gives extensive information about the health status, risk behaviors, and access to care and insurance for different age groups, including young adults. Information is also gathered regarding usual sources of health care, insurance coverage, and employment status according to age categories including ages 18–24, so it is particularly useful in measuring indicators related to successful transition. States may add questions to obtain data on particular health conditions (e.g., asthma, diabetes, depression) and additional information on health care costs and barriers to the BRFSS.

Youth Risk Behavior Surveillance System

http://www.cdc.gov/healthyyouth/yrbs

The Youth Risk Behavior Surveillance System surveys seventh, ninth, and eleventh graders on health risk behaviors exploring behavioral risk factors associated with the most important causes of mortality and morbidity in youth and adults.

Improving the Health of Adolescents
and Young Adults: A Guide for States and Communities

http://nahic.ucsf.edu/index.php/companion/index/

Improving the Health of Adolescents and Young Adults: A Guide for States and Communities is a companion document to *Healthy People 2010*. The document is designed to help communities and individuals translate the *Healthy People 2010* objectives that are key to adolescent health and safety into a vision for improving adolescent health and well being. It provides a framework for helping communities to establish priorities, take collective action, and measure progress toward the shared goal of improving the health, safety, and well being of their adolescents and young adults.

Monitoring the Future

http://www.monitoringthefuture.org

Yearly national surveys of 50,000 students in eighth, tenth, and twelfth grades and follow-up of a sample of high school graduates is conducted to gather data on tobacco, alcohol, and drug use; attitudinal correlates of drug use; positive attitudes; and life experiences. These surveys examine at-risk behaviors for all teens. The National Institute on Drug Abuse funds this project, located at the University of Michigan.

National Health Interview Survey and National Health Interview Survey on Disability

http://www.cdc.gov/nchs/nhis.htm

The National Center for Health Statistics (NCHS) is responsible for compiling national data pertaining to health issues. NCHS oversees the collection of population data and data pertaining to children and adults with disabilities. Population data are collected using the National Health Interview Survey on Disability (NHIS-D) through personal interviews or examinations. Other population data are collected from vital and medical records. More detailed information about NHIS-D can be found on the NCHS web site, including access to the latest year of the Health United States survey, which summarizes health surveys. The NHIS-D is a telephone survey of a randomized sample of children and adults with developmental disabilities, specific health conditions, behavior problems, sensory loss, or physical disabilities. The survey contains questions related to medical home, transition, screening, and access to community-based services. Although data are provided at a regional level, some states have "purchased" additional data collection efforts to acquire state-level data.

Medical Expenditure Panel Survey

http://www.meps.ahrq.gov

The Medical Expenditure Panel Survey (MEPS) uses a nationally representative subsample drawn from households that participated in the prior year's National Health Interview Survey. The MEPS provides annual estimates for a variety of measures of health status, health insurance coverage, health care use and expenditures, and sources of payment for health services. The panel design of the survey, which features several rounds of interviewing covering 2 full calendar years, makes it possible to determine how changes in respondents' health status, income, employment, eligibility for public and private insurance coverage, use of services, and payment for care are related.

National Survey of Children's Health

http://www.cdc.gov/nchs/about/major/slaits/nsch.htm

This national survey is conducted to examine the physical and emotional health of children ages 0–17 years of age. Special emphasis is placed on factors that may relate to the well-being of children, including medical homes, family interactions, parental health, school and after-school experiences, and safe neighborhoods. State and local area integrated telephone survey methodology is used in this survey.

National Maternal Child Health Clearinghouse

http://childstats.gov

This web site offers easy access to federal and state statistics and reports on children and their families, including population and family characteristics, economic security, health, behavior and social environment, and education. Reports of the Federal Interagency Forum on Child and Family Statistics include *America's Children: Key National Indicators of Well-Being*, the annual federal monitoring report on the status of the nation's children.

National Adolescent Health Information Center

http://nahic.ucsf.edu/

The overall goal of the National Adolescent Health Information Center (NAHIC) is to improve the health of adolescents by serving as a national resource for adolescent health information and research and to ensure the integration, synthesis, coordination, and dissemination of health information. NAHIC also houses the National Initiative to Improve Adolescent Health by Year 2010. The program development resource, *Using Data to Shape Health Programs for Youth* is available at http://nahic.ucsf.edu/index.php/publications/article/niiah_brief_documents/.

Child Trends

http://www.childtrends.org

Child Trends is a nonprofit, nonpartisan research organization in partnership with the National Adolescent Health Information Center and the Public Policy Analysis & Education Center for Middle Childhood, Adolescent, and Young Adult Health. Child Trends is dedicated to improving the lives of children by conducting research and providing evidence-based information to improve the decision-making, programs, and policies that affect children and their families. The report, *Statistical Portrait of Well Being in Early Adulthood, 2005,* summarizes status of transition of young people in the United States.

Trends in the Well-Being of America's Children and Youth, 2002

http://aspe.hhs.gov/hsp/02trends

This report provides information on 89 indicators within the domains of population, family, neighborhood, economic security; health conditions and health care; social development and behavioral health, including teen fertility; and education and achievement. Indicators are drawn from more than 20 data sources including federally collected data, national surveys, and specific studies from peer-reviewed journals.

National Longitudinal Surveys of Youth, 1979 and 1997

http://stats.bls.gov/nls/home.htm

The National Longitudinal Surveys of Youth (NLSY79, NLSY97) are a set of surveys designed to gather information at multiple points in time on labor market activities and other significant life events. NLSY79 is a nationally representative sample of 12,686 young men and women who were 14–22 years old when they were first surveyed in 1979. These individuals were interviewed annually through 1994 and are currently interviewed on a biennial basis. NLSY97 consists of a nationally representative sample of approximately 9,000 youths who were 12–16 years old as of December 31, 1996. Round 1 of the survey was conducted in 1997. In that round, both the eligible youth and one of that youth's parents received hour-long personal interviews. Sample youth continue to be interviewed on an annual basis.

National Longitudinal Study of Adolescent Health

http://www.cpc.unc.edu/projects/addhealth/

The National Longitudinal Study of Adolescent Health (Add Health) is a school-based study designed to explore the causes of health-related behaviors of adolescents in grades 7–12, with an emphasis on the influence of social context. Add Health postulates that families, friends, schools, and communities play roles in the lives of adolescents that may encourage healthy choices or may lead to unhealthy, self-destructive behavior. Initiated in 1994 under a grant from the National Institute of Child Health and Human Development with co-funding from 17 other federal agencies, Add Health is the largest, most comprehensive survey of adolescents ever undertaken. Data at the individual, family, school, and community levels were collected in two waves between 1994 and 1996. In 2001 and 2002, Add Health respondents, 18–26 years old, were reinterviewed in a third wave to investigate the influence that adolescence has on young adulthood.

Child and Adolescent Health Measurement Initiative

http://www.cahmi.org

The Child and Adolescent Health Measurement Initiative (CAHMI) is a national collaboration whose purpose is to develop and implement a comprehensive set of consumer-centered quality measurement tools. CAHMI is composed of consumer organizations, federal and state policy makers, health care purchasers, researchers and practitioners that influence health care delivery, quality measurement and reporting. On the web site are reports on promoting healthy development and special health care needs.

Annie E. Casey Foundation

http://www.caseyfoundation.org and http://www.caseylifeskills.org

The Annie E. Casey Foundation focuses particularly on programming for emancipating foster youth. A description of the programs implemented throughout the country using the Casey methods can be found on the web site. Assessment tools are also available, including the Annie E Casey Life Skills Assessment and the Ansell-Casey Life Skills Assessment, an on-line assessment for different age youth to determine strengths and areas of need.

KIDS COUNT

http://www.kidscount.org

KIDS COUNT, a project of the Annie E. Casey Foundation, is a national and state-by-state effort to track the status of children in the United States. By providing policy makers and citizens with benchmarks of child well-being, the goal of KIDS COUNT is to enrich local, state, and national discussions concerning ways to secure better futures for all children.

National Center for Educational Statistics

http://nces.ed.gov

The National Center for Educational Statistics is the primary government agency for collecting and analyzing data that are related to education in the United States and other nations.

Commonwealth Fund

http://www.cmwf.org

The Commonwealth Fund is a private foundation that supports independent research on health and social issues and awards grants to improve health care practice and policy. The fund is dedicated to helping people become more informed about their health care, and improving care for vulnerable populations such as children, elderly people, low-income families, minority Americans, and the uninsured. Examples of issue briefs available on the web site include "Quality of health care for children and adolescents: A chartbook" (April, 2004) and "Rite of passage: Why young adults become uninsured and how new policies can help" (May, 2004).

MacArthur Research Network on Transitions to Adulthood and Public Policy

http://www.transad.pop.upenn.edu/about/index.htm

The MacArthur Research Network on Transitions to Adulthood and Public Policy examines the changing nature of early adulthood, and the policies, programs, and institutions that support young people as they move into adulthood. From a developmental perspective, network researchers are examining the traditional milestones in the journey to adulthood—leaving home, entering, or leaving school, finding employment, marriage, and childbearing. They are also exploring how psychological development relates to these social transitions, and how institutions that have typically aided the transition—such as schools and workplaces—might adapt to address the needs of young people in the 21st century.

PUBLIC AGENDA

Publicagenda.org

http://www.publicagenda.org/research/research_reports_details.cfm?list=31

A report of a national survey of young adults examining the decisions they make about work or college can be found on this web site. Findings suggest that the vast majority of young adults, of all races, strongly believe in the value of higher education. However, the study raises questions about the shortage of high school counselors and the economic pressures felt by many young adults, especially minorities. The study also portrays the hit-or-miss career path experienced by those who enter the workforce with a college or technical degree.

The Urban Institute

http://www.urban.org

The Urban Institute studies health, disability, aging, and family health, and produces reports that monitor health issues in the United States.

The Horatio Alger Association

http://www.horatioalger.org

Since 1996, The Horatio Alger Association of Distinguished Americans has conducted a survey of young people between the ages of 13 and 19 to ascertain the issues and feelings of American youth. The report, *The State of Our Nation's Youth, 2005–2006,* contains valuable insights into the lives of teens across the country and what effect our nation's government, culture, and their own relationships have on their lives.

The Adverse Childhood Experiences Survey

http://www.acestudy.org

Adverse Childhood Experiences is a large, ongoing research investigation conducted at Kaiser Permanente in California. This study is examining the dose-response effects of adverse childhood experiences such as abuse and household dysfunction (e.g., growing up with family member in prison, mother treated violently, alcoholic or drug using family member, mentally ill family member) and physical and mental health of adults in their 50s including obesity, cardiac and pulmonary diseases, diabetes, and behaviors such as smoking and sexual practices. This research has implications for youth with disabilities, as they tend to live in poverty with the potential for adverse childhood experiences that might affect their health status and health behaviors in adulthood. Report by Vincent Felitti, 2004, *The relationship of adverse childhood experiences to adult health: Turning gold into lead,* is available at http://www.healthpresentations.org/docs/goldintolead.pdf.

RESOURCES ON YOUTH AND YOUNG ADULTS WITH DISABILITIES

Healthy & Ready to Work National Center

http://www.hrtw.org

Health impacts all aspects of life. Success in the classroom, within the community, and on the job requires that young people with special health care needs stay healthy. To stay healthy, young people need an understanding of their health and to participate in their health care decisions. This web site focuses on understanding systems, access to quality health care, and increasing the involvement of youth including tools for providers and resources needed to make more informed choices.

DisabilityInfo.gov

http://www.disability.gov

DisabilityInfo.gov serves as the U.S. government's gateway to disability information. The user can type "disability statistics" in the search field type for a list of a variety of statistical sources. Health information can be located by clicking on the "Health" tab at the top; one category along the left margin is disability statistics.

Social Security Administration

http://www.ssa.gov or http://www.socialsecurity.gov

The Social Security Administration (SSA) web site contains various reports about SSA beneficiaries and programs for beneficiaries, including use of work incentives.

Office of Special Education and Rehabilitation Services

http://www.ed.gov/about/offices/list/osers/index.html

Information and statistics about special education and special education students are available on this web site. An annual report on the status of U.S. special education programs and special education students can be found at http://www.ed.gov/about/reports/annual/index.html.

National Institute on Disability and Rehabilitation Research

http://www.ed.gov/about/offices/list/osers/nidrr/index.html?src=mr

The National Institute on Disability and Rehabilitation Research provides leadership and support for a comprehensive program of research related to the rehabilitation of individuals with disabilities. Multiple reports focusing on health, education, work, and community participation status of people with disabilities are available. Chartbooks on disability in the United States can be found at http://www.infouse.com/disabilitydata.

National Center for Secondary Education and Transition

http://www.ncset.org

The National Center for Secondary Education and Transition coordinates national resources, offers technical assistance, and disseminates information related to secondary education and transition for youth with disabilities. The purpose of this information is to support educators, providers, youth, and families in creating opportunities for youth to achieve successful futures.

The National Collaborative on Workforce and Disability for Youth

http://www.ncwd-youth.info

The National Collaborative on Workforce and Disability for Youth is a web site source for information about employment and youth with disabilities. The partners—experts in disability, education, employment, and workforce development—strive to ensure the highest quality most relevant information is available for users to access.

National Organization on Disability/
Harris Survey of Americans with Disabilities

http://www.nod.org

Access to the results of national on-line and telephone surveys of people with disabilities compared with people without disabilities on a variety of quality of life indicators since 1986 is available on this web site. The National Organization on Disability/Harris Poll information for 2004 is available with comparisons to previous surveys.

National Longitudinal Transition Study
and National Longitudinal Transition Study 2

http://www.sri.com/policy/cehs/dispolicy/ and http://www.nlts2.org

The National Longitudinal Transition Study (NLTS) reports data on more than 8,000 youth with disabilities from 300 school districts across the nation. Data were collected in 1987 and 1990 from students who were enrolled in secondary schools and in special education in 1985. Data were collected by telephone interviews with parents (and the youth themselves if they were able to respond), surveys of teachers and principals who served them, and analyses of students' school records contributing to a comprehensive look at many aspects of the lives of young people with disabilities. The National Longitudinal Transition Study 2 (NLTS-2), funded by the U.S. Department of Education, is documenting the experiences of a national sample of 3,000 students who were 13–16 years of age in 2000 as they move from secondary school into adult roles. These are the longitudinal studies of students in special education—again focusing on work and participation in society rather than health issues, but helpful in understanding how young adults with special needs are doing.

National Council on Disability

http://www.ncd.gov

The National Council on Disability (NCD) is an independent federal agency that makes recommendations to the President and Congress on issues affecting 54 million Americans with disabilities. NCD is currently working on a series of reports that interrelate with centerpiece initiatives presented in President Bush's New Freedom Initiative. These reports focus on transitioning people from social security income to work, long-term supports and services, the impact of the Americans with Disabilities Act, and financial incentives related to employment and living independently. A report on transition-age youth, "Transition and post-school outcomes for youth with disabilities: Closing the gaps to postsecondary education and employment," published on November 1, 2000, can be obtained by inserting "young adults with disabilities" into the search site.

Measuring and Monitoring of Community-Based
Systems of Care for Children with Special Health Care Needs,
Early Intervention Research Institute, Utah State University

http://eiri.usu.edu/projects/MandM/

Measuring and Monitoring of Community-Based Systems of Care for Children with Special Health Care Needs (M&M project) provides technical assistance and support to the states to enable them to strengthen their measurement capacity via data warehousing, data integration, development of interagency surveys, and simply sharing data results that pertain to the broader population of children with special health care needs.

Disability Statistics Center

http://www.dsc.ucsf.edu

The Disability Statistics Center at the University of California, San Francisco, produces and disseminates policy-relevant statistical information on the demographics and status of people with disabilities in American society. The center's work focuses on how that status is changing over time with regard to employment, access to technology, health care, community-based services, and other aspects of independent living and participation in society. A wide variety of statistical information about people with disabilities is available, including disability statistics reports, disability abstracts, and "Disability watch: Status of people with disabilities in the United States."

Cornell University Rehabilitation Research and Training Center for Economic Research on Employment Policy for Persons with Disabilities

http://www.ilr.cornell.edu/edi/ and http://www.disabilitystatistics.org

Cornell University Rehabilitation Research and Training Center for Economic Research on Employment Policy for Persons with Disabilities coordinates research, training, and dissemination activities aimed at deepening the understanding of policy makers and other stakeholders about how the economy, public policies, and other sociopolitical factors affect the employment and economic self-sufficiency of persons with disabilities. The center's web site offers disability statistics and policy briefs on transitions with special focus on work.

Research and Training Center on Family Support & Children's Mental Health at Portland State University

http://www.rtc.pdx.edu

Research and information on mental health issues for children, youth and young adults is provided on this web site. Focal Point publications are available on the following topics pertaining to transition: Transition (Spring, 2001) and Resilience and Recovery (Summer, 2005).

Substance Abuse & Mental Health Services Administration

http://www.samhsa.gov and http://www.mentalhealth.samhsa.gov/

These web sites contains data on mental health issues in the United States and resources for programming. The Substance Abuse & Mental Health Services Administration Sustainability Tool Kit is intended to help communities that receive federal funding for programs and services for children and youth with serious emotional disturbance and their families to ensure that systems of care continue to be in place long after federal funds are gone. These tools are designed to assist local communities to assess their current status in efforts to sustain critical elements and objectives of systems of care, facilitate the process of completing sustainability strategic plans, and guide communities in raising matching funds to sustain their programs. The tool kit is available at: http://www.nrchmi.samhsa.gov/search/detail.asp?ResID=13459.

PLANNING TOOLS

American Diabetes Association.
Sample Section 504 Plan & Diabetes
Medical Management Plan for a student with diabetes

http://www.diabetes.org/uedocuments/504-plan-2004.pdf

Health Care Transition Workbooks 12–14, 15–17, 18+

http://hctransitions.ichp.ufl.edu/resources.html

Life Maps: Developmentally appropriate transition questionnaires that allow families and young people to identify their own individual needs

http://chfs.ky.gov/#Life

Transition Timeline for Children and Adolescents with Special Health Care Needs

http://depts.washington.edu/healthtr/Timeline/timeline.htm

Index

Page references to figures, tables, and footnotes are indicated by *f, t,* and *n,* respectively.